Kinesiology Foundations for OTAs

Kinesiology Foundations for OTAs

Daniel C. Snyder, MA
LeAnne M. Conner, MEd
Gregory F. Lorenz, MA

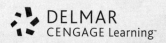
DELMAR
CENGAGE Learning

Australia • Brazil • Japan • Korea • Mexico • Singapore • Spain • United Kingdom • United States

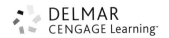
DELMAR
CENGAGE Learning

Kinesiology Foundations for OTAs
Daniel C. Snyder, LeAnne M. Conner,
and Gregory F. Lorenz

Vice President, Health Care Business Unit:
  William Brottmiller

Director of Learning Solutions: Matthew Kane

Managing Editor: Marah Bellegarde

Acquisitions Editor: Sherry Dickinson

Product Manager: Juliet Steiner

Editorial Assistant: Angela Doolin

Marketing Channel Manager: Michele McTighe

Executive Marketing Manager: Jennifer McAvey

Marketing Coordinator: Chelsey Iaquinta

Production Director: Carolyn Miller

Content Project Manager: Kenneth McGrath

Senior Art Director: Jack Pendleton

For product information and technology assistance, contact us at
Cengage Learning Customer & Sales Support, 1-800-354-9706
For permission to use material from this text or product,
submit all requests online at **www.cengage.com/permissions**
Further permissions questions can be emailed to
permissionrequest@cengage.com

ISBN-13: 978-1-4283-3511-0

ISBN-10: 1-4283-3511-0

Delmar
Executive Woods
5 Maxwell Drive
Clifton Park, NY 12065
USA

Cengage Learning is a leading provider of customized learning solutions with office locations around the globe, including Singapore, the United Kingdom, Australia, Mexico, Brazil, and Japan. Locate your local office at **www.cengage.com/global**

Cengage Learning products are represented in Canada by Nelson Education, Ltd.

To learn more about Delmar, visit **www.cengage.com/delmar**

Purchase any of our products at your local bookstore or at our preferred online store **www.ichapters.com**

Printed in the United States of America
5 6 7 13 12 11

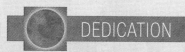

DEDICATION

To my wife, Renee, whose love and support through this endeavor has been lasting and loyal. To my daughters Aubyn and Piper, thanks for your enduring smiles and laughter. To my dogs Buster and Sabrina, for sitting by my side through many hours of hard work.

Daniel Snyder

I would like to dedicate this book to my parents, Jack and Sharon Lorenz, and to my brother Jeff for believing in me and instilling in me a work ethic that allows me to succeed in life. I would also like to dedicate this book to Krislene, who endured many hours of hard work and sacrifice. Thanks!

Greg Lorenz

To LeAnne Conner, whose passion for kinesiology and teaching inspired us through the completion of this textbook.

Dan and Greg

CONTENTS

Preface / xi

PART I GENERAL BACKGROUND INFORMATION

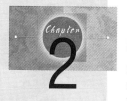

Introduction to Kinesiology / 3

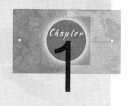

Muscular Anatomy and Physiology / 17

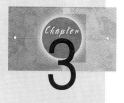

Muscle Characteristics / 33

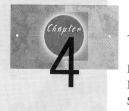

The Nervous System / 53

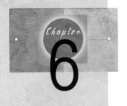

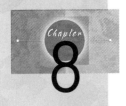
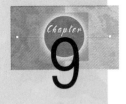

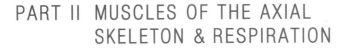

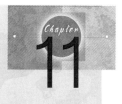

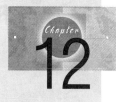

PART III MUSCLES OF THE INFERIOR
APPENDICULAR SKELETON

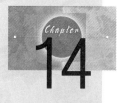

PART IV MUSCLES OF THE SUPERIOR APPENDICULAR SKELETON

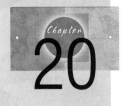
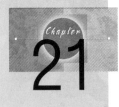

PREFACE

The human body is amazing. All of its structures work together to provide locomotion and support. If you stop and think about how the muscles, joints, bones, soft tissue, and microscopic anatomy function to provide just one simple movement, it is at times overwhelming. Even as you take the time to read this preface, your muscles are hard at work, stabilizing your back, moving your eyes, and even holding your head upright. While you read each chapter in this textbook, take the time to think about how amazing the interactions are between these structures in the human body. It has been our goal to create a kinesiology textbook that combines accurate material, practical applications, and detailed pictures that will allow students and professionals in the field of occupational therapy to understand this difficult subject matter rather than merely memorizing facts. The information in this textbook is provided for professional and student exercise physiologists, personal trainers, physical therapist assistants, occupational therapy assistants, and strength conditioning coaches. This book will suit your needs as a health care professional, and we know that many of your questions about the structures of the human body will be answered.

Kinesiology Foundations for OTAs is designed to describe the structures and functions of muscles, bones, and ligaments of the human body. This textbook further addresses the interactions between these structures and illustrates how movements are performed. All of the needed information is covered so that the health care professional will have the knowledge to perform the duties in his or her chosen field.

 ## WHY WE WROTE THIS BOOK

The purpose for writing this textbook is to provide students, faculty, and health care professionals with a detailed and accurate kinesiology reference guide. The textbook is designed for a one-semester kinesiology course. Material in the textbook follows a natural progression, beginning with a general overview of kinesiology terms and subjects, then progresses to identifying the structure and function of each joint specific to human movement. There are currently very few kinesiology textbooks that incorporate accurate material, practical application exercise experiences, and detailed illustrations in one book. Furthermore, we are aware of kinesiology textbooks that have been written for specific allied health professionals, but there are only a few detailed kinesiology textbooks for health care providers in occupational therapy and the exercise sciences.

ORGANIZATION OF THE TEXT

Kinesiology for OTAs is organized in four different parts to provide a natural progression for learning. Part I consists of a discussion and review of the major systems and concepts that are associated with human movement. Parts II through IV build on the material discussed in Part I, with an in-depth study of the kinesiology concepts of the axial skeleton, the lower extremity, and the upper extremity. Each of the chapters in this textbook is supplemented with kinesiology perspectives from occupational therapists. These reflections aid in applying the material to further understand how disorders, diseases, and accidents affect the everyday movement of patients in the clinical setting. The critical thinking questions and laboratory exercises were developed by physical therapists and occupational therapists to help the students apply the material in this textbook to actual clinical and professional settings.

The information presented in Part I (Chapters 1–7) was designed to provide the foundation concepts for basic human movement. More specifically, Part I begins with a review of anatomical positions, muscle physiology, muscle characteristics, the nervous system, bones, joint structures, and arthrokinematics. Each chapter in Part I concludes with in-depth review questions.

In Part II (Chapters 8–12), the student can take a closer look at the structure and function of the muscles and joints located in the axial skeleton. We begin with Chapter 8 by discussing the head and neck region, move down to the lower back and abdominal regions in chapters 9 and 10, and then combine the concepts discussed in previous chapters and discuss the kinesiology concepts associated with postural assessment. Chapter 12 presents the anatomy and physiology of the muscles that are associated with respiration and discusses the important concepts needed to understand this complex system.

Part III takes the student through an in-depth discussion of the muscles of the lower body that are used for locomotion. It begins with a discussion of major landmarks, joint structures, nervous innervation, and, finally, the muscles of the lower extremities. Part III begins with a discussion of the hip joint in Chapter 13 and then progresses to the structures and function of the knee in Chapter 14 and the ankle joints in Chapter 15, concluding with Chapter 16, which includes a discussion of the kinesiology concepts of gait.

Part IV provides the student with a resource that discusses the difficult components of the upper extremities. Chapter 17, The Shoulder Girdle, provides an introduction to the complex anatomy of the upper extremity. This chapter provides the student with a review of the brachial plexus and continues with the major landmarks, joint structures, and nervous innervation, and how the muscles of the shoulder girdle interact with the muscles of the shoulder joint. The next chapters of Part IV include a discussion of the major landmarks, joint structures, and nervous innervation and are found in Chapter 18, The Shoulder Joint; Chapter 19, The Elbow and Radioulnar Joints; Chapter 20, The Forearm and Wrist; and Chapter 21, The Hand. The final chapter of Part IV, Chapter 22, Movement Analysis, ties together all of the kinesiology concepts discussed in the textbook. In this chapter the students are asked to analyze the movements of all the joints during the motion of throwing a ball and drinking a cup of coffee. We believe that when students learn, understand, and apply the concepts of kinesiology, the analysis of all movements should become routine and easy to understand.

As a student of kinesiology, you will benefit from this book in many ways. First, you will learn by reading the detailed relationships between body components and tissues. Second, you will learn visually by looking at the relationships between components and tissues as shown in the illustrations. Third, you will learn in small groups by completing the activities at the conclusion of each chapter.

FEATURES

Kinesiology Foundations for OTAs is designed with the student in mind. There are many outstanding features to this book. Learning objectives provide an overview of the material that are covered in each chapter. Each chapter begins with an introduction specifying the importance of each topic as it relates to human movement and practical experience. Illustrations are detailed to enable the student to visualize each muscle by itself and in a muscle group as a whole. Following the presentation of the material, key concepts reinforce the importance of the concepts discussed.

ACKNOWLEDGMENTS

We would like to thank Ms. Janice Hinds and Joanna Goldin for their contributions for the physical therapy assistant and occupational therapy assistant boxes. We extend a special thanks to Amy Solomon for writing Chapter 4, The Nervous System. Finally, we extend a thank you to Patty Pernell for her contribution of Chapter 11, Posture Assessment and Intervention.

 REVIEWERS

Dolores Bertoti, MS, PT, PCS
Alvernia College
Reading, PA

David Pavlat, MPE, ABD, HFI, CSCS
Central College
Pella, IA

Michael Nordvall, EdD
Marymount University
Arlington, VA

Kathy Kenna, PT, ATC, MD
Columbia College
Sonora, CA

Martha Branson-Banks, OTR
Lake Michigan College
Niles, MI

Becky Robler, OT
Pueblo Community College
Pueblo, CO

Sandy McIlnay, MS, OTR
Penn Valley Community College
Kansas City, MO

Chris Barrett, PT
Lake Area Technical Institute
Watertown, SD

Ronald De Vera Barredo, PT, MA, GCS, EdD
Kaskaskia College
Centralia, IL

 CONTRIBUTOR

Judi Malek-Ismail, MEd, OT/L
Keiser University
Ft. Lauderdale, FL

Part I
General Background Information

Chapters 1-7

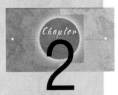

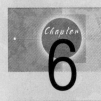

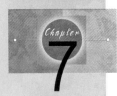

Chapter

1

INTRODUCTION TO KINESIOLOGY

Key Words

anatomical position	inferior	posterior
anterior	infra	posterolateral
anterolateral	kinesiology	posteromedial
anteromedial	lateral	prone
axis	linea alba	proximal
brevis	longus	sagittal axis
caudal	magnus	sagittal plane
cranial	maximus	superficial
deep	medial	superior
distal	medius	supine
dorsal	midline	supra
frontal axis	minimi	transverse plane
frontal plane	minimus	ventral
fundamental position	plane	vertical axis

INTRODUCTION

For many years, mankind was obsessed with understanding the mechanical functions of the human body. The Greek and Egyptian societies provided the first documented studies of human movement as they learned more about the human body. These early studies have provided the bases for the study of human movement. As time elapsed, studies of movements of the human body progressed, giving rise to many of today's professions, including occupational therapy (OT), physical therapy (PT), exercise physiology, massage therapy, and biomechanics among others. To be successful, individuals in these professions must have a sound understanding of the interactions between the bones, joint structures, muscles, and nerves and the principles of physics as they apply to each movement of the human body. **Kinesiology** is the study of human movement and explains the relationships between the complex structures of the human body.

ANATOMICAL TERMS

Occupational therapy assistants (OTAs) must have a strong working knowledge of anatomy and physiology terms in order to identify the various components of the body used in human movement. These terms can then be applied to the kinesiological functions of the human body. For example, OTAs in the field do not say that "something is close to something" or that "something is in front of something." Instead they use anatomical terms to describe the location of a structure on the body. Numerous terms have been defined to provide a universal understanding of the positions of the bones, tendons, ligaments, nerves, and muscles within the human body.

Anatomical Position

In order to describe the movements of the human body, there must be a common starting point on which to reference all movements. This position is called the **anatomical position** and is described as standing erect with the feet flat and the palms facing forward (Figure 1-1). When identifying the bones, joints, ligaments, tendons, origins, insertions, muscles, and the principles of physics, the anatomical position is used as a general reference point to provide a common functional starting point. For example, if we observe the radius and ulna of the forearm in the anatomical position, the radius is away from the body (lateral) and the ulna is toward the body (medial).

Fundamental Position

Another position that may be used as a position of reference is the **fundamental position,** which varies little from the anatomical position. This position is identified as standing erect, with the feet flat and the palms facing toward the sides slightly toward the back. Generally speaking, the fundamental position is the position that humans are in when they are standing in a relaxed position and is often used when describing movements of the upper extremity. However, the fundamental position is seldom used, and, in this text, positioning is based on the anatomical position.

Midline of the Body

Another term that is vital to understanding anatomical reference points is the **midline** of the body. When identifying the midline, imagine a line drawn down the center of the body (see Figure 1-1). The first reference point for the midline is the suture joints found within the cranium that separates the skull into right and left halves. From here, if a continuous line were drawn toward the feet, it would travel down the center of the nose and to the sternum, separating these structures into even right and left halves. From this point on the body, identification of the midline becomes tricky. For example, if a section of yarn or string is extended from the tip of the sternum and attached to the symphysis pubis (where the two pelvic bones come together), the line would continue through the abdominal cavity. In the human body the string actually represents the **linea alba** (white line) that separates the right and left halves of the abdominal muscles. The line then extends to the floor and separates the lower limbs into the right and left legs.

In addition to the anatomical position, the midline of the body also is used as a reference point to describe the location of the bones, joints, ligaments, tendons, origins, insertions, and muscles, and the principles of physics. Using the radius and ulna of the forearm as examples, the radius is more specifically away from the midline (lateral) of the body; whereas the ulna is closer (medial) to it.

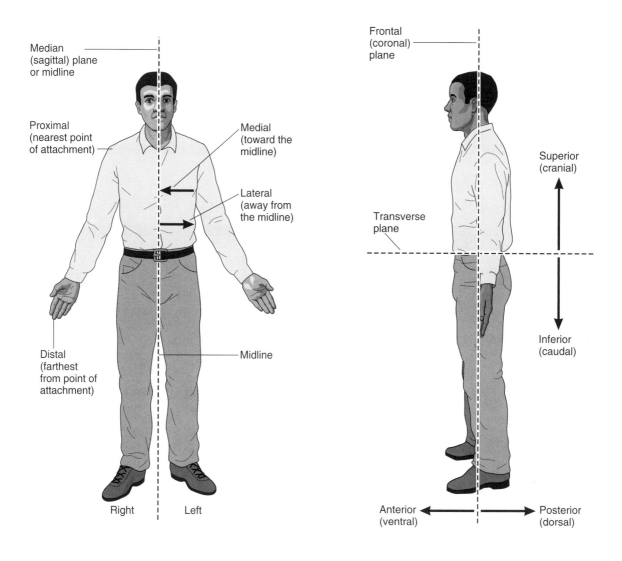

Figure 1-1 *Anatomical Position*

 DIRECTIONAL TERMS

Once the common reference positions have been established from the anatomical position and midline of the body, it is necessary to describe movement using directional terms (it is easiest to remember these terms by pairing each one with its opposite). Using the radius and ulna as examples, it has been established that **medial** and **lateral** are related positions to one another (see Figure 1-1). Therefore, the different reference terms can be broken down into lying down, front/back, near/away, toward the surface/away from the surface, toward the top/toward the bottom, and combination words associated with human movement. A comprehensive understanding of anatomical terms provides a sound background for understanding the terminology associated with human movement.

Anatomical References to Lying Down

When a client is lying down on an examination table, several terms can be applied to the positions in which they lie. The **prone** position is described as lying in a horizontal position with the face down (Figure 1-2A). This position would be used when attempting to palpate the hamstring muscles of the posterior thigh region in an examination setting. The **supine** position

OTA Perspective

The OT perspectives in this textbook will follow OT conceptual models of practice and integrate various treatment approaches from these frames of reference. "Top-down" approaches, or occupational performance-based models of practice, include the Model of Human Occupation (MOHO) and the Occupational Therapy Intervention Practice Model (OTIPM). "Bottom-up" approaches, or impairment or deficit-based and restorative models, include the Biomechanical Model, the Motor Control Model, the Sensory Integration Model, and the Spatiotemporal Adaptation Model. Although it is an occupational therapist's skill and, therefore, responsibility to determine the model(s) of practice that will guide individualized client treatment, the OTA is expected to have an understanding of the theory-treatment relationship. In clinical practice, the OTA should be able to link kinesiology concepts to client treatment to OT theory. An ongoing research and review of the models of practice while studying kinesiology may be beneficial to the OTA student in recognizing the relationships between kinesiology and OT practice.

(opposite of prone) is described as lying horizontally on the back with the face pointing toward the ceiling (Figure 1-2B). This position would be used when the clinician is palpating the quadriceps muscles located on the anterior surface of the thigh.

Anatomical References to the Front and Back

Several anatomical references can be applied to positions of the body when referring to the front and back of an individual. The first two terms, **anterior** and **posterior**, are most often used when referring to the location of an anatomical structure in the human body (see Figure 1-1). Any anatomical structure that is positioned toward the front of the body is referred to as being anterior to another structure serving as a reference point. For example, the pectoralis major (large chest muscle on the anterior surface of the chest cavity) is a powerful anterior muscle that provides forceful movements of the upper limbs. The opposite term of *anterior* is *posterior*, which refers to a structure located toward the backside of the body or in reference to another structure. A muscle of the shoulder region that is located posteriorly would be the latissimus dorsi, which works in opposition to the pectoralis major.

Two other terms also refer to the front and back positions: **dorsal** and **ventral** (see Figure 1-1). With regard to the regions of the human body, these two terms are mainly used when describing positions of the anatomical structures located in the foot, ankle region, and spinal cord. To better understand the term *dorsal*, imagine a shark swimming with its dorsal fin protruding out of the water. In this example, the dorsal fin protrudes out of the water from the shark's back. In the human body, the dorsal surface of the foot is the surface that faces the ceiling. The term *ventral* is the opposite of dorsal and refers to "toward the front." The plantar surface of the foot is opposite the dorsal surface; it is therefore on the ventral surface.

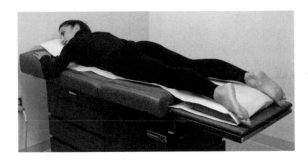

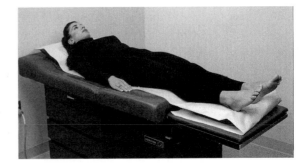

Figure 1-2A Prone Position

Figure 1-2B Supine Position

Anatomical References to Near and Away from the Midline

There are four terms that refer to the proximity of an object to the midline of the body. These terms are important in understanding the positions of anatomical structures that do not lie within the midline of the body or are at a distance away from the midline.

The first two terms, *proximal* and *distal,* refer to the position of bones, muscles, and joints from the midline (see Figure 1-1). **Proximal** refers to an anatomical structure that is closer to the midline of the body or one that is closer to another structure. A simple word device is to remember that when something is in close proximity, it is close to you. For example, the arm is more proximal to the midline of the body than the hand, or the fingers are more proximal to the hand than the chest. The opposite term of proximal is **distal**, which refers to an anatomical structure that is farther away from the midline of the body than another. For example, the hand is more distal from the midline of the body than the arm. Use these terms when learning the positions of anatomical structures in relationship to one another.

The remaining anatomical terms referencing far and away and which were discussed previously in this chapter are *medial* and *lateral.* One example that describes these terms is the location of the eyes and ears. The eyes are always medial compared to the ears, which are always lateral to the midline of the body.

Anatomical References to Toward the Surface and Away from the Surface

Many times, identifying the position of muscles in reference to how close or far they lie from the surface of the body is important in understanding their location within the human body and how easily each muscle is palpated. Therefore, the terms **superficial** and **deep** can be applied to the distance that an anatomical structure lies from the surface (Figure 1-3). Structures that are closer to the surface in relation to another structure are referred to as superficial structures, and those that are further away from the surface or in relation to another structure are deep structures. A simple example of this relationship can be found in the chest region and the relationship between the ribs and the heart. It is a well-known fact that the heart lies under the ribs, making the heart deep to the ribs, which are superficial to the heart. Another example is the relationship between the brain and the skull. In this example, the brain is deep to the skull. The terms *superficial* and *deep* are often used to identify the positions of the muscles in the body.

Anatomical References to Toward the Top and Toward the Bottom

Six terms can be applied to the direction "top" and "bottom." The first two pairs of terms, **superior** and **inferior**, are commonly used to describe the location of a structure when an individual is standing in the anatomical position (see Figure 1-1). The term *superior* refers to an anatomical structure that is toward the head or is above another structure, and *inferior* refers to structures that are toward the feet or below another structure. For example, the skull is a superior structure that is superior to the foot, which is an inferior structure when related to the skull. As muscle regions in the human body are further classified there will be discussions of the muscles of the upper and lower back; abdominal region; superior appendicular skeleton, including the shoulders and arms; and the muscles of the inferior appendicular skeleton, including the hip and legs.

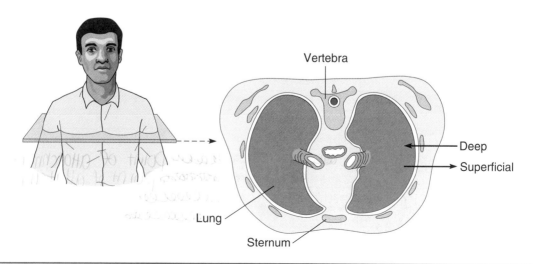

Figure 1-3 *Relationship of Superficial and Deep*

Two more terms that can be applied to the human body are **cranial** and **caudal** (see Figure 1-1). These two terms are seldom used in this book, but it is important to understand them. The term *cranial* refers to an anatomical structure that is located toward the skull, and *caudal* (tail) refers to a structure that is below or toward the bottom or tailbone (coccyx). Further identification of the midline reveals that the imaginary line bisects the body from cranial to caudal.

The last two terms, **supra** and **infra**, are actually derivatives of the terms *superior* and *inferior*. Much like their combined roots, the word component "supra" refers to an anatomical position that is above a structure, with "infra" being below a structure, for example, the supraspinatus muscle and infraspinatus muscles of the shoulder girdle region. The positions of these two muscles are above (supraspinatus) the spine of the scapula and below (infraspinatus) the spine of the scapula, respectively. Table 1-1 provides a summary of directional terms.

Combinations of Anatomical References

Often, the identification of movements and positions of anatomical structures requires the combination of terms to relate their position within the human body. As a result, the combination of two terms to describe the location of an anatomical structure is much like identifying the northwest and southwest directions.

Four terms are generally used in combination when describing anatomical positions; *anterior, lateral, posterior*, and *medial*. When identifying these anatomical positions, the terms *posterior* and *anterior* are used first with an *O* added to the root of the first term, followed by the term *medial* and *lateral*.

The combination of words is a simple endeavor, which should be followed by a simple description of the location of the anatomical structure. The term **anterolateral** refers to a structure that is both anterior and lateral to the midline of the body. The cheekbones are a good example of structures that have an anterolateral position on the body. The other three anatomical combination terms include **anteromedial**, **posterolateral**, and **posteromedial** (Table 1-2). Think of examples for the proceeding terms to help you understand the position of anatomical structures in greater depth.

Table 1-1   *Summary of Directional Terms*

Directional Term	Description
Anatomical Position	Standing erect, palms facing forward, and feet flat
Fundamental Position	Standing erect, palms facing the side of the body, and feet flat
Midline of the Body	Imaginary line bisecting the body into two equal right and left halves
Prone	Lying down with the face toward the ground
Supine	Lying down with the face toward the ceiling
Anterior	Toward the front of the body
Posterior	Toward the back of the body
Ventral	Toward the front of the body
Dorsal	Toward the back of the body
Superior	Toward the head or above another structure
Inferior	Toward the ground or below another structure
Cranial *cephalic*	Toward the head or skull
Caudal	Toward the ground or tailbone
Supra	Above an anatomical structure
Infra	Below an anatomical structure
Proximal	Close to the midline or an anatomical structure *point of attachment*
Distal	Away from the midline or an anatomical structure *point of attachment*
Medial	Close to the midline of the body along a linear line
Lateral	Away from the midline of the body along a linear line
Superficial	Toward the surface or closer to the surface than another structure
Deep	Away from the surface or farther away from the surface than another structure

Table 1-2   *Combination Terms Referencing Anatomical Positions*

Anatomical Combination	Description
Anterolateral	Toward the anterior and lateral surface
Anteromedial	Toward the anterior and medial surface
Posterolateral	Toward the posterior and lateral surface
Posteromedial	Toward the posterior and medial surface

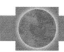 TERMINOLOGY USED TO DESCRIBE SIZE AND LENGTH

One simple technique to use for understanding the name of an anatomical structure is to determine its size in comparison to other structures that are located in a given region of the body. For example, you may notice that certain muscles in a given region are longer or shorter than others. Much like anatomical reference terms, the size of a structure can be divided into further categories, such as physical size and anatomical length.

Physical Size

Many times you will notice that a muscle has a large or small mass. In this case, terms that refer to the physical size of a muscle are given to the muscle of the given region. The terms **magnus** and **maximus** are given to muscles with a large surface area or size, whereas the terms **minimus** and **minimi** are given to muscles of a smaller surface area or size. For example, when identifying the muscles of the gluteal region, the terms *gluteus maximus, gluteus medius,* and *gluteus minimus* are used to describe the size of the muscles in relationship to one another. In this example, the size of the gluteus **medius** is between the size of the gluteus maximus and that of the gluteus minimus. Another example of the size of a structure can be applied to the little finger and little toe, which are both named the digiti minimi.

Anatomical Length

The length of a structure may also be used to describe a structure. The terms **longus** and **brevis** are commonly associated with the length of the structure. *Longus* means that the structure is longer than another structure in the same region, whereas *brevis* refers to a structure that is shorter. For example, the adductor muscle group of the hip region has three muscles that return the leg back to its original position after the leg has been moved away from the midline. These muscles include the adductor magnus, adductor longus, and adductor brevis. When these muscles are discussed further in the text, they can be identified accordingly as being huge (adductor magnus), long (adductor longus), and short (adductor brevis).

 PLANES AND AXES

Anatomists and biomechanists have devised a method to understand the appropriate movements around a specific joint. The terms *planes* and *axes* are applied to the movements of the human body as it moves through a full range of motion. An in-depth discussion of the planes and axes of movement are further provided in Chapter 3.

Anatomical Planes

There are three anatomical **planes** associated with the three dimensions in space. Each plane is at a 90-degree angle, or perpendicular, to the other two planes. The first plane is the **sagittal plane** (Z plane), sometimes called the median plane (Figure 1-4). It is a vertical plane that passes through the body, dividing it into right and left sections. An example of a movement in the sagittal plane would be nodding the head "yes." The second plane is the **frontal plane** (X plane), sometimes called the

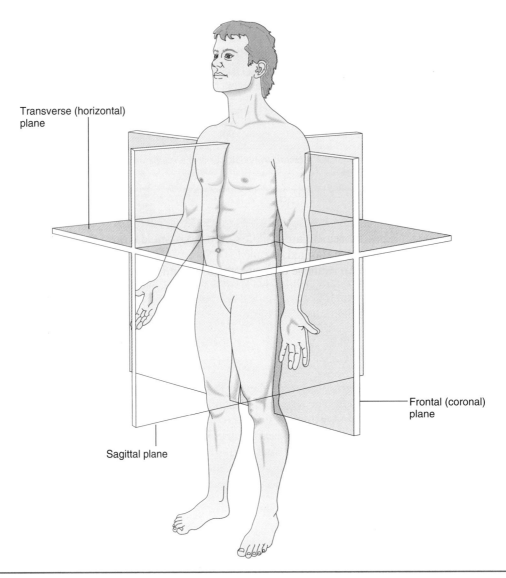

Transverse (horizontal) plane

Frontal (coronal) plane

Sagittal plane

Figure 1-4 *Anatomical Planes*

OTA Perspective

Activity analyses will be emphasized throughout this textbook, because they are a specialty skill area for the OTA. Clinical reasoning questions will be raised, and in order to discuss and answer them, the OTA may need to reference practice guidelines that include state licensure laws, the American Occupational Therapy Association's (AOTA's) Code of Ethics, and Standards of Practice. Examples of interventions to use in client-centered treatment foci are a combination of what is common practice and more innovative concepts. The necessary OTA skills and knowledge will be applied across the life span to various diagnostic categories and in a variety of treatment settings. Language used will generally be from *The Occupational Therapy Practice Framework* (*The Framework*), rather than the *Uniform Terminology-III* it is replacing. Keep in mind that in order to be a true OT practitioner, kinesiology concepts must be integrated within fundamental OT practices.

lateral plane (see Figure 1-4). It is also a vertical plane that passes through the body, dividing it into anterior and posterior sections. An example of a movement in the frontal plane would be jumping jacks. The last plane is the **transverse plane** (Y plane), sometimes called the horizontal plane (see Figure 1-4). This is a horizontal plane that passes through the body, dividing it into superior and inferior sections. An example of a movement in the transverse plane would be twisting the trunk from right to left and back again.

Axes

All movements occur in a plane and around an axis. An **axis** is most easily defined as a rod or rigid bar that passes through the joint that is moving. Because there are three planes of movement, there are also three axes that lie perpendicular to a given plane. The first is called the **frontal axis** (X-axis), which passes horizontally through the body from side to side. An example of a movement around the frontal axis is hip flexion, which is a movement in the sagittal plane around the frontal axis (Figure 1-5). The second axis is called the **sagittal axis** (Z-axis), which passes horizontally through the body from front to back (see Figure 1-5). An example of a movement around the sagittal axis would be arm abduction, which is a movement in the frontal plane around the sagittal axis. The last axis is called **vertical axis** (Y-axis), which passes vertically through the body from top to bottom (see Figure 1-5). An example of a movement around the vertical axis would be shaking the head "no" (lateral rotation), which is a movement in the transverse plane around the vertical axis.

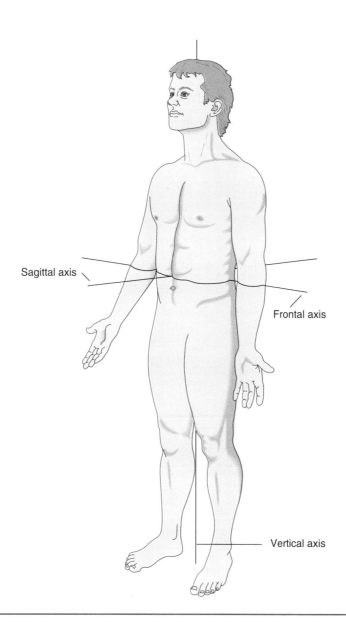

Figure 1-5 *Axes*

KEY CONCEPTS

◼ Kinesiology is the study of human movement and explains the relationships between complex structures of the human body. A strong understanding of kinesiology will aid the OTA in their field of work.

◼ The anatomical position is demonstrated by standing erect, with the feet flat on the ground and the palms of the hands facing forward. This position allows for a common starting point that is used for all directional terms to describe the movements and positions of the human body.

◼ Terminology used to describe size and length shows the relationships between anatomical structures.

◼ Planes and axes are used to describe the movements of the human body as it progresses through range of motion.

BIBLIOGRAPHY

Jones, B. D. (1999). *Delmar's comprehensive medical terminology: A competency based approach.* Clifton Park, NY: Thomson Delmar Learning.

Marieb, E. N. (2003). *Human anatomy and physiology* (6th ed.). Menlo Park, CA: Addison Wesley Longman.

Rizzo, D. C. (2001). *Delmar's fundamentals of anatomy and physiology.* Clifton Park, NY: Thomson Delmar Learning.

Scott, A. S., & Fong, E. (2004). *Body structures and functions.* (10th ed.). Clifton Park, NY: Thomson Delmar Learning.

Taber's cyclopedic medical dictionary (19th ed.). (2001). Philadelphia: F. A. Davis.

WEB RESOURCES

• To learn more about the Model of Human Occupation, go to www.uic.edu.
   Click on Academic Departments
   Click on Occupational Therapy
   Click on MOHO
   or search the University of Illinois at Chicago Web site for Model of Human Occupation, or MOHO.
• To learn more about the field of OTAs, go to www.aota.org.

(These Web addresses were current as of September 2003.)

REVIEW QUESTIONS

Fill in the Blank

Provide the word(s) or phrase(s) that best complete the sentence.

1. The <u>Sagittal</u> plane divides the body into two equal right and left halves.

2. A movement in the sagittal plane occurs around a/an <u>frontal</u> axis.

3. The <u>horizontal</u> plane divides the body into inferior and superior regions.

4. A movement in the frontal plane occurs around a/an _Sagittal_ axis.

5. The _frontal_ plane divides the body into anterior and posterior regions.

Multiple Choice

Select the best answer to complete the following statements.

1. The nose is _____ to the mouth.
   a. lateral
   b. inferior
   c. superior
   d. distal

2. The heart is _____ to the sternum.
   a. superficial
   b. lateral
   c. caudal
   d. deep

3. The radius is _____ to the ulna in the anatomical position.
   a. medial
   b. distal
   c. superficial
   d. lateral

4. Standing erect with the feet flat and the palms facing toward the sides of the body describes the _____ position.
   a. prone
   b. supine
   c. fundamental
   d. anatomical

5. Minimi is to maximus as brevis is to _____.
   a. magnus
   b. caudal
   c. cranial
   d. longus

Matching

Match each of the following descriptions with the appropriate term.

_E_ 1. Closer to the midline

_G_ 2. The white line that is a separation point

_A_ 3. An anatomical structure on the anterior and lateral surfaces

_K_ 4. Referring to the front

_D_ 5. A structure located on the posterior and medial side of the body

_C_ 6. A structure that is considered to be short

_H_ 7. The study of human movement

_B_ 8. Referring to the back

_J_ 9. Lying face down

_I_ 10. Away from the midline

A. Anterolateral

B. Dorsal

C. Brevis

D. Posteromedial

E. Proximal

F. Caudal

G. Linea alba

H. Kinesiology

I. Distal

J. Prone

K. Anterior

Critical Thinking

1. Consider the phrase from a well-known children's game "Put your right arm in, pull your right arm out." Complete an activity analysis of that movement in terms of anatomical positions and planes and axes of movement.

2. List the plane and axis in which each of the following movements occur:
   a. Cervical flexion
   b. Glenohumeral internal rotation
   c. Trunk side bending
   d. Radial and ulnar deviation
   e. Hip abduction
   f. Forearm flexion

3. Demonstrate the joint movement that occurs in each of the following planes:
   a. Transverse
   b. Sagittal
   c. Frontal

4. Using the directional terms learned in this chapter, describe the movement of the right arm (remember to start in the anatomical position). Have your partner demonstrate one, then switch.
   a. Bowling
   b. Eating
   c. Walking
   d. Sweeping
   e. Dusting
   f. Swimming (freestyle)

5. Describe *occupational therapy*. Include a brief description of a model of practice. At this point in your study of OT and kinesiology, do you have a concept of how the models, and which ones, might interact with kinesiology? Write this down and review it at the end of this particular course of study.

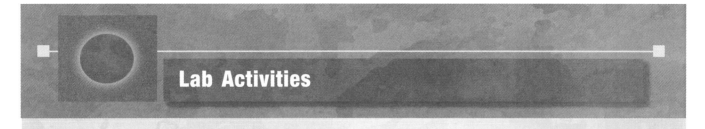

Lab Activities

Lab 1-1: Activity Analysis—Walking

Objective: To identify the movement of the body through planes when walking.

Equipment Needed: A lab partner, pen/pencil, paper

Step 1. Have one person walk across the room slowly.

Step 2. Describe the motion that occurs in the right leg at the hip, knee, and ankle joints in terms of planes and axes of movement in the three different phases:

- Stance phase—the weight is put on the right leg
- Swing Phase—the right leg is in the air
- Heel strike—the right leg makes contact with the ground

Step 3. Switch roles with your lab partner and repeat steps 1 and 2.

Lab 1-2: Anatomical Positions

Objective: To identify the various anatomical positions commonly used in the practice of physical therapy and occupational therapy.

Equipment Needed: A lab partner, pen/pencil, paper

Step 1. Place your partner in the following positions:

- Anatomical position
- Fundamental position
- Prone lying
- Supine lying

Step 2. Switch roles with your lab partner and repeat step 1.

Lab 1-3: Use of Anatomical Terminology

Objective: To identify and describe anatomical terms.

Equipment Needed: A lab partner, pen/pencil, paper

Step 1. Pretend that your partner is your client. Describe the following terms to your client in layman's language. Give a specific example for each using anatomical examples.

- Medial
- Lateral
- Distal
- Proximal
- Superior
- Inferior
- Anterior
- Posterior
- Dorsal
- Ventral
- Cranial
- Caudal

Step 2. Switch roles with your partner and repeat step 1.

Chapter 2

MUSCULAR ANATOMY AND PHYSIOLOGY

Objectives

Upon completion of this chapter, the reader should be able to:

- Identify the three types of muscle tissue.
- Describe the macroscopic anatomical structure of muscle.
- Identify the structures of the sarcolemma and the contributing roles of each structure to muscle contraction.
- Describe the functional unit of muscle and identify the components that make up this structure.
- Describe the myofilaments and their relationship to the function of the sarcomere.
- Discuss the role of calcium in the regulation of muscle contractions.
- Define the role of adenosine diphosphate and adenosine triphosphate in muscle contractions.
- Describe the anatomy of the neuromuscular junction.
- Describe the physiological functions that occur at the neuromuscular junction.
- Provide an understanding of the complex physiological steps involved in the Sliding Filament Theory.

Key Words

acetylcholine (ACh)
actin filament (F-actin)
adenosine diphosphate (ADP)
adenosine triphosphate (ATP)
anaerobic glycolysis
anisotropic band (A band)
ATP-phosphocreatine system
basal lamina
calcium ion
cardiac muscle
endomysium
epimysium
fasciculus
globular actin (G-actin)
heavy myosin chain
inhibitory troponin I (TnI)
innervate
insertion
isotropic band (I band)
light myosin chain
motor end plate
motor neuron
muscle fiber
myofibril
myosin
neuromuscular junction
origin
perimysium
sarcolemma
sarcoplasm
sarcoplasmic reticulum
skeletal muscle
smooth muscle
terminal cisternae
transverse tubule
tropomyosin
troponin C (TnC)
troponin complex
troponin T (TnT)
Z disk

INTRODUCTION

Imagine all of the different movements the body makes. The heart beats to pump blood throughout the body (cardiac muscle), the arteries contract to help the heart move blood throughout the cardiovascular system, the intestines use peristalsis to move food for digestive purposes (smooth muscle), and skeletal muscles contract to allow the extremities to move through a full range of motion. Contractions of the various muscles in the body are provided by a specific tissue makeup of organs and body regions.

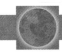

MUSCLE TISSUE

The body consists of three types of muscle tissue: smooth, cardiac, and skeletal. Each type of tissue provides a specific function for the region of the body in which it is located.

Smooth Muscle

Picture what would happen if you had to consciously think about contracting the muscles in your intestines and arteries at all times during the day! This would be extremely difficult and would probably give you a headache by just thinking about these movements. Fortunately, the organ structures that move substances through the body are made up of **smooth muscle** (muscle that is unmarked by any striations), and their actions are strictly involuntary. The actions and cell shape of smooth muscle distinguish it from other types of muscle tissue (Figure 2-1). Often termed *nonstriated muscle*, smooth muscle has a simple shape and is found running parallel to the long axis of the specific organ in which it is located. This parallel arrangement allows the contracting muscle to propel substances throughout the organs.

Cardiac Muscle

Cardiac muscle tissue is only found in the heart. Although cardiac muscle is involuntary, the muscle cells are striated, which means that they have alternating areas of light and dark bands with a structural appearance similar to that found in

OTA Perspective

OT practitioners treat clients with diagnoses that directly or indirectly affect muscle function and, thereby, occupational performance. Nervous system diseases, including degenerative diseases such as Parkinson's disease and multiple sclerosis, congenital diseases such as cerebral palsy and muscular dystrophy, and musculoskeletal diseases or impairments such as systemic lupus erythematosus (SLE) and hand function impairments, all affect muscle function. In order to treat the client's functional goals in an occupational performance context, the OTA must have an understanding of the diseases or injuries that affect the muscles, hence the reason for the study of kinesiology! Although the focus will be on the study of movement—performance skills and client factors—refer to *The Framework* for other aspects within the domain of OT. It is further suggested that a resource on human diseases be available to help you understand the relationship between OT, kinesiology, and human disease and pathology.

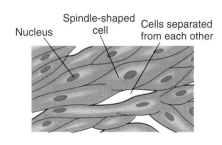

Nucleus

Spindle-shaped cell

Cells separated from each other

Figure 2-1a Smooth Muscle

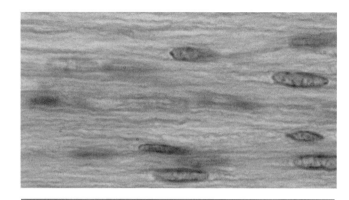

Figure 2-1b Smooth Muscle

skeletal muscle. However, cardiac muscle tissue is branched, and the distances between the striations are further apart (Figure 2-2).

Skeletal Muscle

The third type of muscle tissue found in the human body is **skeletal muscle** tissue (Figure 2-3). Skeletal muscle is voluntary, is arranged in long rod-like bundles of muscle fibers that possess a striated appearance, and allows the extremities to move through a full range of motion. The striations found in skeletal muscle, unlike cardiac muscle, are uniform and arranged in long bands. The study of human movement is directly related to the structure and function of skeletal muscle.

 MUSCLE

To understand the true fundamentals of human movement, the OTA must first understand the complex anatomical and physiological relationships that occur between the largest and smallest skeletal muscle structures. The OTA must also realize that muscle contractions are dependent on the complex interactions between the muscular and nervous systems. Therefore, muscle contractions are a complex series of events rooted in the anatomical and physiological structures of the muscular and nervous systems.

When individuals think of muscle tissue, they often picture large, bulky muscles that are identified by name or location, such as the gastrocnemius, pectoralis major, and biceps brachii. In the study of kinesiology, one must understand that the macroscopic and microscopic anatomical structures of muscles in the body have common characteristics and that the arrangements of these structures allow the complex physiological processes to occur during muscle contraction. To get away from thinking about specific muscles, we begin our study of muscle anatomy and physiology by investigating the general macroscopic anatomical structures of muscle and then studying the complex physiological processes that occur between the

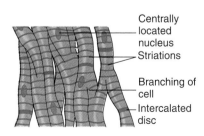

Centrally located nucleus

Striations

Branching of cell

Intercalated disc

Figure 2-2a Cardiac Muscle

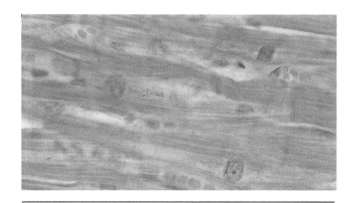

Figure 2-2b Cardiac Muscle

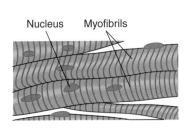

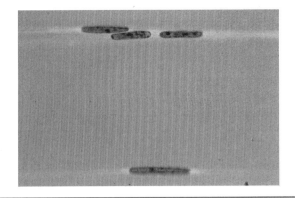

Figure 2-3a   *Skeletal Muscle*   *Figure 2-3b*   *Skeletal Muscle*

microscopic structures. Once these anatomical structures and physiological processes have been explained, we will take an in-depth look at the relationships between the nervous and muscular systems and the Sliding Filament Theory.

The Macroscopic Structure of Skeletal Muscle

Every skeletal muscle in the human body has a similar macroscopic structural arrangement (Figure 2-4). When a muscle is dissected to smaller levels of organization, it shows that the muscle possesses universal characteristics throughout. Muscle is specifically bundled together into functional groups of tissue and is distinguished from the macroscopic and microscopic levels of organization by these grouping as shown in Table 2-1 and Table 2-2.

A distinct feature of skeletal muscle is that (in most cases) it possesses two tendons that firmly attach it to a bone. One tendon, usually the more stable, is the **origin**, and the other tendon is the **insertion**, which is connected to the bone that is moving. Tendons are continuous with the muscle and during a contraction pull the origins and insertions together as the muscle shortens, decreasing the joint angle. The concept of origin and insertion is discussed further in Chapter 3. This concept becomes increasingly important as the muscles are described in each chapter.

The outermost muscle tissue that covers the entire belly of the muscle is a dense, fibrous overcoat tissue called the **epimysium**. The epimysium holds the muscle firmly in place and is continuous with the muscle tendon. A cross-sectional cut of the epimysium and muscle belly would reveal many bundles of muscle fibers, which are called **fasciculi**. A second connective tissue sheath, called the **perimysium**, covers each fasciculus and distinguishes each one from the next. A final deep connective tissue, the **endomysium**, covers each individual muscle fiber. The fibrous connective tissues found in muscle provide support and reinforcement for the muscle during each contraction.

The Microscopic Structure of Skeletal Muscle

The **muscle fiber** (Figure 2-5) is the cell of the muscle that covers the entire length of the muscle. For example, a muscle fiber in the sartorius muscle, the longest muscle in the body, could be close to 1 1/2 to 2 feet long. Although muscle fibers are

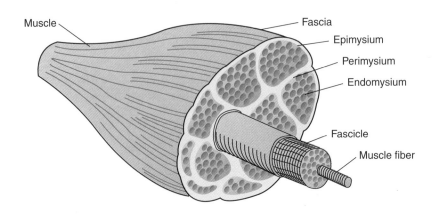

Figure 2-4   *Macroscopic Structure of Muscle*

Table 2-1 *Functional Group of Muscles at the Macroscopic Level*

Functional Group	Description
Epimysium	Outer tissue surrounding all muscular components
Perimysium	Tissue surrounding each fascicular bundle
Endomysium	Tissue surrounding each fascicle
Fasciculus	A bundle of muscle fibers

Table 2-2 *Functional Group of Muscles at the Microscopic Level*

Functional Group	Description
Muscle Fiber	Microscopic structure containing the physiological components that cause muscle contraction
Sarcolemma	Tissue that covers the muscle fiber and allows nervous stimulation to cause muscle contraction
Myofilaments	Contractile units within the muscle fiber, including the sarcomere, actin, and myosin

long, their circumference is only between 10 and 100 micrometers; therefore, it is necessary to use a microscope to see their structural components. Muscle fibers are important to muscle contractions because they contain the contractile structures that allow the complex physiological processes to occur during the contraction.

Each muscle fiber is made up of hundreds to thousands of rod-like **myofibrils** that span the entire length of the muscle fiber. These rod-like structures contain thousands of actin and myosin molecules that line up lengthwise along the long axis of the muscle fiber and are responsible for muscle contraction. Surrounding the myofibril groupings of a muscle fiber is the **sarcolemma**, which is the cell wall of the muscle fiber.

The Sarcolemma
The sarcolemma has several unique structures that are involved in transmitting the nervous stimulation and nutrients deep inside the muscle fiber to cause muscle contraction and to nourish the muscle cell. Immediately deep to the sarcolemma is the gel-like liquid cytoplasm of the muscle fiber called the **sarcoplasm**. The sarcoplasm suspends the myofibrils and ensures the delivery of **calcium ions** and nutrients to the interior regions of the muscle fiber (intrasarcoplasmic).

The importance of the sarcolemma to muscle contractions is twofold (Figure 2-6). First, each sarcolemma is found next to the terminal portion of the **motor neuron** (nerve) that **innervates** (stimulates) the muscle fiber and forms the neuromuscular junction. This close proximity allows nervous stimulation to move from a motor neuron to the muscle tissue. Second, embedded within the sarcolemma are three structures that are responsible for transmitting the impulse deep into the myofibrils and stimulate the contractile units of the microscopic muscle tissue. These important structures include the transverse tubules, sarcoplasmic reticulum, and terminal cisternae (triad).

Transverse Tubules. An extensive network of **transverse tubules** (T-tubules) runs perpendicular to the myofibrils and extends from the superficial layers of the sarcolemma to the deepest myofibrils. The T-tubules carry an action potential from a stimulated sarcolemma and deliver the stimulation to the deepest myofibrils. T-tubules also provide a pathway to deliver glucose, oxygen, proteins, and ions to the sarcoplasm to be used for cellular and metabolic processes.

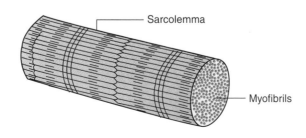

Figure 2-5 *The Muscle Fiber*

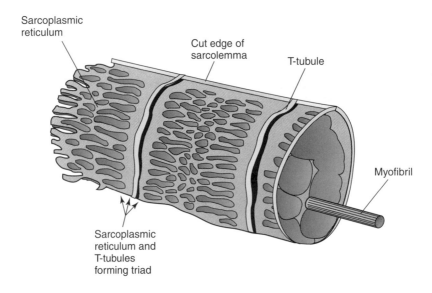

Figure 2-6   *Anatomy of the Sarcolemma*

Sarcoplasmic Reticulum. Superficial to the myofibrils is a second complex series of tubes called the **sarcoplasmic reticulum** (SR). The SR are found deep to the sarcolemma and run parallel to the myofibril. Each SR contains a reservoir of calcium ions and its close proximity to the myofibrils is important to the release and binding of calcium to the contractile units of the sarcomere.

Terminal Cisternae. The distal end of the SR that articulates with the T-tubules is the **terminal cisternae**. The surface membranes of the terminal cisternae contain hundreds of calcium-gated ion channels that regulate the intrasarcoplasmic calcium concentration. When an action potential from the T-tubules reaches the terminal cisternae, the ion channels of the terminal cisternae release calcium from the SR into the sarcoplasm. The release of calcium into the sarcoplasm creates the first intrasarcoplasmic processes that cause a muscle contraction.

Each terminal cisternae has "junction feet" that articulate with the adjacent T-tubules. When an action potential reaches the terminal cisternae, either electrical stimulation or chemical stimulation opens the calcium-gated ion channels and release additional calcium ions into the sarcoplasm. However, this action is yet to be fully identified. Following the action potential, excess calcium ions are taken back into the terminal cisternae via active transport with the use of **adenosine triphosphate (ATP)**.

Sarcoplasm The sarcoplasm is a gel-like substance that surrounds each of the individual myofibrils and provides nourishment for the organelles of the muscle fiber. Following the action potential, calcium is released into the sarcoplasm and binds to the contractile unit of the myofibrils, causing the ensuing muscle contraction. The sarcoplasm also contains metabolic substances that include ATP, the oxygen-binding compound myoglobin, and stored glycogen, which are all important for providing energy for the muscle contraction. In addition, the sarcoplasm contains proteins, which are used to build muscle, and minerals, which nourish the muscle cell.

The Sarcomere The functional unit of muscle is a microscopic structure called the sarcomere (Figure 2-7). It has been estimated that each myofibril has approximately 1,500 to 2,000 individual sarcomeres that connect with one another and that extend the full length of the long axis of the myofibril.

Each sarcomere is made up of several distinct myofilaments, including actin, myosin, Z disks, and titin filaments. The Z disks are commonly referred to as the anchor point for the sarcomere and distinguish one sarcomere from the next. **Actin filaments (F-actin)** are "thin" filaments that firmly attach to the **Z disk**. The functional purpose of actin is to provide a binding site for the **myosin** ("thick" filaments) during the muscle contraction. A third important component of the sarcomere is the "thick" myosin filament. During a contraction, a major portion of the myosin molecule pulls on the actin, causing the actin filament to slide over the myosin molecule. This pulling on the actin fiber causes the shortening of the sarcomere. The shortening of the Z disks at the microscopic level results in a decreased joint angle at the macroscopic level.

The striated appearance in skeletal muscle is caused by the anatomical position of the actin and myosin in the sarcomere. Two distinct color bands can be identified when a muscle fiber is magnified under an electron micrograph. The dark bands in the sarcomere are composed of the myosin filament and the non-Z disk ends of the actin filaments. Because of the

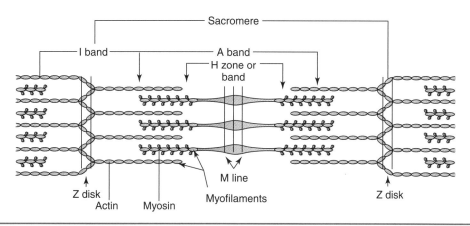

Figure 2-7   *The Sarcomere*

position of these components, this area does not polarize light; it is termed the **anisotropic band (A band)**. A second area, which polarizes light, is the **isotropic band (I band)**. The I band contains the Z disk portion of the actin and the Z disks. During the muscle contraction, the I band area decreases as the sarcomere shortens.

The Myofilament   The contractile structures of the sarcomere are the myofilaments, which consist of the F-actin, G-actin, troponin complex, tropomyosin, myosin molecule, heavy myosin chain, and light myosin chain. Each of these components plays an important role in each muscle contraction.

Actin Myofilament.   The actin myofilament is composed of a complex series of protein structures including the actin filament, globular actin, tropomyosin, and troponin. Each of these components plays an important role in the muscle contraction and structure of the sarcomere.

The actin filament (F-actin) is a double helix structure made up of small oval-shaped polymerized **globular actin (G-actin)** proteins (Figure 2-8). Each F-actin protein has approximately 13 G-actin molecules per helical revolution. The G-actin structure is important to muscle contraction because each contains one molecule of **adenosine diphosphate (ADP)**, which is the active site that attracts the myosin head to cause a muscle contraction.

Troponin Complex.   The **troponin complex** is a series of three protein structures that are bound to the G-actin and tropomyosin positioned next to the active site on the G-actin molecules (see Figure 2-8). During resting conditions, the troponin complex allows the tropomyosin strands to cover the active sites on the G-actin molecules. Each troponin structure provides a separate physiological function that is important to muscle contraction.

The protein compound **troponin C (TnC)** has a strong attraction for calcium ions, and each TnC has the ability to bind with up to four calcium ions. When the intrasarcoplasmic concentration of calcium ions increases, the calcium ions bind to the TnC and cause the troponin complex to go through a conformational change that cause the complex to shift and tug on the tropomyosin. A second troponin molecule is **troponin T (TnT)** which is bound to the tropomyosin strands. When the complex goes through a conformational change, TnT tugs on the tropomyosin, exposing the binding sites on the G-actin molecules. The third troponin protein is **inhibitory troponin I (TnI)**, which binds the troponin complex to the G-actin. During a muscle contraction, the TnI pivots further to help expose the active site on the G-actin.

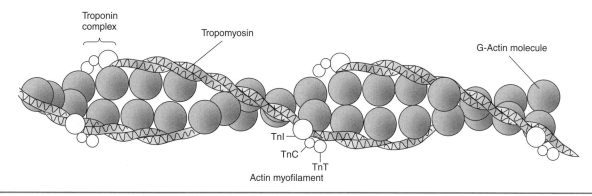

Figure 2-8   *The Actin Myofilament*

Tropomyosin. Tropomyosin is a long strand structure that wraps around the entire length of the F-actin. The tropomyosin strand is unique because it is not directly attached to the actin. This relationship allows the tropomyosin to rest on the active site and shift when the troponin complex shifts. During a muscle contraction, the tropomyosin shifts off the G-actin active sites when the troponin complex goes through its conformational change. More specifically, when TnC shifts because of the increase in intrasarcoplasmic calcium concentrations, the TnT tugs on the tropomyosin. The action causes the tropomyosin to shift off the active site, allowing the myosin head to attach to the active site on the G-actin and causing the actin to slide over the myosin.

Myosin Molecule. Myosin is the second major myofilament found in the sarcomere (Figure 2-9). The myosin structure is made up of several hundred myosin molecules. Myosin provides the cross-bridge and physical powerstroke that pulls the actin filaments toward the center of the sarcomere.

Heavy Myosin Chain. Each myosin molecule is made up of two types of polypeptide chains wrapped in a double helix formation. The first of these chains is the myosin body, which is more commonly referred to as the **heavy myosin chain** (Figure 2-10). The myosin body is a double helix structure and is the base of support for the mechanical events provided by the myosin head. The heavy chain myosin provides an arm that extends the myosin outward to attach to the active site. Numerous myosin bodies make up the physical appearance of the myosin molecule.

Light Myosin Chain. The **light myosin chain** (myosin head) is a structure made up of four small polypeptide chains (see Figure 2-10). The myosin head provides the cross-bridge and attaches to the active site on the G-actin molecule. As a result, the myosin head pivots and pulls on the active site.

The myosin head has several important distinguishing characteristics that are important for the physical events that occur during a muscle contraction. First, the myosin head is attracted to the ADP on the G-actin active site. Once troponin shifts off the active site, the exposed ADP attracts the myosin head. This allows the myosin head to attach to the active site, providing the cross-bridge. Second, each myosin head is spaced 120 degrees from the previous head. This allows the heads to "move" the actin while pulling the actin structures toward the center of the sarcomere. Finally, each myosin head has a binding site for ATP, and deriving the energy for the contraction from this high-energy compound.

 ## ENERGY FOR THE MUSCLE CONTRACTION

The energy derived for muscle contractions comes from the formation of ATP from stored creatine phosphate, glycogen, fat, and protein. ATP, used in muscle contractions, is derived from chemical reactions that break down the stored fuel sources in the sarcoplasm and mitochondria of the muscle fiber.

ATP-Phosphocreatine System

The initial energy for the muscle contraction is provided by the **ATP-phosphocreatine system**. During power events and initiation of exercise, creatine kinase breaks down phosphocreatine to provide the necessary ATP for the muscle contraction. Figure 2-11 shows reaction for this.

Anaerobic System

During exercise that lasts from 1 to 5 minutes, ATP is provided through the breakdown of glycogen stored in the liver and skeletal muscle cells. The process through which glycogen is broken down is called **anaerobic glycolysis**. Anaerobic glycol-

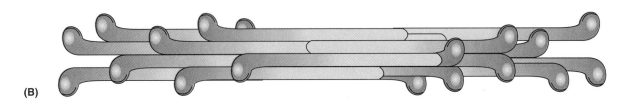

(B)

Figure 2-9   *The Myosin Myofilament*

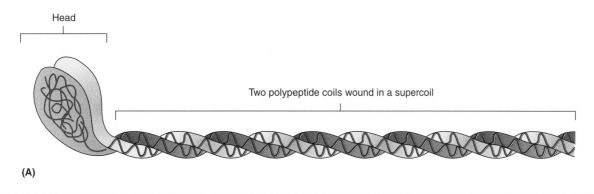

Figure 2-10   *The Anatomy of the Myosin Molecules*

ysis occurs as one molecule of glycogen is broken down without the use of oxygen to provide the body with two ATP molecules. The end result of anaerobic glycolysis is the formation of lactic acid, which is commonly associated with this system. However, during periods of extended exercise, glycogen is broken down aerobically and is the initiation point for metabolism during sustained exercise.

The third metabolic pathway requires oxygen to break down fats and carbohydrate for the production of ATP. Fat is specifically broken down in the mitochondria of the muscle fibers and provides large quantities of ATP for the muscle contraction. During periods of sustained exercise, mainly aerobic, the fat in the body is mobilized and delivered to the muscle fiber to provide large quantities of energy.

THE NEUROMUSCULAR JUNCTION

Nerves that innervate skeletal muscles originate from the cranial nerves or motor nerves of the anterior horns of the spinal cord. These nerves can extend from several inches, for example, those that innervate the muscles in the back, to 1 meter, such as those that originate from the lumbosacral plexus in the pelvic region and innervate the muscles that move the big toe.

Each motor neuron that innervates a skeletal muscle terminates at the **motor end plate**, or synapse, found at the **neuromuscular junction** (Figure 2-12). It is important to know that a gap is formed between the distal end of the motor neuron and the sarcolemma of the muscle that the nerve innervates (the two tissues never touch). As a result, the synaptic cleft is formed and chemical neurotransmitters must be present to carry the action potential from the motor neuron to the sarcolemma. The terminal end of the motor neuron at the neuromuscular junction is made up of several unique structures that are required for the nervous stimulation to pass from the motor neuron to the innervated muscle.

Contained in each motor end plate are thousands of small sac structures called synaptic vesicles that house the chemical neurotransmitter **acetylcholine (ACh)**. With each action potential, approximately 300 synaptic vesicles fuse with the end plate and release ACh into the synaptic cleft. ACh is an important neurotransmitter because this chemical messenger carries the action potential from the motor neuron across the synaptic cleft to the ACh receptor site found on the sarcolemma of the innervated skeletal muscle. As a result, the action potential travels along the sarcolemma and down the T-tubules to cause the release of calcium ions from the terminal cisternae.

Immediately following an action potential, additional ACh is rapidly resynthesized by the cytoplasm of the motor end plate and absorbed by the synaptic vesicles. Remaining ACh in the synaptic cleft is broken down by the enzyme acetylcholinesterase.

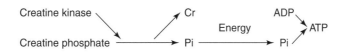

Figure 2-11   *ATP Phosphocreatine System*

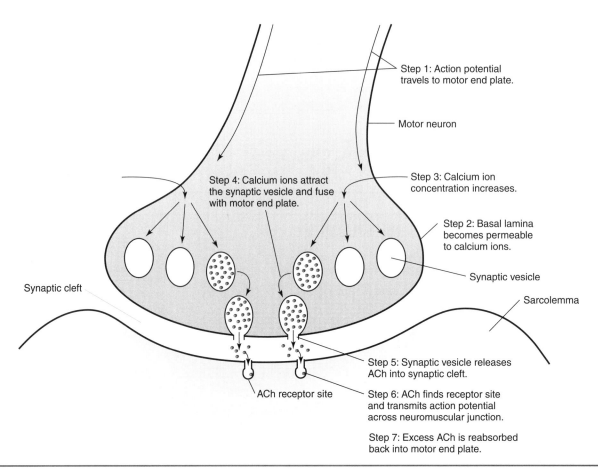

Figure 2-12 *The Neuromuscular Junction*

The **basal lamina** is connective tissue also found in the distal end of the motor neuron. During the action potential, the lamina becomes highly permeable to extracellular concentrations of calcium ions. Once the permeability of the lamina changes, the inside of the motor neuron floods with calcium ions. This increase in calcium causes the synaptic vesicles to fuse with the distal end of the motor end plate, resulting in the release of ACh into the synaptic cleft.

OTA Perspective

OT practitioners employ a variety of therapeutic treatment techniques that focus directly on muscular deficit, namely, range of motion (ROM) and strengthening exercises: soft tissue massage; prolonged stretch, including splinting and serial casting; postural control and alignment exercises; physical agent modalities; and work simplification activities and education. Focusing on muscular deficit, the OTA employs concepts and treatment techniques from the "bottom-up" models, a treatment focused on occupational performance, and then utilizes concepts and interventions from "top-down" models for changes in functional ability that may be caused by muscular deficits. Not only does the OTA need to understand the treatment techniques and how they integrate into an occupation performance context, matching the client's goals, but he or she also needs to understand the effect of that intervention on the disease process.

THE SLIDING FILAMENT THEORY

In the early 1950s, Hubert Huxley first devised the theory that explains the physiological events that occur during a muscle contraction. His theory is still taught today and continues to be the best explanation of the physiological steps that cause a muscle contraction.

Before its attachment to the active site, the myosin head is in its high-energy state (Figure 2-13). During this state, ATP is broken down into ADP and an inorganic phosphate ion (Pi), resulting in the creation of potential energy. After the myosin

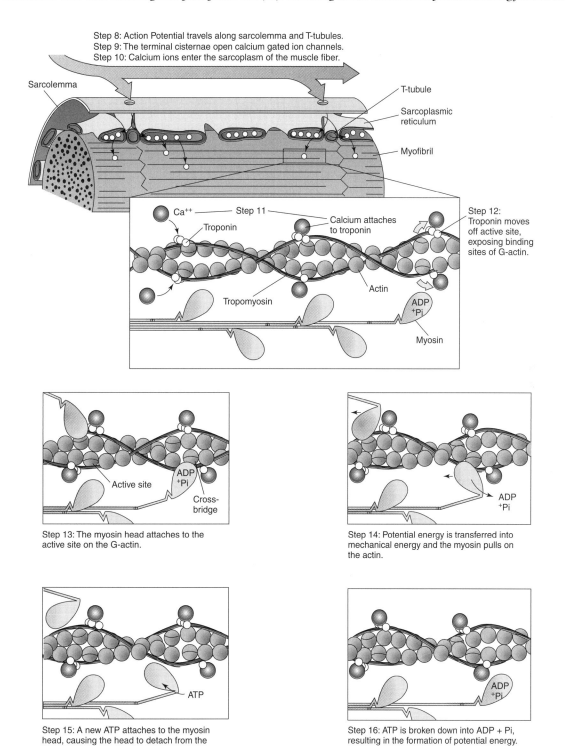

Figure 2-13 *The Events of the Sliding Filament Theory*

head attaches to the active site on the G-actin, the potential energy from the ADP + Pi is released and converted into mechanical energy. This transfer of energy causes the myosin head to pull on the actin and shorten the sarcomere. After the ADP + Pi energy is released, the myosin head converts to its low-energy state.

Following the mechanical events of the myosin head, a new ATP molecule attaches to it. Once attached, the myosin head detaches from the active site and the myosin is relaxed. The enzyme ATPase then hydrolyzes the ATP molecule, breaking it into ADP + Pi. The result of this transformation is the conversion of the myosin head back to its high-energy state. After these processes occur, the myosin head is ready for the next action potential and muscle contractions.

Each myosin head is anatomically spaced 120 degrees from the previous myosin head. Mechanically speaking, the placement of the heads allows the myosin head to "move" the actin filament and pull with greatest mechanical force. During the muscle contraction, only one out of three myosin heads is attached to the active site on the G-actin. This allows the myosin head to keep tension on the actin. For example, imagine the Egyptians moving a large stone of the pyramids. To keep the tension, some of the people had to keep constant tension on the rope while others moved their hand forward. Similarly, several myosin molecules keep tension on the actin molecule while others are moved forward. The 120-degree separation allows for the conduction of these mechanical events. Table 2-3 summarizes the steps that lead to a muscle contraction.

Table 2-3 *Summary of the Physiological Steps that Lead to the Muscle Contraction*

The Neuromuscular Junction (see Figure 2-12)	
Step 1.	An action potential travels down a motor neuron to the motor end plate.
Step 2.	The basal lamina becomes highly permeable to calcium ions.
Step 3.	The concentration of calcium ions inside the motor end plate increases.
Step 4.	Calcium ions attract the synaptic vesicle to fuse with the motor end plate.
Step 5.	The synaptic vesicles release ACh into the synaptic cleft.
Step 6.	ACh finds the ACh receptor site on the sarcolemma and the action potential transmits across the neuromuscular junction.
Step 7.	Acetylcholinesterase breaks down the remaining ACh in the synaptic cleft and reabsorbed back into the motor end plate.
The Sarcolemma (see Figure 2-13)	
Step 8.	The action potential travels along the sarcolemma and down the adjacent T-tubules.
Step 9.	After reaching the terminal cisternae, the action potential causes it to open calcium gated ion channels.
Step 10.	Calcium ions from the sarcoplasmic reticulum enter the sarcoplasm of the muscle fiber.
The Myofilaments (see Figure 2-13)	
Step 11.	Calcium attaches to the TnC of the troponin complex. Up to four molecules of calcium attach to each TnC.
Step 12.	The troponin complex goes through a conformational change, tugging on the tropomyosin. The movement of the tropomyosin exposes the binding sites on the G-actin.
Step 13.	The myosin head, attracted to the active site, flips up and attaches to the active site on the G-actin.
The Sliding Filament Theory (see Figure 2-13)	
Step 14.	Potential energy from the ADP + Pi is transferred into mechanical energy and the myosin pulls on the actin.
Step 15.	After the myosin head cocks, it is in its low-energy state. A new ATP attaches to the myosin head and causes the head to detach from the G-actin active site.
Step 16.	ATPase hydrolyzes the ATP, breaking it down into ADP + Pi, and causing the formation of potential energy. Once ATP is broken down, the myosin head is in its high-energy state. This process occurs hundreds of times per muscle contraction as myosin attaches, cocks, and pulls on the actin molecule.

KEY CONCEPTS

- The human body consists of three types of muscle: smooth, cardiac, and skeletal. Each provides a specific function for the system that it is associated with. Kinesiology is mainly concerned with the role of skeletal muscle.

- The macroscopic structure of muscle includes the epimysium, perimysium, endomysium, and fasciculus. Each macroscopic layer covers the next, from macroscopic to microscopic.

- The functional unit of muscle is the sarcomere. This structure contains the myofilaments actin and myosin. During a muscle contraction, these structures work together to pull the sarcomere structure together.

- Actin is made up of three compounds: TnT, TnC, and TnI. The TnC compound is excited in the presence of calcium and initiates the physical events that occur during a muscle contraction.

- During a muscle contraction, thousands of calcium ions are released into the sarcoplasm. This release is important to the contraction because the actin myofilaments are attracted to the calcium ions. Because of this attraction, calcium binds to the actin and causes a shift of the actin complex, which exposes the binding site.

- The neuromuscular junction is located at the synapse between the nervous and muscular tissues. Located at the junction is acetylcholine, which transmits the nervous stimulation from the nerve to the muscle tissue.

- Energy for a muscle contraction is provided by ATP. During a contraction, ATP is continuously broken down into the ADP + Pi form. As a result, energy for the contraction is produced.

- During the muscle contraction, hundreds of thousands of muscle coupling events take place between the myosin head and the active spot on the G-actin.

- The theory that explains the physical events that occur during a muscle contraction is known as the Sliding Filament Theory.

BIBLIOGRAPHY

ACSM's resource manual for guidelines for exercise testing and prescription (4th ed.). (2001). Philadelphia: Lea & Febiger.

Baechle, T. R. (2000). *Essentials of strength training and conditioning* (2nd ed.). Champaign, IL: Human Kinetics.

Guyton, A. C. (2000). *Textbook of medical physiology* (10th ed.). Philadelphia: W.B. Saunders.

Hasson, S. M. (1994). *Clinical exercise physiology*. St. Louis, MO: Mosby.

Marieb, E. N. (2000). *Human anatomy and physiology* (6th ed.). Menlo Park, CA: Addison Wesley Longman.

McArdle, W. D., Katch, F. I., & Katch, V. L. (2001). *Exercise physiology—energy, nutrition and human performance* (5th ed.). Philadelphia: Lea & Febiger.

Wilmore, J. H. & Costil, D. L. (1999). *Physiology of sport and exercise* (2nd ed.). Champaign, IL: Human Kinetics.

WEB RESOURCES

- Visit the Web site http://entertainment.howstuffworks.com/muscle.htm to read more about the function of muscles in the body. (This Web address was current as of September 2003.)
- Search for other Web sites that are related to how muscles contract and the physiology of muscle movement.

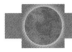 REVIEW QUESTIONS

Fill in the Blank

Provide the word(s) or phrase(s) that best completes the sentence.

1. The _____ muscle tissue covers the external muscle and is continuous with the _____ that connects the muscle to the bone.

2. When looking at a skeletal muscle under an electron microscope, the _____ band is dark and does not polarize light whereas the _____ is light, and polarizes light.

3. A muscle contraction depends on intrasarcoplasmic concentrations of _____ and the high-energy compound _____.

4. The troponin complex is a specialized structure made up of three specific molecules, including _____, _____, and _____.

5. The Sliding Filament Theory was first devised in the early _____ by a researcher named _____.

6. During a muscle contraction, the myosin attaches to the _____ on the _____, resulting in the actin sliding over the _____.

7. The two types of muscle tissue that are strictly involuntary are the _____ muscle and the _____ muscle.

8. The _____ of the sarcolemma contains a reservoir of calcium ions. Following an action potential, the _____ releases the calcium ions into the sarcoplasm.

9. The neurotransmitter _____ is found in the _____ and carries the action potential from the motor neuron to the sarcolemma.

10. Up to _____ calcium ions bind with the troponin C molecule when it is introduced into the sarcoplasm.

Multiple Choice

Select the best answer to complete the following statements.

1. The _____ covers each individual fasciculus.
   a. epimysium
   b. perimysium
   c. endomysium
   d. ectomysium

2. During a muscle contraction, the _____ covers the active site.
   a. troponin complex
   b. G-actin
   c. F-actin
   d. tropomyosin

3. Of the following metabolic pathways, the two that do not require oxygen to break down stored energy are _____ and _____.
   a. ATP-PC
   b. aerobic
   c. anaerobic
   d. oxidative

4. When the myosin is in its high-energy state, _____.
   a. calcium is attached to the myosin head
   b. ATP is bound to the myosin head
   c. potential energy is bound to the myosin head as ATP + Pi
   d. potential energy is bound to the myosin head as ADP +Pi

5. Following an action potential that has traveled down a motor neuron, _____.
   a. the basal lamina becomes permeable to calcium ions
   b. the synaptic vesicles fuse with the motor end plate
   c. the motor end plate floods with calcium ions
   d. acetylcholine is released into the synaptic cleft

Matching

Match each of the follwoing descriptions with the appropriate term.

_____ **1.** Neurotransmitter

_____ **2.** Single component that makes up F-actin

_____ **3.** Fluid substance that suspends organelles

_____ **4.** With oxygen

_____ **5.** Binding site for calcium

_____ **6.** Without oxygen

_____ **7.** Organelle containing contractile units

_____ **8.** Bundles of muscle fibers

_____ **9.** Sarcoplasm

_____ **10.** Carries action potential deep to myofibrils

_____ **11.** Component bound to the tropomyosin

_____ **12.** Binding site for ATP

_____ **13.** Cell wall for the muscle cell

_____ **14.** Covers the fasciculus

_____ **15.** Long strand structure that wraps around F-actin

A. Troponin C

B. Troponin T

C. Tropomyosin

D. Acetylcholine

E. Sarcolemma

F. Sarcoplasm

G. Transverse tubule

H. G-actin

I. Myosin head

J. Anaerobic

K. Aerobic

L. Perimysium

M. Fasciculus

N. Myofibril

O. Cytoplasm

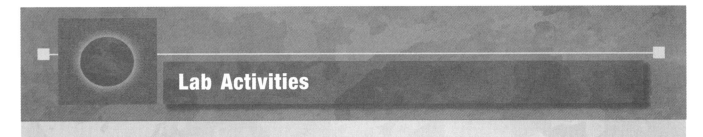

Critical Thinking

1. Choose one of the diagnoses mentioned in the OTA perspective box. What is the muscular impairment of that diagnosis? How does it manifest itself?

2. The diagnoses and treatment techniques discussed in this chapter are not necessarily unique to OT. From what you know about OT and other disciplines such as PT and speech and language pathology, discuss the perspective that each discipline uniquely brings to client treatment. Enlist the expertise of therapists in each of those fields to assist you with the dialogue and further understanding of your program of study as necessary.

3. From what you know about OT treatment, the interventions mentioned in this chapter likely follow which (specific) models of practice? Write a brief paper depicting your thoughts.

Lab Activities

Lab 2-1: Muscle Impairment

Objective: To identify muscular impairments of disease.

Equipment Needed: Pencils and paper, if answers are to be written; resource books or Internet access

Step 1. Choose one of the diagnoses mentioned in the Perspective boxes.

Step 2. Using resource books or the Internet, identify the muscular impairment of the diagnosis you have chosen.

Step 3. Explain the manifestation of the impairment.

Step 4. Record your findings. Be prepared to report your findings to the class.

Chapter 3

MUSCLE CHARACTERISTICS

Key Words

agonist	fusiform muscle	prime mover
antagonist	isokinetic	reversal of muscle pull
attachment site	isometric	rhomboidal muscle
bipennate muscle	isotonic	stabilizer
concentric	length-tension relationship	static stretching
contractility	multipennate muscle	strap muscle
dynamic	multiple heads	synergist
eccentric	neutralizer	triangular muscle
elasticity	oblique muscle	unipennate muscle
excitability	parallel muscle	
extensibility	pennation angle	

INTRODUCTION

From a kinesiology perspective, skeletal muscles serve two important functional purposes. First, muscles stabilize the various joints throughout the body during static (nonmoving) muscle contractions. For example, muscles located in the back contract to stabilize the back while the body resists the force of gravity. Second, skeletal muscles contract and pull on the bones that they are attached to, resulting in rotation of two bones (in most cases) around a joint axis. The combination of these effects allows us to walk down the street, pick up a backpack, throw a baseball, or even sit in a chair.

Learning the intricacies of the specific muscles is difficult enough, not to mention how they function as a whole. This chapter provides a user-friendly method of identifying individual muscles and understanding how they operate together. It also is a comprehensive guide for the general roles and characteristics of muscles and their actions.

CHARACTERISTICS OF MUSCLE

Observing skeletal muscle tissues up close reveals that skeletal muscle possesses unique characteristics that enhance function during human movement. These unique characteristics are contractility, extensibility, elasticity, and excitability.

Contractility

The term **contractility** refers to the ability of a muscle to shorten and move an object when resistance is applied to the muscle. During a muscle contraction, the thin actin myofilaments slide over the thick myosin myofilaments, which shortens the muscle sarcomere. When applying this example to the macroscopic level, note that all of the hundreds of sarcomeres lined up along a myofibril shorten together. As a result of these processes, the entire muscle shortens and moves a bone around a joint axis, causing a specific movement.

Extensibility

During a muscle contraction, the muscle that works in opposition to the muscle that is contracting performs a lengthening movement. The lengthening movement is referred to as **extensibility**. During extension movements, the contracted actin myofilaments slide away from the center of the sarcomere back to the resting position.

Another circumstance of muscle extensibility occurs when the muscle is stretched in a static position and an external force is applied to it. For example, **static stretching** exercises (a movement in which the muscle length stays the same yet responds to tension) performed before, during, or after exercise causes an additional static tension on the actin and myosin myofilaments. Static stretching is one form of exercise used to increase the range of motion about a joint.

Elasticity

An important functional component of muscle is its ability to return to its original shape after contracting or stretching. This ability is referred to as **elasticity** and occurs as a muscle snaps back or recoils to its original position after it has been extended or contracted. One example of elasticity is when a rubber band is pulled, it may be stretched 10 to 12 inches. After the rubber band is snapped, it returns to its original shape.

Excitability

Chapter 2 identified the neuromuscular junction and the electrical events that cause a muscle contraction. The ability of the muscle cells to respond to multiple stimuli is an extremely important component of skeletal muscles. Many muscle activities rely on the ability of the muscle to react to increased and multiple stimuli; this is referred to as **excitability**. Therefore, the extent to which the muscle responds to nervous stimulation increases its ability to function efficiently. Imagine a marathon runner, the length of a marathon (26.2 miles), the numerous times that muscles contract during a race, and the number of times a stimulus causes a muscle contraction. Indeed, excitability is an important characteristic of muscle tissue!

NAMING MUSCLES

Initially, it can be overwhelming to memorize each muscle in the body without an organized plan. In most cases, muscles are named based on seven distinct identification categories: location, shape, action, size, number of attachment sites, number of heads, and direction of fibers. Use these identification categories as a tool to learn the names of the muscles and to understand them in greater depth.

In the following chapters, each muscle of a specific joint region is discussed in depth. Immediately following the discussion, the important concepts of each muscle are provided for clear understanding and review. The review breaks down each muscle into its origin (O), insertion (I), nerve (N), action(s) (A), and palpation (P).

Location

The simplest tool for learning the names of the muscles is to recognize the muscle name by location. Take, for instance, the tibialis anterior muscle. The tibia is located in the leg, and "anterior" means "toward the front." Therefore, the tibialis anterior muscle is located on the anterior side of the tibia (Figure 3-1).

Shape

When the ancient Greeks began naming individual muscles, they often based it on the shape of the muscle. For example, palpate the large muscle in the shoulder. This muscle is shaped like an upside-down triangle and is named the deltoid muscle (Figure 3-2). The Greek letter delta (Δ) is shaped like the deltoid muscle. Another example of a shaped muscle is the serratus anterior muscle. This muscle is located on the anterolateral surface of the ribs. The serratus muscle receives its name because of the jagged shape it possesses, much like a serrated knife.

Action

The action that a muscle provides can aid in learning its name and where it is located. This is especially true of the muscles of the wrist, hand, ankle, and foot (Figure 3-3). For example, the extensor digitorum longus muscle extends the digits of the toes, and the flexor hallucis longus muscle flexes the big toe.

Another clue to help identify a muscle is combining the action and location of the muscle or muscle group in the body. For example, observe the extensor muscles of the forearm and hand. The muscles that cause extension movements of the hand are located on the posterior surface of the radius and ulna. In similar fashion, the muscles that cause flexion of the hand are located on the anterior surface of the radius and ulna.

Size

The size of a muscle may also be incorporated into its name, for example, the adductor muscle group around the hip joint. This muscle group has three muscles that are each named by size: the adductor magnus, adductor longus, and adductor brevis (Figure 3-4). In this example, the adductor magnus is large, the adductor longus is long, and the adductor brevis is short. Use the size of the muscle to help identify the different muscles when comparing the different regions of the human body. Table 3-1 summarizes the terminology used when describing size of muscles.

Number of Attachment Sites

Muscles may have two or more attachment points corresponding with the origin and insertion of a muscle. The origin is usually the more proximal attachment that provides the base of support for the movement. The insertion is usually distal and moves toward the origin during a contraction. In many circumstances, these **attachment sites** help identify the muscle from other muscles in a region being studied. A sound example of this arrangement is the sternocleidomastoid muscle located in the neck region (Figure 3-5). Break the name of this muscle down into three separate components and recognize that the sternocleidomastoid muscle has three attachment points: the sterno (sternum), cleido (clavicle), and mastoid (mastoid process).

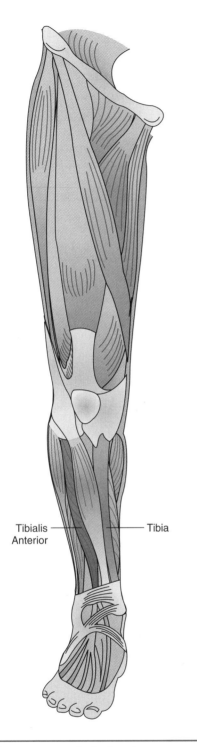

Figure 3-1   *Naming Muscles by Location*

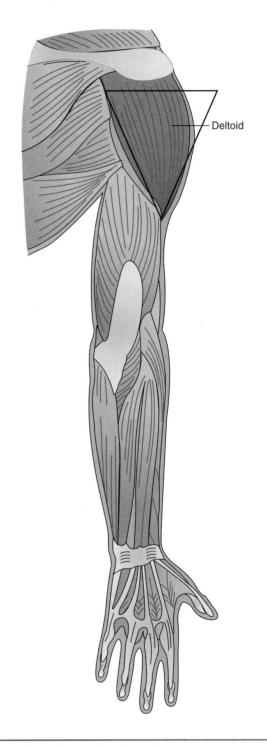

Figure 3-2   *Naming Muscles by Shape*

Table 3-1   *Terminology of a Muscle that Denotes Its Size*

Word	Meaning	Example
Brevis	Short	Extensor Corpi Radialis Brevis
Minimi	Small	Extensor digiti minimi
Longus	Long	Extensor Carpi Radialis Longus
Magnus	Large	Adductor magnus

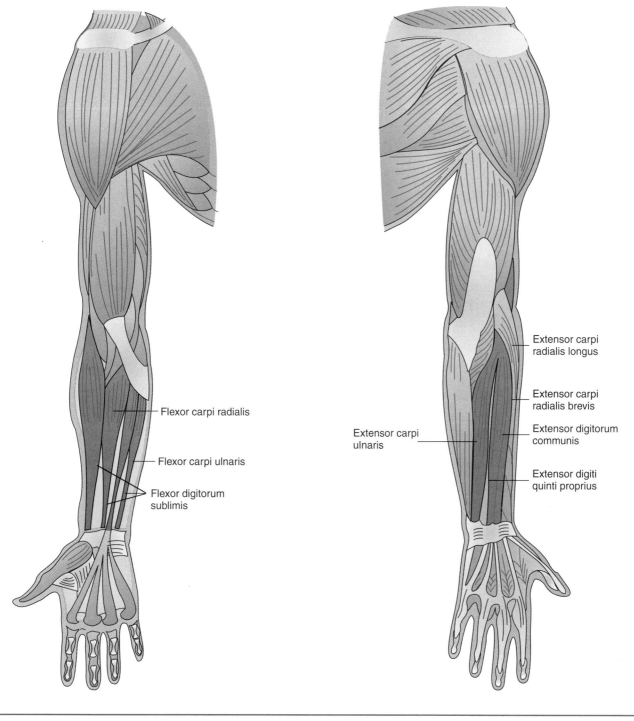

Figure 3-3 *Naming Muscles by Action*

Extensor carpi radialis longus

Extensor carpi radialis brevis

Extensor carpi ulnaris

Extensor digitorum communis

Extensor digiti quinti proprius

Flexor carpi radialis

Flexor carpi ulnaris

Flexor digitorum sublimis

Number of Heads

Certain muscles have **multiple heads** that can be identified when observations of their structures are made. Realize that each of these heads typically originates from its own origin, centralizes into a common tendon, and attaches to a common insertion. For instance, observe the three heads of the triceps brachii (Figure 3-6). Each head has its own origin, either on the scapula or humerus, runs into a central tendon, and inserts into the olecranon process of the ulna. Another example of this would be the two heads of the biceps brachii. Observe a picture of the biceps brachii and note the origin, central tendon, and common insertion.

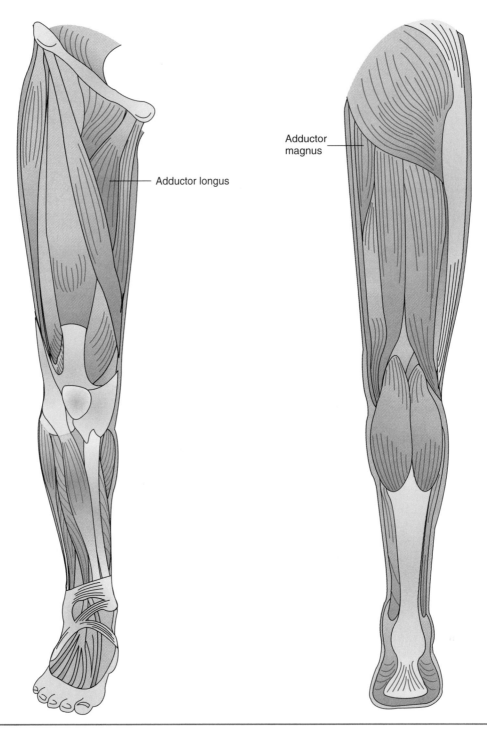

Figure 3-4 *Naming Muscles by Size*

Direction of Fibers

When learning the different muscles of the human body, determine the different directions that the muscle fibers run. This simple clue, in many cases, helps identify the name of the muscle. The direction of the fibers may run vertically to other muscles and bones, such as the rectus (straight) abdominis (Figure 3-7). Others, however, may run at diagonal angles to other muscles and bones, such as the internal and external oblique muscles.

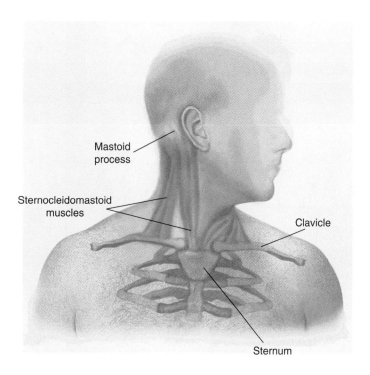

Figure 3-5　Naming Muscles by Attachment Sites

 FIBER-TYPE ARRANGEMENT

Look closely at pictures of the muscles in the human body (refer to Figure 3-1). Note that each muscle in the body has a specific structure and shape. Some muscles are large with a round shape, whereas others are short with a flat shape. The structure of a muscle can be determined by a few variables. Some of these variables are the size of the area or the space where the muscle is located. Sometimes a muscle has a limited area or space in which it can work. For instance, the muscles of the forearm and hand are designed so that they can operate the fingers and wrist like the strings on a puppet. If the muscles of the forearm and hand were large and bulky, they would greatly inhibit the function of the limbs, and movement would be compromised.

The structure of a muscle can also be determined by its specific purpose. Muscles have fibers that run in specific directions. The direction that the fiber of a muscle runs often dictates the specific action of that muscle. Some muscles are designed for range of motion and stabilization, whereas others are designed for maximal force production.

There are many variations of the muscles that exist within the body, such as muscle fiber length, number of muscle fibers, and direction of fibers. (This certainly can vary from individual to individual but is extremely similar for most people.) These specific variations can affect the function and strength of the specific muscle or muscle group. In general, there are two distinct types of muscle fibers that are based on fiber arrangements: parallel and oblique.

Parallel Muscles

The muscle fibers found within **parallel muscles** run parallel to the long axis of the bone. They are advantageous to human movement because of their length and ability to shorten through a full range of motion. This, coupled with the fact that muscles can shorten up to half of their resting length, makes the parallel arrangement beneficial for movements that require a large range of motion. However, the downside to the greater range of motion potential is that parallel muscles have a smaller amount of muscle fibers in a given area. Fewer muscle fibers equate to lower force production even though they can shorten over a greater distance. Therefore, parallel muscles have a relatively high range of motion potential but low force production capability. There are four types of parallel muscles: strap, fusiform, triangular, and rhomboidal.

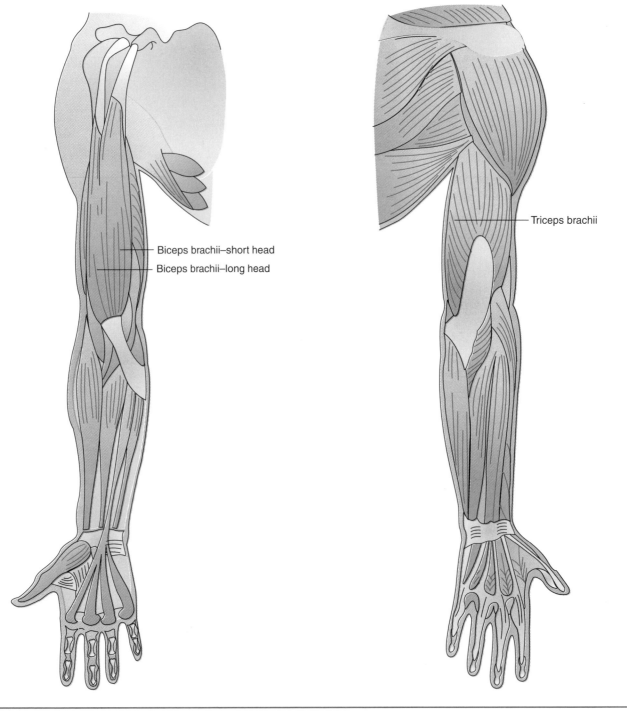

Biceps brachii–short head
Biceps brachii–long head
Triceps brachii

Figure 3-6   *Naming Muscles by Number of Heads*

Strap Muscles   Parallel muscle fibers that have a long, thin, and flat fiber arrangement running the entire length of the muscle are classified as **strap muscles**. During human body dissection, strap muscles remind one of belts that run throughout the body. An example of a strap muscle is the sartorius muscle found on the anterior surface of the thigh. Figure 3-8A shows the sartorius muscle, which is long, thin, and flat, and runs from the anterior superior iliac spine of the pelvis to the anterior medial surface of the tibia. In addition, the fibers of the sartorius muscle run parallel to the femur found deep to the muscle. The sartorius is a great example of a muscle with extremely long fibers that allows the body to move through a full range of motion but does not generate a large amount of force generation during human movement.

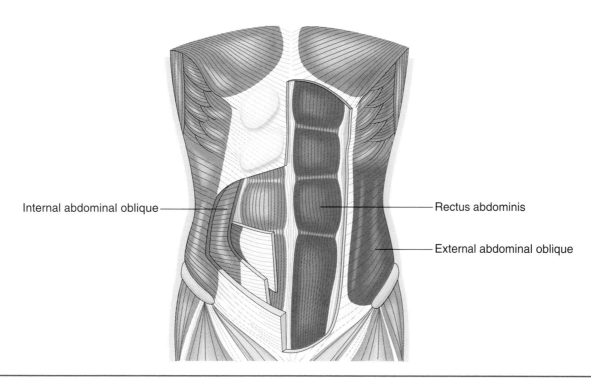

Internal abdominal oblique —

— Rectus abdominis

— External abdominal oblique

Figure 3-7 *Naming Muscles by Direction of Fibers*

Fusiform Muscles The **fusiform muscle** is common in areas that require a large range of motion, such as the shoulder, elbow, hip, and knee joints. Fusiform muscles are spindle shaped with two narrow tendons that give rise to a thick muscle belly. For instance, observe the biceps brachii in Figure 3-8B. Each of the biceps' heads originates from the scapula via a narrow tendon. The muscles then give rise to a large muscle belly and then insert to the radius via a narrow biceps tendon into the radial tuberosity. The arrangement of the fusiform tendons increases the number of muscle tendons that can pass over a given joint region.

OTA Perspective

OT practitioners combine knowledge from multiple contexts—the client's status and goals, frames of references, assessment results, the environment in which the client functions, and a supervisor or colleague's point of view, just to name a few. All of these and more are combined with what the practitioner also knows about the client from a kinesiology perspective—what movements are anticipated because of who the client is and the disease or injury, or the need for a wellness and prevention program that has resulted in an OT "eval and treat" physician's order.

So given that occupational therapists and OTAs both consider the "big picture" and deal in minutia, how does one decide what assessments and interventions best suit a particular client? All that knowledge and ability are imparted via a clinical reasoning process. In subsequent chapters, when we consider the detailed study of movement of a particular muscle group, we will also examine some of the details that go into OT decision-making and the ensuing treatment.

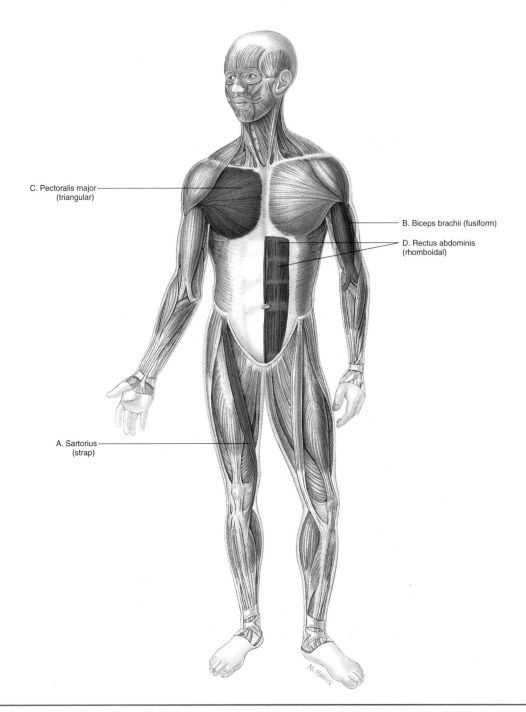

C. Pectoralis major
(triangular)

B. Biceps brachii (fusiform)

D. Rectus abdominis
(rhomboidal)

A. Sartorius
(strap)

Figure 3-8 *Parallel Muscle Fiber Arrangements: (A) Strap; (B) Fusiform; (C) Triangular; (D) Rhomboidal*

Triangular Muscles Muscles in the human body that are fan shaped are named **triangular muscles**. Triangular muscles have a broad origin and a muscle belly that gives rise to a narrow insertion tendon. Figure 3-8C shows the pectoralis major, which is located in the chest. The origin of the pectoralis major is large and broad with the muscle covering most of the superior chest region. The muscle then narrows into a smaller tendon that inserts into the medial lip of the intertrabecular groove. The broad-based fiber arrangement increases the force generation capabilities of triangular muscles.

Rhomboidal Muscles The final parallel muscle arrangement consists of muscles that are four-sided, short, flat, and resemble the shape of a square or rectangle (see Figure 3-8D). Both the origin and insertion of **rhomboidal muscles** are broad and are connected by a thick area consisting of strong muscle fibers. The arrangement of these fibers strongly increases the amount of force that can be produced by these muscles. For example, the rectus abdominis muscle of the abdominal region originate on the vertebral border of the scapula and insert on the vertebrae. As the muscles contract, they stabilize the scapula and increase its stability as the humerus moves through a full range of motion and pulls on the scapula.

Oblique Muscles

The second type of muscle fiber arrangement runs at an angle or in an oblique direction to the long axis of the bone and is defined as the **pennation angle**. The structures of **oblique muscles** are similar in appearance to a bird feather and are thus named pennate muscles, which, in Latin means "feathers." The muscle fibers of the oblique muscle are short, resulting in a smaller number of muscle fibers in a given area. The oblique muscles cannot shorten over a very large distance because of the short length of muscle fibers. However, they have more muscle fibers packed into a specific cross-sectional area, resulting in a greater production of force. For example, compare the difference between the muscle arrangements of the biceps brachii (parallel) and triceps brachii (oblique). As the biceps muscles provide a greater range of motion, the triceps muscles generate a larger force because of the larger amount of muscle fibers within the muscle. There are three types of oblique muscles: unipennate, bipennate, and multipennate.

Unipennate Muscles **Unipennate muscles** have the shape of a feather that has been cut along the sagittal line, or midline. This shape produces a broad origin that firmly attaches the unipennate muscle to the bone for most of its distance. From the origin, the muscle fibers run at angles to the bone and centralize into one common narrow tendon. A prime example of a unipennate muscle is the tibialis anterior (Figure 3-9A). The origin of the tibialis anterior is extremely broad and located on the superior two-thirds of the lateral surface of the tibia. The muscle fibers are found running at angles to the tibia and insert into a common tendon, which inserts into the superior surface of the navicular bone. The advantage of this fiber arrangement is that it increases the force production that is allowed in this area and the strength of the dorsiflexion movement.

Bipennate Muscles The muscle fiber-type arrangement that also resembles a bird feather is classified as a **bipennate muscle**. The origin of bipennate muscles is similar to that of the unipennate muscles. These muscles also have fibers that run diagonally to the bone and into a narrow central insertion tendon. For example, observe the rectus femoris of the anterior thigh in Figure 3-9B. The muscle fibers of the rectus femoris run at angles to the femur and attach to a central tendon, which inserts into the tibial tuberosity.

Multipennate Muscles The last muscle classification is that of **multipennate muscles**. Picture a large bundle of feathers from the tail of a peacock bundled together at the stem of a feather. Multipennate muscles resemble numerous bipennate feathers bundled together. Study the picture of the serratus anterior muscle in Figure 3-9C. This muscle has numerous broad attachments on the clavicle and scapula and runs into a common central tendon, which inserts into the scapula.

 ROLES OF MUSCLE

In order to understand the complete function of muscles, an understanding of the various roles of muscles is necessary. It is important to point out that, many times, the same muscle may have more than one role. For instance, a muscle may provide the force to cause movement (concentric action), and at a different moment the same muscle will provide the force to resist movement (eccentric action). This is a very common occurrence within the human body. Muscles have a variety of roles and it is imperative to understand these roles. The roles of muscles are those of agonist, synergist, antagonist, stabilizer, and neutralizer.

Agonist

The most common and easiest muscle role to understand is that of the **agonist**. When a muscle assumes the role of the agonist, it is acting as the "main mover," or "**prime mover**," causing the motion. For example, if flexion of the elbow is the desired action, the biceps brachii acts as the agonist.

Synergist

Synergists are muscles that assist the agonist in providing a desired muscle action. For example, the biceps brachii muscle group causes elbow flexion, but the brachioradialis muscle group acts as a synergist, or "helper," in this movement.

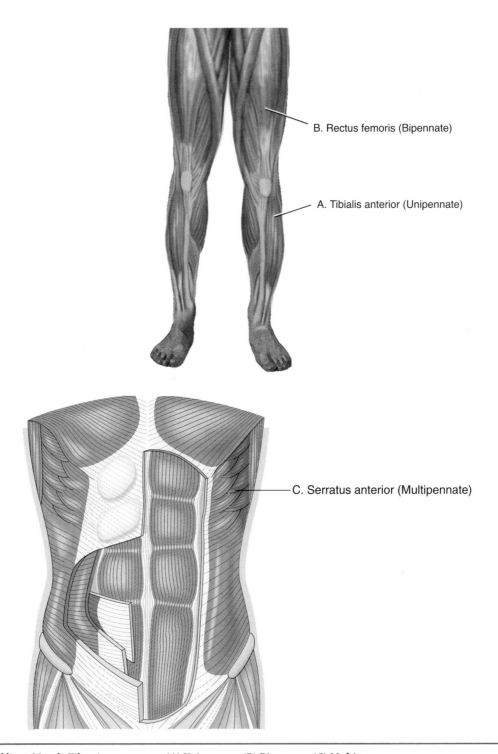

Figure 3-9 *Oblique Muscle Fiber Arrangements: (A) Unipennate; (B) Bipennate; (C) Multipennate*

Antagonist

Another muscle role that is opposite the agonist is the **antagonist**. The antagonist muscle is located on the opposite side of the joint from the agonist. Often, while the agonist is active, the antagonist is stretched, retaining a relaxed condition. In the same example of elbow flexion, the biceps muscle is the agonist, whereas the triceps muscle is the antagonist. In the scenario, the triceps is being stretched while the biceps contracts and vice versa.

Stabilizer

In some circumstances, antagonists contract, providing resistance to stabilize the joint movement. **Stabilizer** muscles or muscle groups assist the agonist by steadily contracting to "balance" the body or body part against the force of contracting muscles or gravity and helping the agonist to act more effectively.

Neutralizer

Neutralizer muscles act to prevent unwanted movements. A muscle does not know direction but acts based on the angle of pull on it. A neutralizer allows a muscle to perform more than one action. This is commonly seen in the muscles of the limbs. These muscles can flex and extend while also supinate and pronate. If only one of these actions is needed, then the opposing action is counteracted and ruled out.

TYPES OF MUSCULAR ACTIONS

All muscles have the capability to produce an action. The word "action" is emphasized because the word "contraction" denotes shortening of the muscle. Muscles have the potential to shorten, lengthen, or remain unchanged.

Isometric Contractions

Isometric, or static, contractions can be best defined as "producing tension within the muscle without a change in length of the muscle fiber." For example, attempt to push open a locked door. This action will produce tension within the triceps muscle but the muscle fibers will not shorten (Figure 3-10). This would be the case as long as there was no change in the joint angle between the forearm and humerus. During an isometric contraction, the myosin cross-bridges attach to the actin, yet they do not slide past one another to cause a reduction in the joint angle. Isometric muscular contractions are common, especially within the muscles that aid in maintaining our posture. Imagine standing at the bus stop. All of the muscles that are supporting the body weight, including the erector spinae muscle group located in the back, the abdominal muscles, and the calf muscles, produce a static or isometric action to stabilize the posture.

Often isometric exercise is used as a mode of resistance training. Because static actions produce tension within a muscle but do not cause any joint movements, they are an ideal way to improve muscular strength without risking damage to the joint. If isometric movement is the desired goal in a sport, then isometric exercises may not be the resistance training

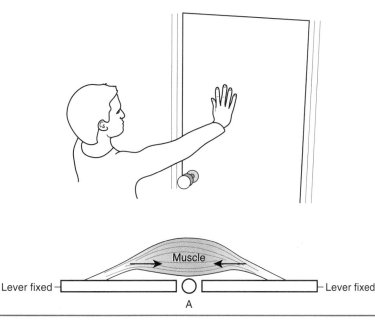

Figure 3-10 *Isometric Contractions*

mode of choice. For example, when athletes desire to train the muscles to act quickly and through a full range of motion, isometric exercise would prevent the muscles from moving through the full range of motion. This concept is beneficial in a rehabilitation setting. If a muscle or joint is not capable of moving through a full range of motion but needs to be strengthened, an isometric exercise would be beneficial.

Dynamic Contractions

If the fibers in a particular muscle either shorten or lengthen, they are said to be acting dynamically. **Dynamic** muscular actions can encompass a variety of contraction types, including isokinetic and isotonic, which can be subdivided further.

Isokinetic Actions *Iso* means "equal" and *kinetic* means "motion." Therefore, a rough interpretation of the term **isokinetic** would be "equal movement." Isokinetic actions are usually facilitated by an external piece of equipment such as a Cybex or hydraulic machine. During isokinetic contractions, the joint angle changes throughout the movement, but the angular velocity or speed of shortening remains equal or unchanged (Figure 3-11). For example, in rehabilitation settings, a knee extension exercise could be performed at a joint angular velocity or speed of 30 degrees of flexion/extension per second. This would be beneficial for a few reasons. Isokinetic movements often decrease the risk for hyper-flexion or extension of the joint putting undue stress on ligaments and tendons. At the same time, the knee flexors and extensors are strengthened through a full range of motion.

Isotonic Actions

The prefix *iso* equates to "equal" and *tonic* equates to "tonus" or "tension." Therefore, the term **isotonic** translates into "equal tension." That is, during an isotonic muscle action, equal tension is produced throughout the range of motion. This term, however, is often misleading because the tension exerted on muscle changes at different joint angles, especially when lifting a constant resistance as opposed to a variable resistance.

The two types of isotonic muscle actions are **concentric** and **eccentric**. A concentric action refers to shortening of the muscle fibers. For example, if the biceps brachii acts in a concentric fashion, then the hand and forearm will move closer to the humerus. The key to remember is that the muscle fibers are shortening and the actin and myosin cross-bridges are sliding past one another. In different terms, the force that the muscle is generating is greater than the resistive force, or force to be overcome. If a 15-pound weight is placed in the hand, the biceps brachii muscle group must exert a force greater than 15 pounds to move the weight concentrically (Figure 3-12).

A muscle can also elongate, or lengthen, which is called an eccentric contraction (Figure 3-13). Eccentric contractions generally occur when gravity is being resisted and the movement of a muscle around a joint is slow and controlled. During

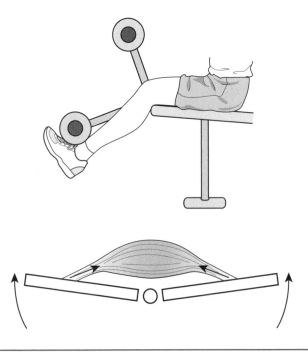

Figure 3-11 *Dynamic Contractions (Isokinetic)*

OTA Perspective

Injury to a muscle is termed a *strain*. Muscle strains are classified according to their severity. A *mild* strain is defined as a tearing of a small number of muscle fibers but the fascia remains intact. A *moderate* strain is defined as a tearing of a larger number of muscle fibers and is caused by a more severe injury. The fascia is still intact but there is a substantial amount of bleeding that is contained within the muscle itself. A *severe* strain of the muscle involves more muscle fibers and severe bleeding. The fascia may be torn and the bleeding will spread out over a large area. The most severe injury is a *complete rupture*. This is caused by a major trauma, and a gap can be felt in the muscle itself. Active contraction of the muscle is not possible in this case.

an eccentric action, the force produced by the muscle is less than the resistive force. Take the previous example of holding a 15-pound weight in the hand in a flexed position. If the biceps muscle produces a force of 14.9 pounds or less, the muscle fibers will lengthen and the elbow will extend. In many cases, there are exceptions to the statement that "eccentric actions occur in slow and controlled motions." For example, imagine a person throwing darts. In this example, the triceps brachii muscle is concentrically acting to produce elbow extension. Because this movement is very quick and rapid, the elbow joint risks injury (hyperextension) if the movement is not slowed down toward terminal extension at the elbow. The biceps brachii contracts eccentrically to provide a braking movement during elbow extension and serves as an antagonist. This example illustrates that eccentric actions often help protect joints from excessive flexion or extension.

As stated earlier in this chapter, the origin is the muscle attachment point that is typically more stable and located closer to the trunk of the body. The insertion is usually attached to the more movable segment and is generally located farther (or distal) from the trunk. During normal muscle contraction, the insertion moves toward the origin. Sometimes the insertion becomes fixed and the origin moves toward the insertion, which is termed **reversal of muscle pull**. An example of reversal of muscle pull occurs when one performs a pull-up exercise. The insertion points, radius and ulna, are fixated by holding the bar, and the origin moves toward the insertion during flexion of the elbow.

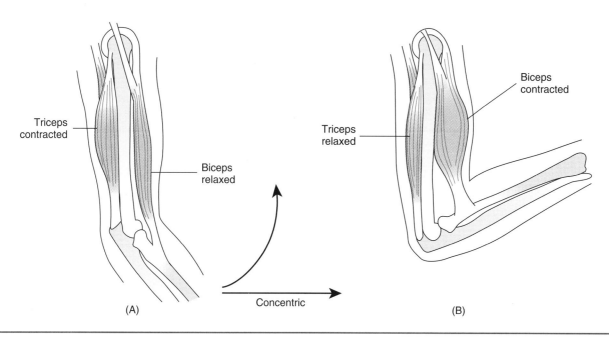

Figure 3-12 *Concentric Contractions*

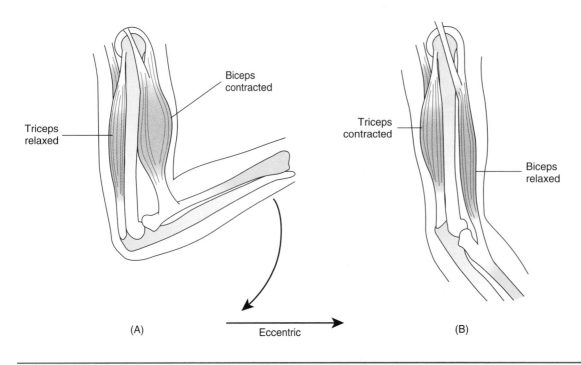

Figure 3-13 *Eccentric Contractions*

 THE LENGTH-TENSION RELATIONSHIP

It is not enough for students of kinesiology to just understand names, roles, and types of muscles if they want to be successful. Other factors or variables occur in real life activities that need further explanation. The **length-tension relationship** is one of those factors that is essential to understand movement within the human body.

Tension is a force developed within a muscle. The length-tension relationship simply states that there is a direct relationship (to a point) between the length of a muscle or muscle fiber and the tension it is able to develop. Furthermore, there is an optimal length where in a muscle is capable of developing maximal force, which is specifically 1.2 times the resting length of the muscle. The length-tension curve (Figure 3-14) is divided into three distinct regions: ascending, plateau, and descending.

The amount of force generated in a muscle is dependent on the number of cross-bridge formations that occur at the sarcomere level. At the plateau region of the curve or the optimal length of muscle for maximal force generation, the actin and myosin filaments are positioned so that the maximal number of cross-bridges can be formed. In the ascending region of the curve, force output is not maximal because the actin filaments from one side of the sarcomere form a double overlap with the actin filaments from the opposite side of the sarcomere. This inhibits the maximal number of cross-bridge formations that can occur. In the descending region of the curve, there is less overlap between the actin and myosin filaments and less number of cross-bridge formations contributing to a decreased force output.

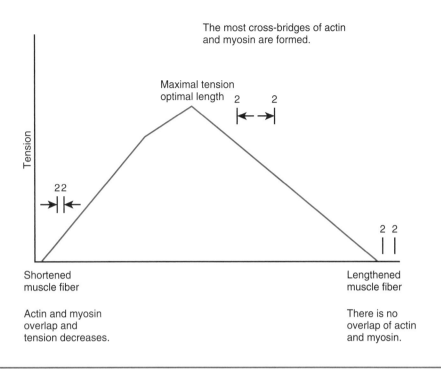

Figure 3-14 *Length-Tension Curve*

■ Four unique characteristics of muscle are described in this chapter. Contractility refers to the ability of a muscle to shorten and move an object when resistance is applied. Extensibility refers to the muscle's ability to extend or lengthen. Elasticity refers to the ability of a muscle to return to the original resting position after contraction or extension. Excitability is a characteristic of muscle that refers to its ability to respond to electrical stimuli, more specifically nerve impulses.

■ The ability to identify muscles is vital for success in the field of OT. There are numerous ways to name a muscle. These methods include naming muscles by shape, action, size, attachment sites, number of muscle heads, and direction of fibers.

■ Fiber-type arrangement is strategically important in the design of the human body. In many areas of the body, muscles do not have much surface area to utilize so the multiple arrangements of fiber types are critical. The direction of muscle fibers can assist in identifying the actions of specific muscles. Furthermore, the direction of muscle fibers allows the body and body segments to perform a wide variety of movements.

■ Studying the direction and arrangement of muscle fiber types will show that some muscles are designed for range of motion, some for stability, and some for power.

■ The forms of muscle actions occurring in the body include static, or isometric, and dynamic. Static actions occur when tension is generated within a muscle but there is no movement of the muscle. Dynamic actions include isokinetic and isotonic actions. Isokinetic actions relate to joint movements that are equal or consistent through the full range of motion. Isotonic motions can be further subdivided into concentric and eccentric motions. Concentric motions refer to shortening motions or instances in which the myofilaments move closer together. Eccentric motions occur during lengthening motions. More specifically, during an eccentric contraction, the force produced by a muscle is less than the resistive force.

■ There are general relationships between the locations of the muscles in the human body that cause movement. There is a direct relationship between the length of a muscle and the tension it is able to develop.

BIBLIOGRAPHY

A.D.A.M. interactive anatomy. (1997). Atlanta, GA: A.D.A.M. Software.

Ehrlich, A. (2000). *Medical terminology for the health professions* (4th ed.). Clifton Park, NY: Thomson Delmar Learning.

Levangie, P. K. (2000). *Joint structure and function* (3rd ed). Philadelphis: F. A. Davis.

Marieb, E. N. (2003). *Human anatomy and physiology* (6th ed.). Menlo Park, CA: Addison Wesley Longman.

Norkin, C. C., & Levangie, P. K., (2001). *Joint structure and function: A comprehensive analysis* (3rd ed.). Philadelphia: F. A. Davis.

Rizzo, D. (2001). *Delmar's fundamentals of anatomy and physiology.* Clifton Park, NY: Thomson Delmar Learning.

REVIEW QUESTIONS

Fill in the Blank

Provide the word(s) or phrase(s) that best completes the sentence.

1. The term _____ refers to a short muscle.

2. An example of a muscle that is named by its action is the _____ muscle.

3. The triceps brachii is named by the _____ origin attachments that it contains.

4. Muscles that are classified as _____ move through a large range of motion but do not create as large a force as the _____ muscle classification.

5. Muscles that assist the agonist muscle during a contraction, such as the brachialis and brachioradialis, provide a _____ contraction.

6. The type of muscle contraction existing when you push against a wall with no binding of the cross-bridges is named a _____ contraction.

7. Dynamic muscle contractions encompass a variety of contractions that are either _____ or _____ .

8. Generally, when the actin slides over the myosin and the sarcomere lengthens, the result is a/an _____ contraction.

9. Generally, when the actin slides over the myosin and the sarcomere shortens, the result is a/an _____ contraction.

10. The tibialis anterior is a _____ muscle because its fibers resemble half of a _____.

Multiple Choice

Select the best answer to complete the following statements.

1. The primary mover is known as the _____.
   a. antagonist
   b. synergist
   c. stabilizer
   d. agonist

2. During the muscle contraction, the antagonist must remain _____ to allow for the muscle contraction.
   a. contracted
   b. stabilized
   c. excited
   d. relaxed

3. The ability of a muscle to shorten and move an object when weight is applied to the muscle is referred to as _____.
   a. contractility
   b. extensibility
   c. excitability
   d. elasticity

4. The ability of a muscle to retain its original shape after being stretched is referred to as _____.
   a. contractility
   b. extensibility
   c. excitability
   d. elasticity

5. During a/an _____ contraction, the muscle length remains unchanged.
   a. isometric
   b. isotonic
   c. concentric
   d. dynamic

Matching

Match each of the following muscles with the proper fiber classification.

_____ 1. Pectoralis major   A. Fusiform

_____ 2. Pronator quadratus   B. Parallel

_____ 3. Subscapularis   C. Strap

_____ 4. Supraspinatus   D. Rhomboid

_____ 5. Biceps brachii   E. Unipennate

_____ 6. Gluteus maximus   F. Bipennate

_____ 7. Peroneus brevis   G. Multipennate

_____ 8. Gracilis

_____ 9. Serratus anterior

_____ 10. Sternocleidomastoid

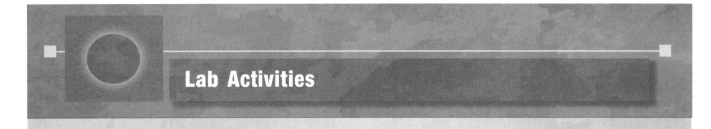

Critical Thinking

1. Review "clinical reasoning" and how that learning process begins for new OT practitioners. Review *The Occupational Therapy Practice Framework* and *Uniform Terminology-III* (as indicated per academic program) as an example of a "big picture" and "attention to detail," along with fundamental OT practice. Within those parameters, review and discuss where kinesiology fits into OT practice.

2. Define the term *fascia* and describe its role in the body.

3. The sartorius muscle is the longest muscle in the body. Research its origin and insertion and how it derived its name.

Lab Activities

Lab 3-1: Muscle Movement

Objective: To demonstrate concentric, eccentric, and isometric movements.

Equipment Needed: A lab partner, pen/pencil, paper

Step 1.   Demonstrate concentric action of the hamstring muscles. Record your findings.

Step 2.   Demonstrate eccentric action of the hamstring muscles. Record your findings.

Step 3.   Demonstrate isometric action of the hamstring muscles. Record your findings.

Step 4.   Demonstrate concentric action of the quadriceps muscles. Record your findings.

Step 5.   Demonstrate eccentric action of the quadriceps muscles. Record your findings.

Step 6.   Demonstrate isometric action of the quadriceps muscles. Record your findings.

Step 7.   Switch roles with your partner and repeat the steps above. Record your findings.

Lab 3-2: Movie Lab

Objective: Compare and contrast portrayals of movement with scientific knowledge of movement.

Equipment Needed: Video and viewing equipment, paper and pencils for writing reaction paper

Step 1.   View a movie that depicts a central character's struggle with movement. Along with discussing Hollywood's portrayal of the person and the disease or injury, discuss movement disabilities in kinesiology terms.

Step 2.   Respectfully mimic the movements addressed and, as indicated, the change in ability pre- and post therapy intervention.

Step 3.   Write a position paper on the movie you chose to watch.

Chapter 4

THE NERVOUS SYSTEM

Objectives

Upon completion of this chapter, the reader should be able to:

- Describe the cellular structure of the nervous system, including the structure of neurons and glial cells.

- Describe the physiology of the action potential, neural transmission, and its role in the communicative functions of the nervous system.

- Draw and describe the structures of the central nervous system and their anatomy, and explain the functions of their anatomical divisions.

- Given a list of brain and spinal cord structures, create a schematic of their relationships to and effects on one another.

- Describe the structures and functions of the peripheral nervous system.

- Describe the structures and functions of the autonomic nervous system, including the effects and functions of the sympathetic and parasympathetic divisions.

- Explain the stretch reflex and the deep tendon reflex and how their interaction maintains posture and position.

Key Words

abducens nerve
accessory nerves
action potential
adrenaline
affective language area
afferent
all-or-none response
amitotic
amygdala
anterior median fissure
arachnoid mater
ascending nerves
association fibers
association neuron
astrocytes
autonomic, or involuntary, system
axon
axon hillock
axonal terminal
basal nuclei
blood-brain barrier
brachial plexus
brainstem
Broca's area
Brodmann's areas
cauda equina
caudate nucleus
cell body
central canal

central nervous system (CNS)
central sulcus
cerebellum
cerebral aqueduct
cerebral cortex
cerebral hemispheres
cerebrospinal fluid (CSF)
cerebrum
cervical plexus
choroid plexus
commissural fibers
commissures
conus medullaris
corpus callosum
corpus striatum
cranial nerves
decussation of the pyramids
deep tendon reflexes
dendrite
denticulate ligaments
depolarization
dermatome
descending nerves
diencephalon
dopamine
dorsal horn
dorsal ramus
dorsal root
dorsal root ganglion

dura mater
dural sinuses
efferent
endorphins
ependymal cells
epidural space
epinephrine
facial nerves
falx cerebelli
falx cerebri
filum terminale
first-order neurons
foramen magnum
free dendritic endings
frontal eye fields
frontal lobe
functional systems
ganglion
general interpretation area
glial cells
globus pallidus
glossopharyngeal nerve
gnostic area
Golgi tendon organs
graded potential
gray commissure
gyri
Hilton's law
hippocampus
homunculus

Objectives (continued)

■ Describe the four plexuses, their function, and how they are formed.

■ Demonstrate an understanding of the innervations of the body, including the dermatomes, the visceral innervations, and the nerve supply of skeletal muscle.

■ Demonstrate an understanding of the sensory mechanisms of the body.

Key Words (continued)

hypoglossal nerves
hypothalamus
inferior colliculi
insula
integration center
internuncial neuron
interventricular foramen
intrafusal fibers
joint kinesthetic
   receptors
jugular foramen
kinesthesia
lateral aperture
lateral fissure
lateral horns
lentiform nucleus
limbic system
longitudinal fissure
lumbar plexus
median aperture
medulla oblongata
   (medulla)
Meissner's corpuscles
meningeal branch
meninges
Merkel's disks
microglia
midbrain
middle cerebellar
   peduncles
mixed nerves
monosynaptic reflex
motor nerves
muscle spindles
myelin
nerve
neuroglia
neurolemma
neurolemmocytes
neuron
neurotransmitter
nodes of Ranvier
nucleus
occipital lobe
oculomotor nerve
olfactory cortex
olfactory nerves
olfactory tract

oligodendroglia
optic chiasma
optic foramen
optic nerves
pacinian corpuscles
parasympathetic system
parietal lobe
perikaryon
peripheral nervous sys-
   tem (PNS)
pia mater
pineal gland
polarized state
polysynaptic reflex
pons
pontine nuclei
postcentral gyrus
posterior median sulcus
postganglionic neuron
postsynaptic neuron
precentral gyrus
prefrontal cortex
preganglionic neuron
premotor cortex
presynaptic neuron
primary sensory cortex
projection fibers
proprioception
proprioceptors
putamen
pyramidal tract
red nucleus
reflex
repolarization
resting or membrane
   potential
reticular activating
   system (RAS)
reticular formation
Ruffini's corpuscles
sacral plexus
Schwann cells
second-order neurons
sensory nerves
sensory receptors
septa
septum pellucidum
serotonin

skull
sodium-potassium pump
soma
somatic, or voluntary,
   system
somatosensory associa-
   tion area
somatotopy
spinal cord
spinal dural sheath
spinal ganglion
spinal nerves
stimuli
stretch reflex
stylomastoid foramen
subarachnoid space
substantia nigra
sulci
superior cerebellar
   peduncles
superior colliculi
superior orbital fissure
sympathetic ganglia or
   sympathetic chain
sympathetic system
synapse
synaptic cleft
synaptic vesicles
telodendria
temporal lobe
tentorium
terminal ganglia
thalamus
third-order neurons
third ventricle
tract
trigeminal nerve
trochlear nerve
vagus nerve
ventral horn
ventral ramus
ventral root
ventricles
vertebral column
vestibulocochlear nerve
Wernicke's Area

INTRODUCTION

Imagine the fastest, most efficient, state-of-the-art computer available. It can process hundreds of signals at once, interpret and make sense of them, interface with other information in a nanosecond, and execute accurate responses and output in about the same amount of time. It regulates, controls, and modifies hundreds of functions simultaneously. This "computer" is the human nervous system.

The nervous system is responsible for receiving and interpreting messages from the environment, coordinating them, and directing appropriate responses to them. When you respond to a dangerous situation, interpret and solve a complex problem, or execute a precise athletic feat, it is your nervous system that oversees and directs those actions. Conversely, when an illness or injury damages the nervous system, its control over bodily functions and actions is altered, and daily activity is affected. The result of such an insult depends on the extent and location of the injury.

As an OTA, understanding both the normal and atypical functions of the nervous system will assist you in carrying out your professional role. As a student of kinesiology, a functional approach to the study of the nervous system will support your ability to understand how the healthy nervous system and its impairment influence the movement needed for daily activities.

This chapter explores how the human nervous system functions as it relates to the control and execution of movement. Rather than provide an in-depth discussion of neuroanatomy and neurophysiology, this chapter focuses on elements from both of those disciplines that play a part in human movement. Using everyday activities as examples, you will gain an understanding of and appreciation for the complexities of this body system as well as some of the changes that occur in the event of illness or injury.

ORGANIZATION OF THE NERVOUS SYSTEM

In order to lay the foundation on which the nervous system functions, we will first examine its basic organization and significant structures. The nervous system is divided into two major parts: the **central nervous system (CNS)** and the **peripheral nervous system (PNS)**. The PNS is further divided into efferent and afferent mechanisms and autonomic and somatic, or voluntary, sections.

The Central Nervous System

The central nervous system (CNS) consists of the brain and spinal cord, which are those structures of the nervous system that are encased in the bony protection of the skull and vertebral column, respectively (Figure 4-1). The primary functions of the CNS are controlling and integrating functions, as well as regulating consciousness, maintaining awareness, interpreting stimuli, and executing thought. Different parts of the CNS exert different types of influence over these functions. Together, the orchestrated effect is one of smooth and coordinated movement for daily activities. Damage to the CNS can result in impaired regulation and direction of movement, bodily functions, and cognitive and emotional processes. The location of the insult or injury affects the way in which an activity is performed, depending on the mechanism that is influenced.

The Peripheral Nervous System

The peripheral nervous system (PNS) consists of the nerve cells that are outside the CNS and are found from their origin in the brain or spinal cord to the tissues of the body (Figure 4-2). Under the regulation and control of the CNS, they transmit the impulses that regulate functions such as muscle contraction, organ performance, and hormonal activity.

Functionally, the PNS is divided into the **afferent** and **efferent** systems. The afferent system carries impulses *toward* the CNS and transmits sensory information, such as heat, cold, pain, sharpness, or dullness, to the brain from sensory receptors in the muscles, skin, joints, and organs of the body.

The efferent system carries impulses *away* from the CNS and activates and controls muscles, organs, and glands.

The PNS carries neural impulses to and from the CNS, via **cranial nerves**, which carry impulses to and from the brain, and **spinal nerves**, which carry impulses to and from the spinal cord.

The PNS is further divided into two sections: the **somatic, or voluntary, system**, and the **autonomic, or involuntary, system**. The autonomic system is then separated into the **sympathetic system** and **parasympathetic system**.

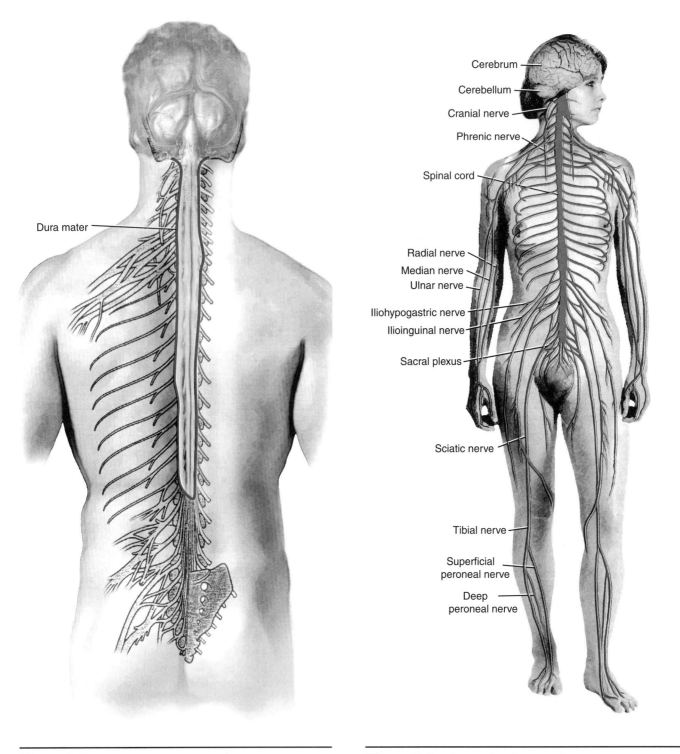

Figure 4-1 *The Central Nervous System*

Figure 4-2 *The Peripheral Nervous System*

The Somatic, or Voluntary, System The somatic (voluntary) system is the portion of the PNS that supplies the skeletal muscle. It is the part of the nervous system that controls conscious movement, hence the name *voluntary*. The spinal nerves that innervate skeletal muscle comprise the voluntary nervous system. Walking, picking up the telephone, and making a face are examples of movements controlled by the voluntary system.

The Autonomic, or Involuntary, System The autonomic (involuntary) system regulates those bodily functions over which we do not exercise conscious control. Functions that fall into this category include the workings of visceral organs, glands, and cardiac muscle. The autonomic system is subsequently divided into two functional subdivisions: the *sympathetic* and *parasympathetic* systems. These two functional subdivisions generally operate in complementary fashion to one

OTA Perspective

Multiple sclerosis (MS) is a neurological disease that affects the myelin sheath within the CNS. In MS, the myelin is lost and replaced by scar tissue; these damaged areas are called plaques, which interfere with normal nerve conduction. The exact cause of MS is unknown but is thought to be an autoimmune disease; other potential factors include gender, environmental triggers such as viruses, and genetics.

Because diagnosis cannot be made with a single test, several tests and procedures are performed, including an examination of the patient's nervous system function, an MRI of the brain to detect plaques, and a spinal tap to analyze the CSF. The patient must present with signs of the disease in different parts of the nervous system and two separate flare-ups of symptoms.

Symptoms of MS are extremely varied, as is the course of the disease. Some patients present with symptoms that continue to worsen with little respite, whereas other patients have relapses and remissions. The most common symptoms include balance problems, bladder and bowel dysfunction, dizziness, spasticity, fatigue, and vision problems.

Treatment consists of disease-modifying drugs, rehabilitation, and alternative medicine.

another. While one stimulates function, the other inhibits it, thus balancing opposite reactions and contributing to the maintenance of homeostasis. The neural structures that regulate the autonomic nervous system are located in the PNS.

TISSUE AND STRUCTURE OF THE NERVOUS SYSTEM

Although there is some variation across the entire nervous system depending on the specialization of a particular neural element, the basic structures and their purposes remain consistent. As with all tissues, nervous tissue is specialized for its function, which, in this case, is to support the transmission of afferent and efferent impulses.

The Basic Structural Component: The Neuron

The specialized cells of the nervous system are known as **neurons**. Although the basic structure of all neurons is the same, they are specialized depending on their location and function.

Neurons differ characteristically from other cells in that they may last a lifetime, use significantly more energy than other cells, and do not possess the ability to divide. Whereas other cells die and are replaced, most neurons do not have this capacity. In order to survive, neurons require a large amount of oxygen and glucose, dying in only a few minutes if deprived of these energy sources.

The main function of a neuron is to transmit signals, or impulses, through the body to regulate bodily functions, including those of movement and those that maintain organ function. They also transmit sensory information to the brain.

In general, a neuron has three major parts: the **dendrite**, which receives impulses; the **cell body**, which processes impulses; and the **axon**, which conducts impulses on to the next neuron, or, in some cases, to an organ, gland, or muscle (Figure 4-3). Together, the dendrites and axons are structures known as processes. Impulses traveling toward the cell body through the axon are termed afferent and impulses traveling away from the cell body are termed efferent.

The dendritic portion of a cell may consist of numerous fibers and spiny extensions that receive impulses from other neurons. From the dendrite or dendritic region, the impulses travel on to the cell body. A dendrite may have numerous branches, each receiving incoming signals from other neurons. The numerous processes allow the dendritic region of the neuron to receive numerous messages, thus increasing a neuron's ability to gather information. The signals that are received and transmitted to the cell body by the neuron are termed a **graded potential**. It is not considered a nerve impulse until it reaches the axon hillock, at which time it becomes an **action potential**.

The cell body, also called the **soma** or **perikaryon**, is the center of the neuron and carries out primary cellular functions. Because neurons are **amitotic** (they do not possess the ability to divide), the cell body contains the organelles typical of other cells, except for centrioles, which play a role in cell reproduction. Cell bodies that are clustered in the CNS are termed a **nucleus** (plural = *nuclei*). Although clusters of cell bodies in the PNS are less common than in the CNS, they do exist and are known as a **ganglion** (plural = *ganglia*).

Once in the cell body, or *soma*, the impulse is sent to the **axon hillock**, where, if the signal is strong enough, it is sent to the *axon*. The axon's two primary functions are to generate and conduct a nerve impulse. At this point (and only if strong enough), the signal becomes a nerve impulse, and an action potential is created.

The axon carries the impulse to another neuron, to an organ or a gland, or to a muscle. At the end of the axon are multiple branches called **telodendria** or **axonal terminals** (also known as synaptic knobs or boutons). The many branches of the axonal terminals represent the junction of the axon with another neuron, an organ or a gland, or a muscle. At the axon terminal, the action potential or nerve impulse causes the secretion of a **neurotransmitter**, a chemical that is synthesized in the cell body and released at the axonal terminals. A neurotransmitter is responsible for initiating a response in the adjacent neuron, organ, or muscle. Bundles of axons in the CNS form a **tract**; in the PNS, the same bundle is referred to as a **nerve**.

An axon may have a coating, known as **myelin**, which is a fatty substance that coats the axon and serves a dual role in neural function. It increases the speed of neural transmission along the axon and provides insulation from the electrical activity of neighboring neurons. The myelin sheath is sometimes referred to as the **neurolemma**. In the PNS, myelin is created by **Schwann cells** or **neurolemmocytes**.

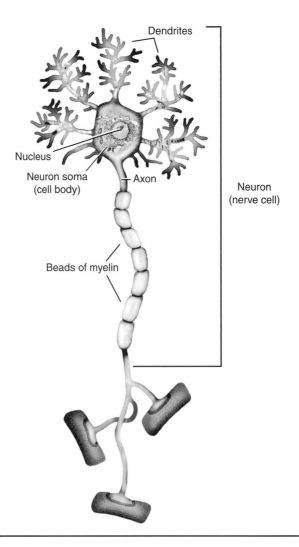

Figure 4-3 *Structure of a Neuron*

Classification of Neurons Neurons may be classified according to structure or function. For the purposes of applied anatomy and kinesiology, we will focus on functional classification because the functional characteristics of neurons relate to clinical practice. However, because the structure of neurons clarifies some of the more specialized functions (such as the senses), an overview of the structural classifications are discussed as well.

Functional Classification. Functionally, neurons are classified according to the direction of their impulses in relation to the CNS. Neurons that carry impulses *toward* the CNS are termed afferent, and neurons that carry impulses *away from* the CNS are known as efferent. Because both of these terms can refer to the direction of signals traveling to and from a neuron's cell body, it is important to differentiate the two applications.

An **association neuron** is named as such because it forms connections between different parts of the brain within the CNS. A neuron that performs this same function in the spinal cord is called an **internuncial neuron**. An association neuron travels and transmits impulses between parts of the brain and the spinal cord. In doing so, various parts of the brain and the spinal cord are able to exert their influence and control over movement and function. An internuncial neuron transmits signals between parts of the spinal cord.

Structural Classification. Depending on where they exist in the body and on their particular function, neurons, although possessing the same basic structures, differ in their configurations. The three major types of neurons are multipolar, bipolar, and unipolar.

Multipolar neurons are characterized by many dendrites (three or more) and a single axon. They are common in the human body and are the primary type of neuron in the CNS. Multiple dendritic processes allow a greater amount of information to be communicated from other neural structures.

Bipolar neurons are found in the sense organs (retina of the eyes, the inner ear, and in the olfactory mechanism) and allow for the processing of sensory input. Bipolar neurons have one dendrite and one axon.

Unipolar neurons are primarily sensory neurons that are located in the ganglia (group of cell bodies) of the PNS. They have a cell body and a single process, the distal portion of which is typically associated with a sensory receptor.

Nerves

The nerves that originate in the brain and travel to the PNS are known as **cranial nerves,** whereas those that originate in the spinal cord are called **spinal nerves**. A nerve is a group of neurons bundled together within a protective sheath. In other words, neurons are the cells that make up a nerve. Nerves that carry afferent signals to the CNS are termed **ascending** or **sensory nerves**, and those that carry efferent impulses to the periphery of the body are referred to as **descending** or **motor nerves**.

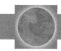 PHYSIOLOGY OF NEURON FUNCTION

The unique physiology of neural tissue enables it to transmit impulses along the axon. Specialized processes allow this to occur. In order to understand how the nervous system enables movement and other functions of the body, it is important to understand the manner in which it functions at the cellular level. To enhance your understanding, keep in mind that thousands of cells functioning in unison allow for daily purposeful activity.

Transmission of Neural Impulses: The Action Potential

Neural impulses must travel from neuron to neuron, and it is the impulse activity that enables the nerves to function. Impulses are electrical and are transmitted by a mechanism called an **action potential**.

In order to better understand the action potential, it is helpful to understand the microanatomy of the membrane of a neuron. Figure 4-4 illustrates the **sodium-potassium pump**. Numerous pumps are located along the cell membrane of the neuron. Reviewing Figure 4-4 as you read the text description may facilitate your understanding.

Positively charged sodium ions (Na^+) are found in greater concentration outside of the neuron, whereas a higher concentration of both positively charged potassium ions (K^+) and negatively charged chloride ions (Cl^-) are found inside the cell. This creates a distribution of electrical charges so that the interior of the neuron is negatively charged in relation to the positive exterior. The purpose of the sodium-potassium pump is to maintain the **resting or membrane potential** of the cell. In this state, there are no impulses traveling along the axon. The sodium-potassium pump maintains this resting state by keeping the balance of Na^+ and K^+ ions inside and outside the cell. The neuron is, thus, in a **polarized state**.

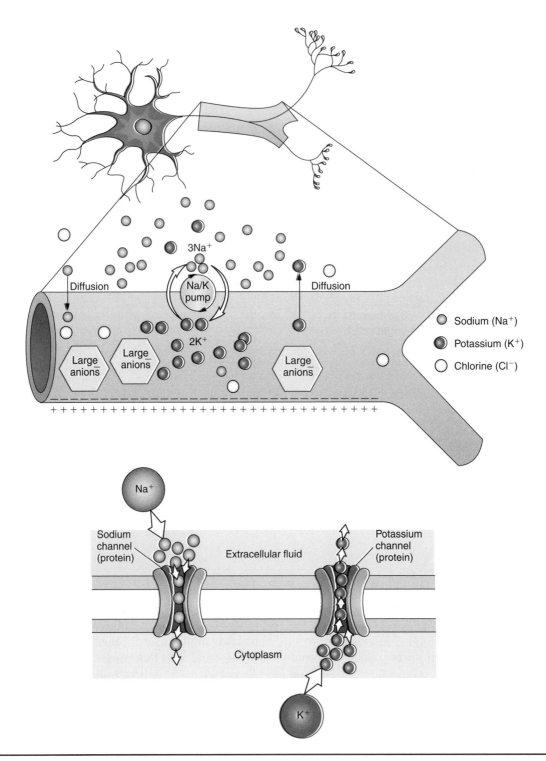

Figure 4-4   *The Sodium-Potassium Pump*

When a nerve impulse occurs in the dendritic region of the neuron, the permeability of the cell membrane changes, allowing Na$^+$ ions to enter the cell in greater concentration. The usually negative interior of the neuron changes to positive, causing a reversal in the electrical charge of the cell. This process is called **depolarization**. This is the beginning of the action potential.

Figure 4-5 illustrates the introduction of the nerve impulse into the dendritic region of the neuron and the resulting action potential. It illustrates the movement of the action potential in a single direction down the axon as well as the **repolarization** of the cell membrane.

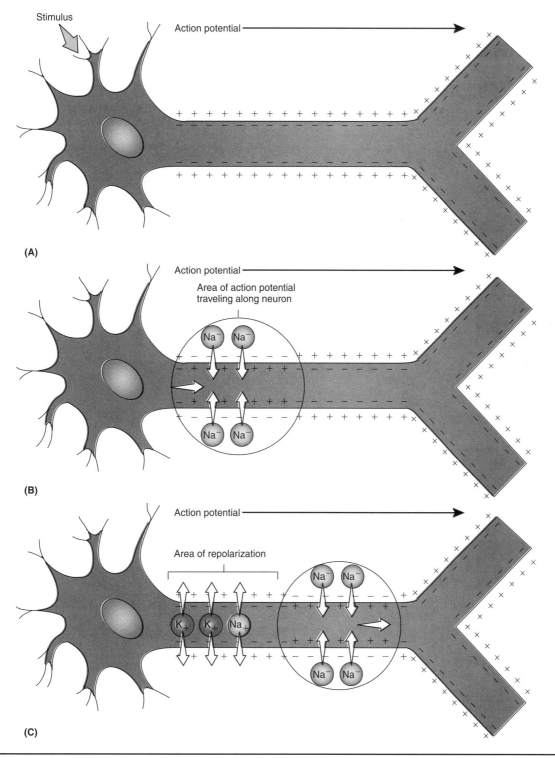

Figure 4-5 *Transmission of a Nerve Impulse*

As the action potential moves down the axon toward the axonal terminal, depolarization occurs along the cell membrane. Concurrently, repolarization occurs behind it as the sodium-potassium pump restores the ion balance and polarization. The action potential continues until it reaches the axon terminal.

A nerve impulse that is not strong enough to initiate the depolarization process will not create an action potential. This is known as the **all-or-none-response**. In other words, all nerve impulses are of adequate and equal strength.

The role of myelin becomes significant in the generation of the action potential. "Gaps" in the myelin sheath are noticeable in the **nodes of Ranvier**. The myelin expedites the transmission of the action potential along the axon by insulating the cell membrane. Because the insulating effect of the myelin prevents depolarization from occurring at covered portions of the cell membrane, the impulse "jumps" along, causing depolarization to occur only at the nodes of Ranvier. This increases the speed of the impulse.

Synaptic Transmission

The junction of a neuron with another neuron or organ of the body is called the **synapse**. Figure 4-6 depicts the synaptic junction. Using the illustration as a guide while you read may be helpful.

At the axon terminal, the nerve impulse is conducted across a small gap known as the **synaptic cleft**. The neuron transmitting the impulse is known as the **presynaptic neuron**, and the neuron (if not an organ) receiving the impulse is called the **postsynaptic neuron**. Essentially, in order for the impulse to continue its movement and reach its ultimate destination, it must cross the synaptic cleft.

Neurotransmitters are chemicals that are released into the synaptic cleft and carry the impulse across it. Acetylcholine is the most commonly used neurotransmitter in the human body. Other neurotransmitters include **adrenalin** or **epinephrine**, **serotonin**, **dopamine**, and **endorphins**. Each has a specific role in various parts of the body.

Neurotransmitters are contained in structures called **synaptic vesicles** located in the axonal terminal. On detection of the neural impulse, the vesicles release the neurotransmitter into the synaptic cleft, allowing the impulse to travel across the cleft to the postsynaptic neuron or organ. To prevent continued discharge, enzymes specific to the neurotransmitter break it down immediately after the impulse is transmitted.

The Brain

The brain is a semisolid mass made up of billions of neurons and supporting cells. To best understand the function of various parts of the brain, we will first examine the types of cells found in each.

Multipolar neurons are the most common type of neurons found in the CNS. As the functions of each of the parts of the brain are discussed, the benefits of this arrangement will become apparent.

In addition to neurons within the brain, there are other cells that serve a supporting role to the neurons. These cells, known as **neuroglia** or **glial cells**, have different names and functions other than transmitting impulses.

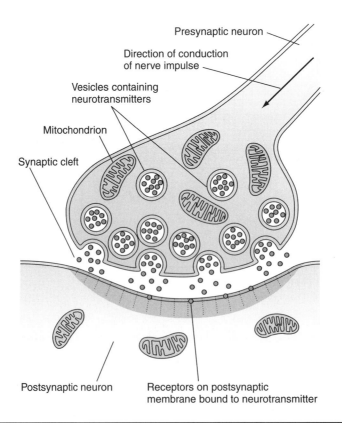

Figure 4-6   *The Synaptic Cleft*

■ **Astrocytes** form a network that supports the neurons of both the brain and spinal cord. They form an attachment between neurons and blood vessels and regulate the nutrients and chemical balance of the nerve cells. They serve a critical role in maintaining the **blood-brain barrier**, which is the mechanism that prevents foreign and potentially harmful substances from entering the brain tissue.

■ **Oligodendroglia** also provide a supportive role as they form a type of connective tissue between neurons in both the brain and spinal cord. They form myelin in the CNS.

■ **Microglia** are phagocytic cells that destroy bacterial cells and cellular debris that occur within the CNS.

■ **Ependymal cells** line the ventricles of the brain and produce **cerebrospinal fluid (CSF)** that bathes and cushions the brain and spinal cord.

The brain is divided into four major parts, each with its own subdivisions and parts. From the lowest (immediately superior to the spinal cord) level to the highest (cerebrum) level, the four major divisions of the brain are:

■ The **cerebrum**, comprised of the **cerebral cortex** and **cerebral hemispheres**

■ The **diencephalon**, comprised of the **thalamus** and **hypothalamus**

■ The **brainstem**, comprised of the **midbrain**, **pons**, and **medulla oblongata, or medulla**.

■ The **cerebellum**

Tract are the ascending and descending axons that carry impulses between the brain and spinal cord. Tracts are made up of **projection fibers**. Tracts are also divided according to the level of the neurons that run from the periphery of the body to the CNS. From distal to proximal, they are **first-order neurons**, which run from the most distal point to the spinal cord; **second-order neurons**, which run from the spinal cord to the thalamus; and **third-order neurons**, which extend from

OTA PERSPECTIVE

Also known as a cerebrovascular accident (CVA), a stroke is a life-threatening event in which a part of the brain suffers from lack of oxygen. There is a huge variance in the amount of damage that can occur. The patient can present with only a minimal deficit and recover completely, or the stroke can be fatal. There are two types of strokes: ischemic and hemorrhagic.

In an ischemic situation the brain does not get enough blood because a blood clot is blocking one of the major arteries leading to the brain. This type of stoke is more common, seen in approximately 80% of stroke patients. The blood clot may be formed within the artery from hardening of the arteries, or it may travel from a distant part of the body and is termed an *embolus*.

A hemorrhagic stroke is caused by excessive bleeding within the brain. This is termed *cerebral hemorrhage* and is often caused by high blood pressure. This type of stroke tends to be more dangerous at the initial onset although the residual damage is often the same.

Risk factors for a stroke include advanced age, high blood pressure, atrial fibrillation, smoking, diabetes, obesity, family history, lack of exercise, or alcohol or drug abuse.

Treatment initially is aimed at stabilizing the patient, preventing further damage, and assessing the damage that has occurred. A CAT scan is usually performed to assess the damage that has occurred. As the patient's condition stabilizes, rehabilitation is commenced. It is often a lengthy process to restore the patient's functional level.

the thalamus to the cerebrum. **Association fibers** transmit impulses within a hemisphere of the brain. **Commissures**, or **commissural fibers** transmit impulses between the hemispheres.

Each of these structures is discussed in terms of their influence on movement. As you read each description, keep in mind the impact on movement that a disease or an injury may affect a particular structure. As an OTA working with physical dysfunction, your clinical skills will be greatly enhanced by critically examining the relationship between a patient's injury or diagnosis and his or her functional skills. It is important to remember that no two individuals are identical neurologically. As a result, each neurological diagnosis that you encounter in practice must be evaluated on an individual basis.

The Cerebrum   When one views the exterior surface of the brain, the cerebral hemispheres are most obvious. The cerebral hemispheres comprise most of the brain's mass. Its primary role in mobility is the control of voluntary movement. Figure 4-7 illustrates the hemispheres of the brain.

Separating the two hemispheres at the midline is the **longitudinal fissure**, which divides the brain into right and left hemispheres. The **lateral fissure** separates the hemispheres into superior and inferior portions. The ridges that are noticeable on the brain's surface are known as **gyri** (singular = *gyrus*) and the grooves are **sulci** (singular = *sulcus*). The **central sulcus** divides the brain into anterior and posterior sections. The **corpus callosum** located deep within the hemispheres is a bundle of neural fibers that communicate between the two hemispheres. There are additional landmarks on the surface of the brain with which you might be familiar; however, for our study of functional movement, we will focus on those listed here because they identify structures that play a major role in the cerebral control of movement. Figure 4-7 illustrates the gyri, sulci, and major fissures of the cerebral hemispheres.

The cerebral hemispheres are divided into lobes, each with its specific function. (Figure 4-8).

The lobes and their primary functions are as follows:

■ The **frontal lobe** is the most anterior portion of the brain and is the part of the brain that allows complex thought processes and is responsible for executive functions, such as decision making and judgment. Damage to this area of the brain results in diminished ability to make reasonable conclusions and effective problem solving. Because the frontal lobe provides conscious control over behavior, the individual with trauma to the frontal lobe may exhibit impulsive behavior.

■ The **parietal lobe**, located directly posterior to the frontal lobe and behind the central sulcus, is the area of the brain that interprets sensory perceptions. Interpretation of touch and spatial perception are functions of the parietal lobe. Deficits in these and other sensory perceptions are frequently noted in individuals with damage to the parietal lobe.

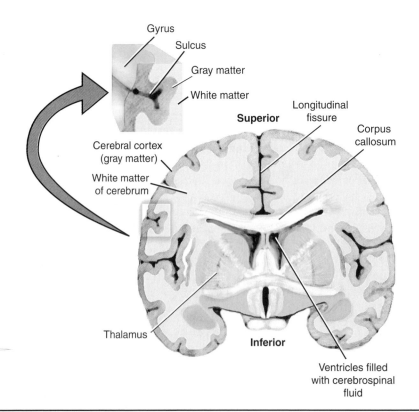

Figure 4-7   *The Right and Left Hemispheres of the Brain*

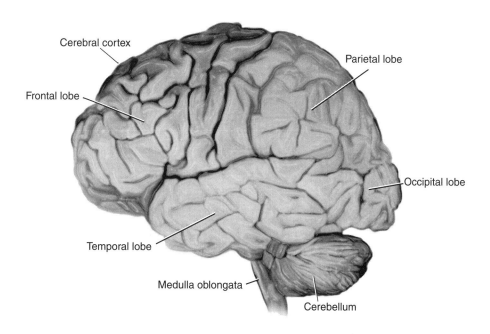

Cerebral cortex

Parietal lobe

Frontal lobe

Occipital lobe

Temporal lobe

Medulla oblongata

Cerebellum

Figure 4-8   *The Lobes of the Brain*

These individuals may have impairment of spatial perception, influencing their mobility in three-dimensional space.

■ The **temporal lobe** lies inferior to the frontal and parietal lobes. The lateral fissure runs along its superior border. The temporal lobe is concerned with hearing and memory processes as well as abstract thinking, which contributes to judgment and other executive functions. The left temporal lobe houses speech centers in most instances. Damage to the temporal lobe may result in impairment of auditory processing, speech (left hemisphere), memory, and may interfere with executive functions because of its involvement with abstract thought processes.

■ The **occipital lobe** is the most posterior of the hemispheric lobes, located inferior to the parietal lobes and concerned with receiving and interpreting visual stimuli. Damage to the occipital lobe typically results in impaired ability to utilize visual input.

■ The **insula** is located deep within the lateral sulcus.

The cerebral hemispheres are covered with a thin layer of gray nervous tissue (cell bodies) called the *cerebral cortex.* It is the structure responsible for consciousness and control of movement as well as the higher cognitive functions of thinking, understanding, and processing complex information and emotions.

Functionally, the cerebral cortex can be divided into three major areas: motor areas, which control conscious movement; sensory areas, which are involved with sensation; and association areas, which integrate information and translate it into purposeful action. Association fibers communicate between the cortical areas within a hemisphere, and commissural fibers communicate between the cortical areas between the hemispheres.

Brodmann's areas are areas of the cortex designated by 52 numbers that correspond to different functional areas. Figure 4-9 illustrates the motor, sensory, and association areas of the cerebral cortex.

Many of the functional areas are self-explanatory as their names suggest. For example, the primary visual cortex is the main area for visual processing, and the visual association area integrates visual input with other sensory and motor information. The result is movement that is coordinated with visual input, for example. The auditory cortex performs the same functions for auditory stimuli.

Other functional areas that are less "obvious" are defined as follows:

■ The primary motor cortex is located on the **precentral gyrus**, which is the gyrus located immediately anterior to the central sulcus. The premotor cortex houses the cell bodies of the neurons that form the corticospinal tract, more commonly known as the **pyramidal tract**, transmits neural impulses from the cortex to the spinal cord. For example, when you throw a ball, the neural signals that direct your arm to throw originate in the cells of the primary motor cortex and travel to the spinal cord via the axons of these cells. From the spinal cord, they are transmitted to the muscles.

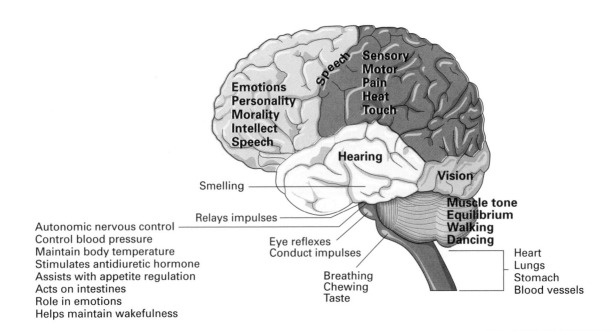

Speech

Emotions
Personality
Morality
Intellect
Speech

Sensory
Motor
Pain
Heat
Touch

Hearing

Vision

Smelling

Muscle tone
Equilibrium
Walking
Dancing

Relays impulses

Autonomic nervous control
Control blood pressure
Maintain body temperature
Stimulates antidiuretic hormone
Assists with appetite regulation
Acts on intestines
Role in emotions
Helps maintain wakefulness

Eye reflexes
Conduct impulses

Breathing
Chewing
Taste

Heart
Lungs
Stomach
Blood vessels

Figure 4-9   *Functional Areas of the Brain*

The primary motor cortex contains a "map" of the body. In other words, each body part is represented in a corresponding area on the primary motor cortex. This is called **somatotopy**. In Figure 4-10, notice that the body (called the **homunculus** in this case) is characterized by parts that are disproportionate to. For example, the hands are larger than the feet. This representation, although disproportionate to the actual body part, is proportionate to the amount of innervation provided to the part. Hands, because of their relationship to purposeful activity, are more highly innervated than the feet. They are, therefore, represented in larger scale on the homunculus.

■ The **premotor cortex** is located directly anterior to the precentral gyrus (primary motor cortex) and controls well-learned motor actions. Its cells also supply impulses to the pyramidal tract. The premotor cortex enables the execution of repetitive and highly familiar actions such as typing or playing the piano.

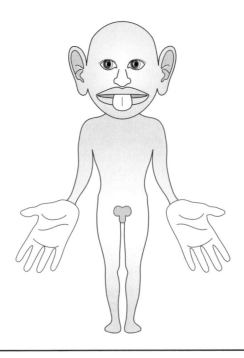

Figure 4-10   *Homunculus*

■ **Broca's area** is located in the temporal lobe and corresponds to Brodmann areas 44 and 45. It is associated with the motor aspects of speech, coordinating the tongue, lips, throat, and voice mechanisms for the act of speaking. It has also been observed to activate during other motor activities and may have a role in other voluntary movements.

■ The **frontal eye fields** are located just anteriorly to the premotor cortex and serve a role in the control of voluntary eye movements.

■ The **primary sensory cortex** is located immediately posterior to the central sulcus in the **postcentral gyrus** of the parietal lobe. It corresponds to Brodmann's areas 1 and 3. The primary sensory cortex is responsible for interpreting sensory stimulation from various body parts. Like the primary motor cortex, the body is represented as a homunculus. Sensory neural distribution patterns are somewhat different than those for motor activity.

■ The **somatosensory association area** is directly posterior to the primary sensory area. Its main function is to integrate various sensory inputs, such as temperature, touch, and pressure, into meaningful information. The somatosensory association area also allows one to remember and use familiar sensory information. For example, when you close your eyes and hold a safety pin in your hand, you know without looking that the object is indeed a safety pin. It is the somatosensory association cortex that controls this ability.

■ The **prefrontal cortex**, located in the anterior frontal lobes, is the portion of the cerebral hemispheres that regulates complex thought and learning and which is associated with cognition. The prefrontal cortex generates abstract thought, provides the foundation for judgment and reasoning abilities, and is the foundation of the conscience. It plays a role in mood and in monitoring emotional responses.

■ The **general interpretation area** (also known as the **gnostic area**) is usually found in the left hemisphere and is responsible for integrating multiple types of input from all sensory areas. It is believed to have a role in storing memories associated with sensation.

■ **Wernicke's area** is one of the language areas thought to be responsible for understanding written and spoken language. It is now believed that comprehension of complex language may occur between the prefrontal cortex and Broca's area, whereas Wernicke's area is more concerned with learning the sounds of new words.

OTA Perspective

The temporal lobe in the cerebral hemisphere is associated with hearing and memory. The cerebral cortex is responsible for processing complex information for thinking and understanding. Broca's area is associated with the motor aspects of speech, with Wernicke's area being associated with understanding language. These are just a few of the CNS functions that contribute to a client's being able to follow directions. If the client does not *hear* what the OTA is instructing him or her to do or if the client does not *understand* what needs to be accomplished or if the client cannot form the thought or language to ask the OTA to repeat or restate the direction, then he or she cannot (does not) comply with direction. Although it is natural for one to speak louder and slow down the rate of speaking, this is not always effective. For example, give your classmate a direction, such as retrieving a certain book from the OT library. Pay attention to the complexity of the direction. How many steps were involved? Did you use hand or facial gestures to augment your verbal directions? Did you use any jargon or slang words in your language? Did your instructions rely on information you assumed your classmate knew (e.g., the location of the OT library)? The study of kinesiology and the nervous system will assist the OTA in recognizing the relationship between specific areas and functions of the brain and the corresponding abilities and, conversely, disabilities. Understanding that relationship will contribute to the OTA's skills to provide quality therapeutic interventions.

■ The **affective language areas** are associated with the emotional components of verbal communication. Tone of voice, inflection, gestures, and other elements of emotional expression are regulated in this area. The affective language areas also allow us to perceive the emotional tone in language that is directed at us.

The **basal nuclei** is a group of nuclei lying within the cerebral hemispheres. Typically, the structures that comprise the basal nuclei are the **caudate nucleus**, the **putamen**, and the **globus pallidus**. Together, the putamen and globus pallidus are known as the **lentiform nucleus**. The lentiform and caudate nuclei as a whole are referred to as the **corpus striatum**. Within the physical configuration of the caudate nucleus is a structure known as the **amygdala**. Functionally, it is part of the limbic system.

The basal nuclei play an important role in the control of movement and may contribute to cognitive abilities. The basal nuclei are thought to have numerous functions including:

■ Starting and stopping movement

■ Monitoring movement directed by the cortex

■ Controlling automatic, stereotypic movements, such as arm movements, that are coordinated with walking

■ Regulating the intensity of movement

■ Inhibiting antagonistic and unnecessary movement

Injury involving the basal nuclei can affect the execution and speed of certain movements, cause tremors and other involuntary movements, and slow movements.

The Diencephalon
Deep within and surrounded by the cerebral hemispheres is the part of the brain known as the diencephalon. It contains the thalamus, hypothalamus, and epithalamus.

The main function of the thalamus is to serve as a sensory relay center. As such, it receives multiple signals from the entire body, sorts the various information, and sends it to the appropriate regions of the cerebral cortex. In addition, the thalamus groups related input together and sends it to the motor cortex, sensory cortex, and sensory association areas. The thalamus also receives and sorts input from the visceral centers, emotional centers, the cerebellum, and the basal nuclei. In doing so, the thalamus plays a significant role in the control of both motor and sensory functions as well as learning and memory. It also controls the function of the hypothalamus.

The hypothalamus, located just inferior to the thalamus and superior to the brainstem, primarily regulates homeostasis and provides control over visceral functions. The pituitary gland is located at the base of the hypothalamus. Hypothalamic functions include:

■ Control of the autonomic nervous system, including blood pressure, force of heart contractions, heart rate, digestive tract function and motility, respiration rate and depth, and adjustment of eye pupil size. In addition, the hypothalamus regulates other automatic responses.

■ Control of emotions and behavior. The hypothalamus is associated with the limbic system and is involved with the perception of pleasure, sexual arousal, fear, and rage. It is related to the physical expression of emotion.

■ Regulation of body temperature. Based on the temperature of the blood, the hypothalamus maintains body temperature by initiating shivering or sweating in response to cold or heat, respectively.

■ Control of food and water intake. The hypothalamus responds to changes in the concentration of body fluid as well as to the nutrient levels of the blood, causing feelings of thirst or hunger when levels reach a certain point. Likewise, the hypothalamus creates feelings of fullness, or satiety, when the appetite is satisfied.

■ Regulation of the sleep cycle. In response to changing light and darkness cues obtained from the visual pathways, the hypothalamus regulates the biological clock.

■ Control of the endocrine function. The pituitary gland (located on the hypothalamus) releases certain hormones. Nuclei in the hypothalamus regulate the release of hormones from other glands.

The epithalamus lies above the thalamus and contains the **pineal gland**. The pineal gland plays a role in the regulation of the sleep-wake cycle and has some influence over mood. The epithalamus also contains **choroid plexus**, a structure that produces cerebrospinal fluid.

The Brainstem
The brainstem is located just superior to the spinal cord and inferior to the rest of the brain. As a whole, the brainstem supports the automatic functions that maintain life, serves as a pathway for spinal tracts, and contains the nuclei for 10 of the 12 cranial nerves. The brainstem has three divisions. Superiorly to inferiorly, they are the midbrain; the pons; and the medulla oblongata or, simply, the medulla. Figure 4-11 illustrates the brainstem and the peduncles, which are the tracts passing through the lower sections of the brain.

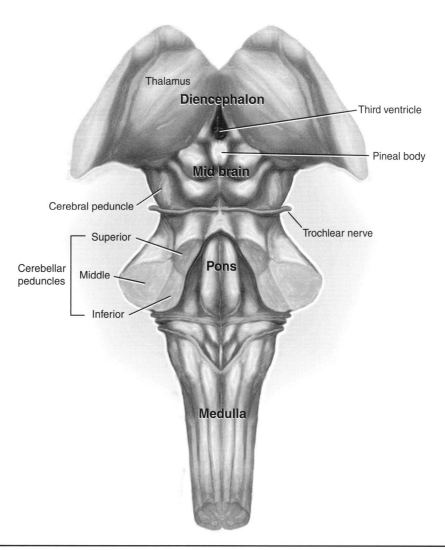

Figure 4-11 *The Brainstem*

The midbrain is the structure located in the most superior part of the brainstem and immediately inferior to the diencephalon. The pyramidal tracts form the cerebral peduncles, which are found on the ventral surface of the midbrain and which connect the cerebrum to the spinal cord. The **superior cerebellar peduncles** connect the cerebellum to the midbrain. Within the midbrain is the **cerebral aqueduct**, which is part of the ventricular system of the brain.

Also contained in the midbrain are the **superior colliculi**, a set of nuclei that coordinates head and eye movements, providing the ability to visually track objects. Another set of nuclei, the **inferior colliculi**, plays a role in the transmission of auditory stimuli to the cortex.

The **substantia nigra**, a large mass of nuclei found in the midbrain, releases the neurotransmitter dopamine, which, with the basal nuclei, regulates movement. Another structure within the midbrain that controls movement is the **red nucleus**, which resides in some of the motor neurons and has a role in controlling limb flexion.

Moving inferiorly, the pons is the next structure in the midbrain. It consists primarily of tracts and contains the **pontine nuclei**, which provide communication between the cerebellum and the cortex. The **middle cerebellar peduncles** connect the pons to the cerebellum. Several of the cranial nerves arise from the pons.

The medulla oblongata, frequently referred to as simply the medulla, is the most inferior structure of the brain, connecting it with the spinal cord. It houses the centers that support critical autonomic life functions, including regulation of heart rate and force, blood pressure, and breathing depth and rate. The hypothalamus exerts its control on the medulla, which, in turn, directly controls the life functions. Other functions controlled by the medulla include vomiting, coughing, sneezing, and swallowing.

In the medulla, the pyramidal tracts cross over one another to the contralateral side of the body at the **decussation of the pyramids**. It is at this point that the left hemisphere exerts its control on the right side of the body, and the right hemisphere on the left. For this reason, individuals who suffer an injury to the left side of the brain experience right-sided deficits, and vice versa.

The Cerebellum   The cerebellum is one of the structures of the brain that is closely related to movement and its control. The cerebellum is located posterior to the brainstem and inferior to the cerebral hemispheres, as shown in Figure 4-12.

The cerebellum provides the unconscious (we do not think about it) timing and coordination of skeletal muscle contraction needed for the smooth execution of movement. The cerebellar peduncles, on their path through the brainstem, originate in the cerebellum and terminate in the cortex. These tracts remain on the ipsilateral, or same, side of the body versus crossing over as do the pyramidal tracts.

The types of information that the cerebellum processes is significant in the study of movement. Impulses from the cortex, as well as the muscles of the body, provide input to which the cerebellum responds. The cerebellum receives input from the following:

◼ The motor association areas of the cortex. When voluntary movement is initiated, the cortex sends impulses to the skeletal muscle via the pyramidal tracts and to the cerebellum.

◼ Proprioceptors in the joints and muscles of the body. Based on the commands from the cortex, the cerebellum regulates the timing and amount of muscle contraction needed to complete the movement with accuracy.

The cerebellum provides information to the following:

◼ The motor cortex so that fine adjustments can be made to the movement

◼ The red nucleus, which helps to regulate muscle contraction

Damage to the cerebellum can affect coordination, muscle tone, and balance as well as the timing and execution of voluntary movement.

Functional Systems of the Brain   There are systems within the brain that are composed of various nuclei and fibers that form a type of network throughout the brain. Because their structure is not of a gross nature that is easily observed, they are known as **functional systems**.

The **limbic system** consists of a group of structures found on the medial surfaces of the cerebral hemispheres. It regulates emotions, and its connections with other areas of the brain allow us to respond with feelings to our environments. The connections between the limbic system and cerebral hemispheres allow us to consciously weigh emotion versus reason. The amygdala and the **hippocampus** of the limbic system are thought to play a role in the storage of information in long-term memory. Figure 4-13 illustrates the neural connections and structures typically associated with the limbic system.

The **reticular formation** is a network of neurons found throughout the brainstem. The axons of these neurons extend throughout the brain and fulfill the role of maintaining general awareness and arousal by transmitting constant signals to brain regions. The axons that extend into the cerebral cortex are called the **reticular activating system (RAS)** and maintain the cortex in a state of alertness. The reticular formation and RAS also filter out unwanted and irrelevant stimuli.

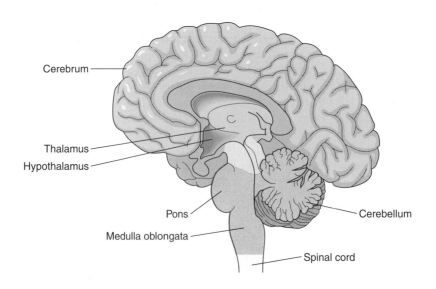

Figure 4-12   *The Regions of the Brain*

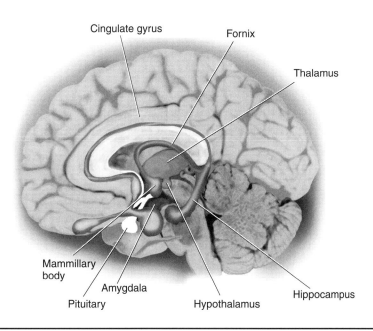

Cingulate gyrus
Fornix
Thalamus
Mammillary body
Amygdala
Pituitary
Hypothalamus
Hippocampus

Figure 4-13 *The Limbic System*

The Ventricular System of the Brain Within the brain are the **ventricles**, the open chambers within the brain. The ventricles of the brain are connected, forming a network of compartments that are continuous with one another and with the **central canal** of the spinal cord.

OTA Perspective

OT and PT practitioners frequently work with clients who have sustained brain damage—whether it is someone with a closed head injury or a person who has an illness such as a cerebral vascular accident (CVA). The location in the brain where the damage has occurred, the results of the natural healing process, and the effects of medication all have an impact on the client's ability to function and the therapy treatment plan. Not only might the ability to move and the quality of that movement be affected, but also so might the client's ability to think and reason—to remember, to problem solve, or to make decisions ("thinking" is termed "cognition"). Therapists typically view therapy as a "patient participation event." This means that in order to participate in a therapeutic regime that involves improving performance skills such as motor skills or physical capacities, the client needs to be able to engage in tasks such as finding his or her way to the therapy room, following directions for engaging in muscle strength and range of motion testing, and remembering the prescribed home exercise program. It is the therapist's responsibility to tailor the treatment to a level that the client can comprehend and, therefore, follow through with. A study of the nervous system within a kinesiology framework will alert the OTA student to the complexities of the brain and how brain dysfunction might make an impact on movement and, therefore, functional abilities.

Parts of the ventricles are lined with ependymal cells that secrete cerebrospinal fluid (CSF). CSF provides buoyancy to the brain and serves as a cushioning agent, protecting the soft tissue of the brain from being bumped and jolted. Figure 4-14 illustrates the ventricles and the circulatory path of CSF.

The ventricles are classified as follows:

■ The lateral ventricles are located deep in the cerebral hemispheres, one in each hemisphere. Anteriorally, they lie close together and are separated by a membrane known as the **septum pellucidum**.

■ The **third ventricle** is within the diencephalon and is connected to the lateral ventricles via the **interventricular foramen**.

■ The fourth ventricle lies posterior to the pons and medulla and is connected to the third ventricle by the cerebral aqueduct in the midbrain. The fourth ventricle is continuous with the central canal that runs down the center of the spinal cord. On the sides of the fourth ventricle are the **lateral apertures**, and in the roof the fourth ventricle, the **median aperture**. These openings connect the ventricles to the **subarachnoid space**, which surrounds the brain. CSF flows into the subarachnoid space as part of its circulation, providing cushioning and protection to the brain.

Although the ventricles have little influence on human movement, conditions that affect their function can have a bearing on it. Conditions such as hydrocephalus or tumors that might impede the flow of CSF through the ventricular system could potentially cause a buildup of fluid, and thus, pressure. Such pressure exerted on the brain structures that control an aspect of movement may have adverse effects on that movement.

Protective Structures of the Brain and CNS Tissue The CNS is protected by several structures. Like the ventricles, the protective structures themselves have little, if anything, to do with functional movement. However, injury to the structures that impact the nervous tissue beneath them has the potential to affect brain function and, therefore, movement.

The brain and spinal cord are encased in the bony protection of the **skull** and **vertebral column**, respectively. Although the hard casing of these structures offers protection, injury to the bone, such as a fracture, can injure the nervous tissue beneath it.

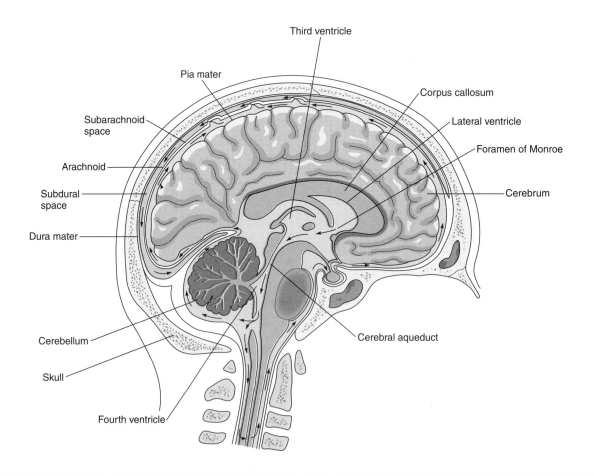

Figure 4-14 *The Ventricles of the Brain*

Between the brain and the skull are the **meninges**, a group of layered membranes that encase the brain and spinal cord. Figure 4-15 illustrates the meninges.

The layers of the meninges are, from external to internal, the **dura mater** (meaning "tough mother"), the **arachnoid mater** (simply called the arachnoid meaning "spider-like"), and the **pia mater** (meaning "gentle mother").

The dura mater is continuous with the periosteum of the skull. It covers the brain but does not extend to cover the spinal cord. The tissue of the dura mater extends into the fissures and sulci of the brain to form **septa** (singular = *septum*), which secure the brain and hold it in place. The septa include the following:

■ **falx cerebri**, which extends into the longitudinal fissure

■ **falx cerebelli**, which extends into the cerebellum

■ **tentorium**, which lies in a horizontal position over the cerebellum

The dura mater also forms the **dural sinuses**, which are reservoirs that collect venous blood for return to the circulatory system via the jugular veins.

Deep to the dura mater is the arachnoid mater, anchored by tiny filaments to the pia mater beneath. These filaments resemble the structure of a spider web, hence the name arachnoid. Directly beneath the arachnoid later is the subarachnoid space, which contains numerous blood vessels and the CSF. The subarachnoid space is continuous with the ventricles of the brain and the central canal of the spinal cord.

The pia mater is the deepest membrane of the meninges. It fits tightly over the surface of brain, following the convolutions of the sulci and gyri. It is supplied with abundant blood vessels.

Whereas the skull and meninges provide physical protection, protection from certain substances is provided by the blood-brain barrier. The blood-brain barrier consists of specialized capillaries, cell junctions, and neuroglia that are selectively permeable. It maintains stable homeostasis in nervous tissue by allowing only certain materials and substances to enter. Because nervous tissue is characterized by a narrow range of acceptable conditions, it is the most susceptible tissue in the body to alterations in its homeostasis. The blood-brain barrier maintains acceptable conditions for the function of nervous tissue.

The configuration of the meninges of the spinal cord is somewhat different from that of the brain, although the function remains the same. The spinal cord is covered by a membrane known as the **spinal dural sheath**, underneath of which is the **epidural space**. The epidural space contains a layer of fatty tissue and veins. As with the brain, CSF fills the space between the arachnoid and pia mater. The meninges of the spinal cord extend below the termination of the spinal cord, forming a reservoir of spinal fluid at the base of the cord.

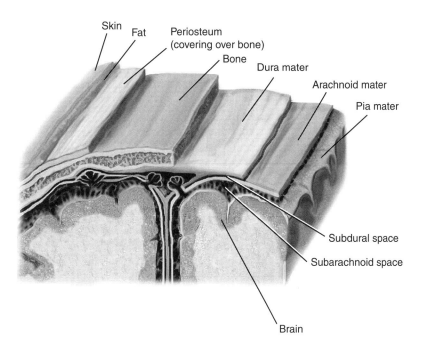

Figure 4-15 *The Meninges*

The Spinal Cord

Extending inferiorly from and continuous with the medulla of the brain is the **spinal cord**. It is primarily composed of tracts that communicate afferent and efferent impulses to and from the brain. The spinal nerves, which supply the periphery of the body, exit along the length of the spinal cord through the intervertebral foramina of the vertebral column. Sensory impulses from the periphery of the body enter the CNS via the spinal cord. In addition, reflex activity that plays a significant role in muscle contraction is moderated at the level of the spinal cord.

Gross Anatomy of the Spinal Cord In addition to its protective coverings and major anatomical features, the spinal cord is divided into segments that correspond to the vertebrae in which it is encased. The levels of the spinal cord, from superior to inferior, are cervical, thoracic, lumbar, and sacral. Figure 4-16 depicts the spinal cord and illustrates its levels and major features.

The levels of the spinal cord are significant in communicating movement dysfunction relative to injuries of the spinal cord. For example, an individual with a spinal cord injury at level T6 (sixth vertebra in the thoracic segment) will have deficits below that level. Understanding which muscles and parts of the body are innervated by the levels below T6 will help determine the functional deficits that this individual may be expected to have.

The other major anatomical structures and functions of the spinal cord are as follows.

■ **Conus medullaris**: The distal and terminating end of the spinal cord found at approximately level L1. The spinal nerves that exit through vertebral levels L2 through S5 travel distally through the CSF contained within the subarachnoid space. These nerve fibers form a bundle known as the **cauda equina**, or "horse's tail," because that is what it resembles.

■ **Filum terminale** ("terminal filament"): An extension of the pia mater that anchors the spinal cord to the coccyx.

■ **Denticulate ligaments**: Tiny extensions of the pia mater found along the edges of the spinal cord, that anchor the spinal cord to the vertebral canal along its length. These ligaments are named for their shape, which resemble tooth-like structures.

■ **Cervical and lumbar enlargements**: Lateral bulges in the cord tissue of the cervical and lumber regions of the cord. Because these areas innervate the upper and lower extremities, innervation density is higher than at other regions of the body. The cervical and lumbar enlargements reflect a greater density of nervous tissue in these densely innervated areas.

Tracts The tracts of the spinal cord are composed of white matter, the axons of neurons. Tracts run in two directions: ascending, or from the body periphery to the central nervous system; and descending, or from the central nervous system to the periphery. Ascending tracts are also known as sensory tracts (they transmit sensory input) and descending tracts are known as motor tracts (they direct and control motor responses).

The tracts are described here with the goal of addressing their role in functional movement. A key point to bear in mind is that injury to a tract (such as a spinal cord injury) will interrupt the neural messages carried by that tract. For motor tracts, this results in disruption of the control exerted via that tract from the CNS. In the case of sensory tracts, sensory input is disrupted. Because movement is regulated by sensory input, disruption in the sensory systems will influence movement. It is also important to recognize that although we can gain a general idea of the deficits that can occur in either of these instances, the complex communication network of the nervous system can be affected in many ways.

Following are some general assumptions that can be made regarding the tracts and their function:

■ Each tract is represented bilaterally; that is, there is a pair of each of the tracts on the right- and left-hand sides of the spinal cord.

■ Tracts consist of first-order neurons (generally extending from the periphery of the body to the spinal cord), second-order neurons (within the cord itself), and third-order neurons (extending from the cord to the brain).

■ The tracts are organized in a methodical manner with specific areas corresponding to specific areas of the body. (This is similar to the systematic arrangement of the motor and sensory cortices of the cerebral cortex.)

■ Most of the tracts decussate (cross over) as do the pyramidal tracts in the medulla of the brainstem. Consequently, below certain points, a given tract will control the opposite side of the body. Some of the tracts cross more than once, meaning that they will influence different sides of the body depending on the level in the spinal cord.

To appreciate the significant influence of the tracts on functional movement, it is helpful to develop a clear understanding of the functions of both the sensory and motor tracts. Table 4-1 summarizes the sensory tracts of the spinal cord, and Table 4-2 summarizes the motor tracts.

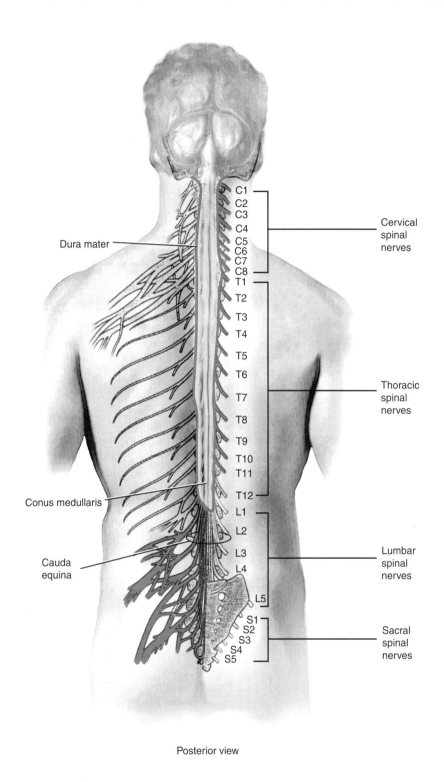

Posterior view

Figure 4-16   *The Spinal Nerves*

Note: *The tracts represented in Table 4-1 and Table 4-2 are those that contribute mainly to daily movement and activity. Refer to the chapter references for more in-depth information.*

Table 4-1 *Ascending (Sensory) Tracts of the Central Nervous System*

Ascending (Sensory) Tract	Location in Spinal Cord and Description	Function
Fasciculus Cuneatus Fasciculus Gracilis	Located in the posterior white matter of the spinal cord. The tract enters the spinal cord at the dorsal root and travels in tract on the ipsilateral side to the medulla. The fibers cross over at the level of the medulla. Fibers ascend from the medulla to the thalamus via the medial lemniscal tract. In the thalamus, they synapse with third-order neurons that travel to the contralateral somatosensory cortex.	Transmit sensory impulses from the receptors of the skin and the proprioceptors of the joints. These impulses are interpreted as discriminative touch and provide a sense of the body's position in space. Fasciculus cuneatus transmits from the upper trunk and extremities and the neck; fasciulus gracilis transmits from the lower body.
Lateral Spinothalamic	Located in the lateral aspects of the white matter of the spinal cord. Neurons of this tract originate in the posterior horn of the cord and cross to the contralateral side before ascending. The neurons of the lateral spinothalamic tract synapse in the thalamus and are, in turn, transmitted to the somatosensory cortex.	Transmits sensations of pain and temperature. Impulses are interpreted by the opposite somatosensory cortex.
Anterior Spinothalamic	Located in the anterior white matter of the spinal cord. The tract originates in the association neurons of the dorsal horn of the cord and crosses over to the contralateral side before ascending. These neurons synapse in the thalamus and are relayed to the somatosensory cortex.	Transmits sensations of crude touch and pressure to the opposite somatosensory cortex for interpretation.
Posterior Spinocerebellar	Posterior portion of the lateral white matter of the spinal cord. Fibers of this tract originate in the ipsilateral posterior horn and ascend to the cerebellum without crossing to the contralateral side.	Transmits impulses related to proprioception from one side of the truck and lower extremities to the cerebellum. Sensations are not consciously registered; it provides the sense of proprioception on a subconscious level.
Anterior Spinocerebellar	Anterior portion of the lateral white matter of the spinal cord. Fibers originate in the neurons of the contralateral posterior horn and cross over to the opposite side in the pons. They terminate in the cerebellums	Provides proprioceptive input from the ipsilateral side of the body; input occurs on a subconscious level.

Cross Section Anatomy of the Spinal Cord A cross-sectional view of the spinal cord displays an orderly and systematic arrangement (Figure 4-17).

Examination of the cross-sectional diagram reveals structures that are significant in the function of the spinal cord. The spinal cord is divided into right and left portions by the **anterior median fissure** and the **posterior median sulcus**.

The gray matter of the spinal cord resembles the letter "H" or a butterfly and is comprised of the cell bodies of neurons. It lies interior to the white matter, which is the reverse of the arrangement in the brain. The gray matter is divided into the **ventral** (or anterior) **horns** and **dorsal** (or posterior) **horns**. Right and left aspects of the horns are joined through the center of the cord by the **gray commissure**. The central canal, which contains CSF, runs through the center of the gray commissure. The **lateral horns** are significant at the thoracic and lumbar segments of the cord.

The ventral and dorsal horns each play a role in the processing of motor and sensory impulses. The ventral horns primarily contain cell bodies of motor neurons and innervate the muscles. They exit the spinal cord via the **ventral roots**, and are responsible for transmitting impulses that direct voluntary movement. A look at the gray matter at different levels of the spinal cord reveals larger ventral horns in the segments of the cord innervating the upper and lower extremities. These nerve cells are associated with the descending, or motor, tracts.

The dorsal horns are associated with sensory neurons that transmit sensory information from the periphery to the CNS where it is interpreted. The sensory neurons have a slightly different arrangement from that of the motor neurons. As these neurons enter the spinal cord, their cell bodies form an enlarged area known as the **dorsal root ganglion** or **spinal ganglion** at the **dorsal root**. The axons of the sensory neurons synapse with several other neurons at different locations within the cord to exert sensory influence via the various tracts.

Table 4-2 *Descending (Motor) Tracts of the Central Nervous System*

Descending (Motor) Tract	Location in Spinal Cord and Description	Function
Lateral Corticospinal (pyramidal)	Located in the lateral white matter of the spinal cord. Originates in the motor cortex of the cerebral cortex; neurons decussate (cross over) at the level of the medulla in the brainstem. Terminates at the interneurons in the anterior horn of the spinal cord.	Transmits neural impulses from the motor cortex to the skeletal muscle. Controls voluntary movement on the contralateral side of the body relative to the cerebral cortex from where the impulse originated.
Anterior Corticospinal (pyramidal)	Located in the anterior white matter of the spinal cord. Originates in the motor cortex of the cerebral cortex. Neural fibers decussate at the spinal level and terminate in the anterior horn of the spinal cord.	Functions the same as the lateral corticospinal tract.
Tectospinal (formerly known as the extrapyramidal tract)	Located in the lateral white matter of the spinal cord. Originates in the midbrain of the brainstem. Fibers decussate to the opposite side of the spinal cord and terminate in the anterior horn.	Conducts impulses from the midbrain that coordinate eye and head movements.
Vestibulospinal	Located in the anterior white matter of the spinal cord. Originates in the vestibular nuclei of the medulla of the brainstem. The fibers descend on the ipsilateral side and terminate in the anterior horn of the spinal cord.	Conducts neural impulses that control muscle tone. Impulses also activate limb and trunk extensor muscles on the ipsilateral side of the body and control head movements. Contributes to maintaining balance while standing and during movement.
Rubrospinal	Located in the lateral white matter of the spinal cord. Originates in the red nucleus of the midbrain of the brainstem and contains fibers that cross over just inferiorly to the red nucleus. Fibers terminate in the anterior horn of the spinal cord.	Transmits neural impulses that regulate muscle tone (primarily that of the flexor muscles) on the contralateral side of the body.
Reticulospinal	Located in the anterior and lateral white matter of the spinal cord. Originates in the reticular formation of the brainstem and contains both crossed and uncrossed fibers. They terminate in the anterior horn of the spinal cord.	Impulses control visceral functions and muscle tone primarily and are thought to be involved with unskilled movements.

The lateral horns exert their influence on the autonomic nervous system via the ventral root. They exert influence on the organs of the body via the autonomic system.

Spinal Reflex Arcs
A **reflex** is a predictable and stereotypic response to a stimulus brought about by an unconscious and involuntary neural reaction. Reflexes play a role in the maintenance of muscle tone and contraction, and these specific types of reflexes are discussed in the PNS section. Because neurons in the gray matter significantly affect reflexes, basic action within the spinal cord that supports reflex activity are discussed here.

The basic elements of a reflex arc and their functions are shown in Figure 4-18.

Many reflexes occur at a subconscious level, and we are never aware of their actions. Some occur strictly at the spinal cord level without influence from higher brain structures, whereas others are moderated by input from the brain.

The evaluation of reflexes, as most of us are familiar with during physical examinations, provides the examiner with information about the general health and function of the nervous system. If a reflexive response is atypical, the nature of the response can provide information regarding the possible nature of any dysfunction of the nervous system.

The steps of the spinal reflex are as follows.

◾ The stimulus is received by the sensory receptor at the site of stimulation.

◾ The afferent impulse travels along the sensory neuron to the dorsal root of the spinal nerve at the spinal cord.

◾ On entering the dorsal horn of the cord, the impulse reaches the **integration center**, where the afferent neuron synapses with a motor neuron. In some cases, there may be several synapses before the impulse reaches the motor neu-

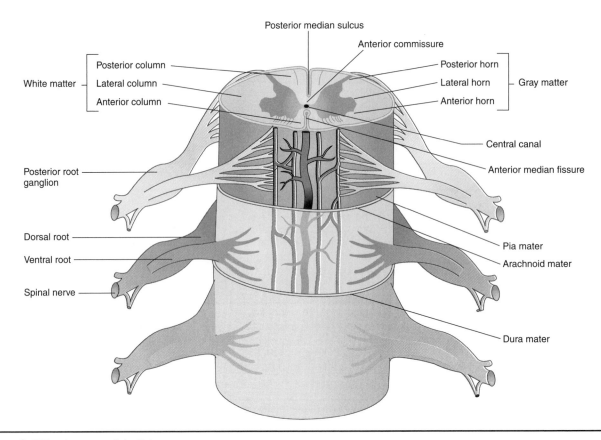

Figure 4-17　*Anatomy of the Spine*

ron. When one synapse is involved, the reflex is called a **monosynaptic reflex**, and when more than one synapse is present, the term **polysynaptic reflex** is used.

■ The motor neuron transmits impulses to the muscle or organ and elicits the reflexive response.

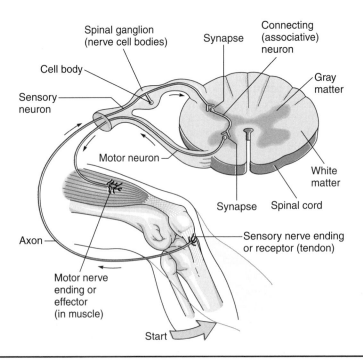

Figure 4-18　*The Reflex Arc*

THE PERIPHERAL NERVOUS SYSTEM

To illustrate the function of the PNS, let us use an everyday example. Suppose you place your hand on a hot stove. The sensation of the heat from the stove is recognized by the sensory receptors in your hand. The impulses registered from that sensation travel along the afferent pathways through the spinal cord to the brain. At the brain, the sensory impulses are interpreted and modified in different ways at different levels of the brain. The brain responds to the sensation of heat with a command to the muscles to execute a response and sends the message, "move your hand!" to the motor neurons that control movement of the hand. You withdraw your hand. At the same time, various brain structures are monitoring and adjusting factors, such as your reaction speed, precision of your movement, and its timing. The speech centers may moderate the utterances of selected expletives. An analysis of this reaction and the structures that enable it illustrates the components of the PNS.

The PNS includes all neural structures outside the CNS. In addition to the peripheral nerves and sensory receptors, the PNS includes the sympathetic and parasympathetic components of the autonomic nervous system as well as certain reflex activity that occurs in the muscles.

The Autonomic Nervous System

The autonomic nervous system is part of the efferent division of the PNS. Although some control is exerted by the CNS, most of its anatomical structures are located in the PNS. The autonomic nervous system is comprised of two parts, the sympathetic and parasympathetic systems, that complement one another's function. Most organs of the body are innervated by both of these systems, with each system exerting a different effect on each organ. Generally (there are a few exceptions), the sympathetic system activates organs and the parasympathetic system provides a calming effect.

Anatomy of the Autonomic System Figure 4-19 A and B illustrate the anatomy of the autonomic nervous system and its effects on selected organs of the body. It will be helpful to refer to the diagrams while reading.

The sympathetic division arises from the thoracic and lumbar regions of the spinal cord. The sympathetic system consists of a short **preganglionic neuron**; the **sympathetic ganglia**, or **sympathetic chain**; and the **postganglionic neuron**. The preganglionic neuron originates in the anterior horn of the spinal cord, and synapses in the sympathetic ganglia, or sympathetic chain, which extends parallel to the thoracic and lumbar regions of the spinal cord. The postganglionic neurons arise from the ganglia and terminate in the various organs of the body. Sympathetic postganglionic neurons release the neurotransmitter norepinephrine to the effector organ.

Examples of the function of the sympathetic system are best illustrated by the "fight or flight" reaction, which include increased heart rate, rapid breathing, and sweating.

The parasympathetic division arises from the brainstem and sacral regions of the spinal cord. Its anatomical structure is essentially the opposite of that of the sympathetic division. The parasympathetic preganglionic neuron runs from the brainstem and sacral areas to the organ and synapses in the **terminal**, or intramural, **ganglia** that lie in the effector organ. The postganglionic neuron is short and extends into the effector organ. The parasympathetic postganglionic neuron releases the neurotransmitter acetylcholine in the effector organ.

Signs of relaxation are examples of the effects of the parasympathetic division, which include decreased blood pressure, lowered heart rate, and normally dilated pupils.

Spinal Nerves and Dermatomes

Thirty-one pairs of spinal nerves arise from each side of the spinal cord. Each nerve is comprised of thousands of neural fibers. The spinal nerves innervate all parts of the body except the head and neck, which are innervated by the cranial nerves.

The spinal nerves are formed as the dorsal and ventral roots merge just distal to the dorsal root ganglia and shortly before exiting through the intervertebral foramina of the vertebrae. Because each nerve contains both sensory and motor fibers, they are referred to as **mixed nerves**, as opposed to being strictly motor or sensory. Spinal nerves at the superior portions of the cord run fairly horizontally as they exit the vertebral column; those in the lumbar and sacral regions run in the distal direction toward the cauda equina before exiting the vertebral column.

Shortly after a nerve exits, it divides into branches known as the **ventral ramus** and the **dorsal ramus** (plural = *rami*). One small branch known as the **meningeal branch** returns to the spinal cord to innervate the meninges. The ventral ramus branch innervates the anterior aspects of the body, and the dorsal ramus branch innervates the posterior aspects. At the thoracic level, the nerves exit, divide into rami, and for the most part, travel laterally to innervate areas close to the level where they emerge from the cord. At the cervical, lumbar, and sacral levels, the nerves form plexuses (singular = *plexus*).

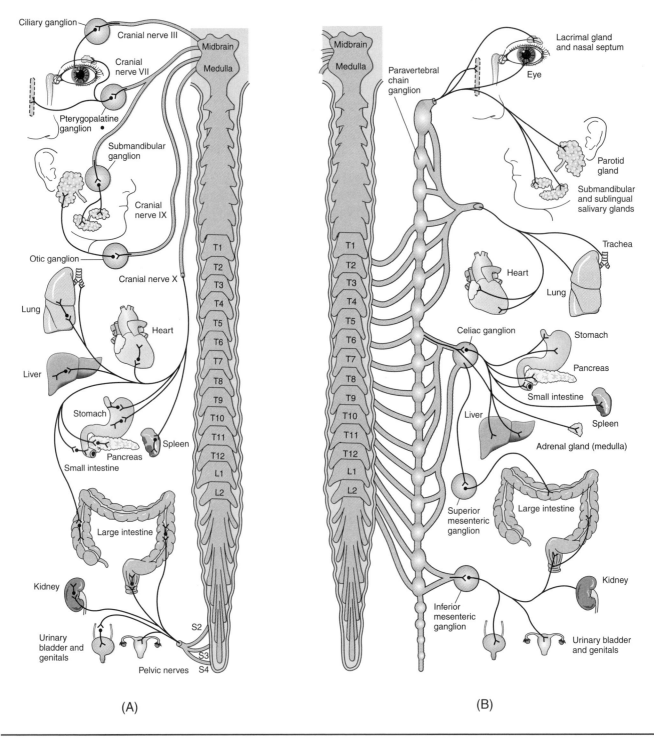

Figure 4-19 *Autonomic Nervous System. (A) Parasympathetic; (B) Sympathetic.*

Spinal nerves are named according to the level where they exit the vertebral column. The nerves are named according to the region of the vertebral column from which they emerge and are numbered superiorly to inferiorly within the corresponding regions. From superior to inferior, the regions and numbered spinal nerves are:

■ Cervical (8 pairs) designated as C1–C8

■ Thoracic (12 pairs) designated as T1–T12

■ Lumbar (5 pairs) designated as L1–L5

■ Sacral (5 pairs) designated as S1–S5

■ Coccygeal (1 pair) designated as C_0

Figure 4-20 illustrates the locations and corresponding names of the spinal nerves.

The nerve that exits immediately inferior to a vertebra assumes the name of the vertebra above it. For example, thoracic nerve 6 (T6) exits the vertebral column just below the sixth thoracic vertebra. The exception is C8 (cervical nerve 8), which exits below C7 and above T1.

The motor fibers of each of the spinal nerves innervate specific muscles in the body. Briefly, the cervical and upper thoracic nerves innervate the upper extremities and upper torso, and the lower thoracic and sacral nerves innervate the lower

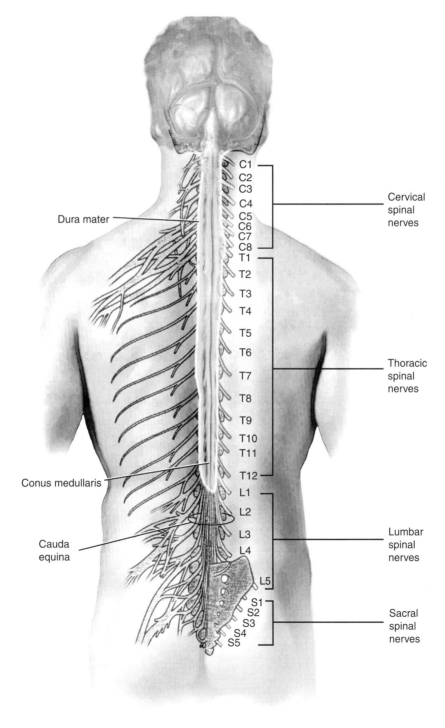

Posterior view

Figure 4-20 *The Spinal Nerves*

torso and lower extremities. In working with patients who have endured an injury to the spinal cord, understanding the innervation of the major muscles will enable you to understand the extent of their injuries. Table 4-3 outlines the major muscles of the body, their innervations, and the function that will be impaired in the event of an injury. Remember that an injury to the spinal cord will have effects on the movement and functions controlled distal to the point of injury.

The regions of the skin are innervated by the cutaneous branches of specific spinal nerves. Each spinal nerve, with the exception of C1, has a corresponding area of the skin it innervates. The area innervated by a particular nerve is called a **dermatome** and is identified by the name of the spinal nerve providing its innervation. Figure 4-21 illustrates the dermatomes of the body.

The joints of the body are innervated by the same nerves that innervate the muscles that produce movement at that joint. This is known as **Hilton's law**.

Plexuses

A plexus is an interlacing of neural fibers that is formed by the ventral rami as they extend distally from the spinal cord. Fibers from several of the spinal nerves intertwine and interweave so that as the peripheral nerves branch toward the periphery of the body, they are influenced and controlled by more than one level of the spinal cord. In the event of injury, damage to one segment of the spinal cord will not cause total paralysis.

There are three major plexuses in the nervous system: the **cervical plexus**, the **brachial plexus**, the **lumbar plexus**, and the **sacral plexus**. They consist of only the ventral rami of spinal nerves. The four plexuses are illustrated in Figure 4-22.

Plexuses begin with the ventral rami, called roots (only in regard to the plexuses, however). Fibers from the roots branch and interweave to form trunks, and fibers from the trunks intertwine to form divisions. In turn, fibers from the divisions form cords. The cords combine to form nerves that innervate the periphery.

The cervical plexus, located in the neck, supplies the neck with primarily cutaneous nerves. It gives rise to the phrenic nerve, which innervates the diaphragm and is instrumental in respiration.

Table 4-3 *Muscle Groups, Innervation, and Loss of Function*

Major Muscle Name	Muscle Innervation	Functional Impairment
Sternocleidomastoid	Accessory nerve	Neck flexion and rotation
Pectoralis Major	Pectoral nerves	Horizontal adduction, shoulder extension
Deltoid	Axillary nerve	Shoulder abduction
Biceps Brachii	Musculocutaneous nerve	Shoulder flexion and elbow flexion
Triceps Brachii	Radial nerve	Shoulder extension and elbow extension
Forearm Flexors	Median and ulnar nerves	Wrist flexion
Forearm Extensors	Radial nerves	Wrist extension
Latissimus Dorsi	Thoracodorsal nerve	Shoulder adduction and external rotation
Rectus Abdominis	Intercostal nerves	Abdominal flexion
Gluteus Maximus	Gluteal nerves	Hip extension
Adductor Muscle Group	Obturator nerve	Hip adduction
Biceps Femoris	Sciatic nerve	Hip extension and knee flexion
Semimembranosus	Sciatic nerve	Hip extension and knee flexion
Semitendinosus	Sciatic nerve	Hip extension and knee flexion
Rectus Femoris	Femoral nerve	Hip flexion and knee extension
Vastus Intermedius	Femoral nerve	Knee extension
Vastus Medialis	Femoral nerve	Knee extension
Vastus Lateralis	Femoral nerve	Knee extension
Gastrocnemius	Tibial nerve	Knee flexion

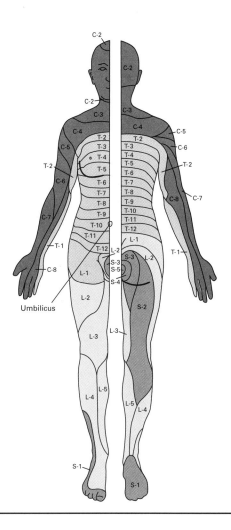

Figure 4-21 *Dermatomes*

The brachial plexus arises from the lower cervical levels and upper thoracic levels of the cord, typically C5–T1. Its major nerves are the axillary nerve, musculocutaneous nerve, median nerve, ulnar nerve, and radial nerve. The nerves of the brachial plexus innervate the upper extremity.

The lumbar plexus is formed by the ventral rami L1–L5. It innervates the lower extremity and forms the femoral nerve and obturator nerve.

The sacral plexus emerges from L4–S4. Because it overlaps considerably with the lumbar plexus, the two are frequently referred to together as the lumbosacral plexus. The sacral plexus innervates the pelvis, the buttocks, and perineum and contributes to the innervation of the lower extremity.

The Cranial Nerves

The cranial nerves innervate the head and neck primarily and arise from the brainstem. One originates in the forebrain, and the other one extends to the abdomen. There are 12 pairs of cranial nerves, each with a name that typically reflects its function and also is identified by a Roman numeral. They are numbered beginning with those that arise from the anterior aspects of the brain to those arising from the posterior aspects. Most of the cranial nerves are mixed nerves, although those that are specialized for sensory function are strictly sensory. Impulses of the mixed cranial nerves originate in the brain and travel to the exterior; the impulses of sensory cranial nerves originate in sense organs and travel to the internal aspects of the brain. Figure 4-23 illustrates the cranial nerves and their origins from the brain.

From anterior to posterior, the cranial nerves are as follows:

I. The **olfactory nerves** are sensory nerves that carry impulses related to the sense of smell. They arise from receptor cells and enter the skull through the cribiform plate of the ethmoid bone. They travel to the **olfactory cortex** as the **olfactory tract** inferior to the frontal lobe and through the cerebral hemispheres.

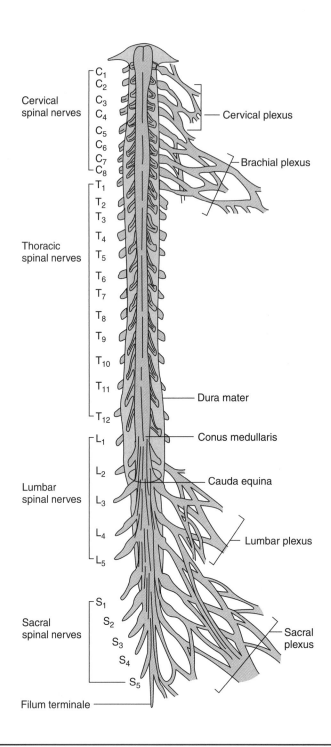

Figure 4-22   *Spinal Plexuses*

II. The **optic nerves** originate in the retina of the eye and pass through the **optic foramen** to the interior aspect of the skull. The optic nerves transmit visual input to the brain and are strictly sensory. The fibers cross at the **optic chiasma** and enter the thalamus as optic tracts. In the thalamus, they synapse with other neurons that continue to the visual cortex.

III. The **oculomotor nerves** originate in the ventral midbrain and exit the skull at the **superior orbital fissures**. The oculomotor nerves are mixed nerves but primarily serve a motor function. They control the inferior oblique and the superior, medial, and inferior rectus muscles, four of the six extrinsic eye muscles that are responsible for moving the eye-

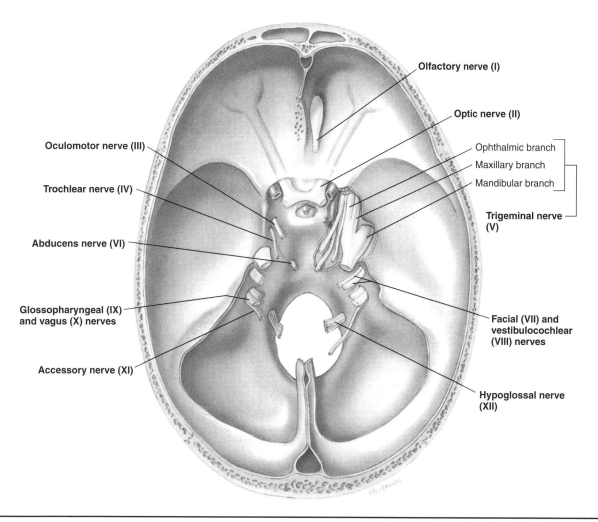

Figure 4-23 *The Cranial Nerves*

ball and raising the upper eyelid. In addition, the oculomotor nerves carry parasympathetic fibers to the pupil, causing it to constrict, and to the lens of the eye, controlling its shape to allow the eye to focus. Its sensory function is to transmit proprioceptive impulses.

IV. The **trochlear nerves** originate in the dorsal midbrain and also exit the skull through the superior orbital fissures. The trochlear nerves are mixed nerves and their function is to innervate the superior oblique muscle, one of the extrinsic eye muscles. Its sensory function is largely proprioceptive in nature.

V. The **trigeminal nerves** originate in the pons. They are the primary sensory nerves of the face. The trigeminal nerves branch into three divisions: ophthalmic, maxillary, and mandibular. The major function of the ophthalmic branch is to transmit sensations of touch, pain, and temperature from the anterior scalp, upper eyelids, nose, nasal cavity, and parts of the eye. The maxillary branch provides the motor fibers to the nose, palate, upper jaw, upper lip, and lower eyelid. The mandibular branch innervates the tongue (except the sense of taste), the lower jaw, and the chin and provides the motor control and sensory input for chewing.

VI. The **abducens nerves** originate in the pons and travel anteriorly, exiting the skull through the superior orbital fissure. They supply motor fibers to the lateral rectus muscle, one of the extrinsic eye muscles, and transmit proprioceptive information from that muscle to the brain.

VII. The **facial nerves** originate in the pons near the abducens nerve and travel though the temporal bone and inner ear before exiting the skull through the **stylomastoid foramen**. They innervate the lateral aspects of the face, providing the motor fibers for facial expressions. The facial nerves carry parasympathetic fibers to the lacrimal (tear) glands, nasal glands, palatine glands, and the submandibular and sublingual salivary glands. They also carry taste sensation from the anterior section of the tongue.

VIII. The **vestibulocochlear nerves** originate in the inner ear near the temporal bone. Their fibers travel to the border of the pons and medulla. The vestibulocochlear nerves are strictly sensory and transmit impulses concerned with hearing and balance, providing the sense of equilibrium.

IX. The **glossopharyngeal nerves** arise in the medulla and exit the skull at the **jugular foramen** of the throat. The glossopharyngeal nerves are mixed nerves and their motor functions include aiding swallowing and moderating the gag reflex. Their sensory roles include conducting taste and other sensory impulses from the throat and posterior tongue. They also help regulate the respiratory rate and heart rate by monitoring the oxygen and carbon dioxide levels of the blood.

X. The **vagus nerves** originate in the medulla of the brainstem and descend through the neck into the thoracic and abdominal regions. They are the only cranial nerves that leave the head and neck areas. The vagus nerves are mixed nerves and most of their fibers are associated with the sympathetic innervation of the heart, lungs, and abdominal organs. The vagus nerves are also concerned with swallowing, regulating heart rate, breathing, blood pressure, and digestive activity.

XI. The **accessory nerves** have two origins: one on the lateral portion of the medulla and one at the cervical level of the spinal cord. The two roots merge near the **foramen magnum**, but separate soon thereafter. The cranial fibers join the vagus nerves and the spinal fibers innervate the neck muscles. Motor fibers of the accessory nerves innervate the larynx, pharynx, soft palate and the trapezius and sternocleidomastoid muscles.

XII. The **hypoglossal nerves** originate in the medulla and provide innervation to the tongue. Their primary function is to control the movements of the tongue that are associated with speech and the mixing of food.

Sensory Receptors

The afferent division of the PNS has specialized cells that sense and respond to changes in the environment and that we experience as changes in temperature, touch, or pressure. The specialized cells are called **sensory receptors** and the environmental changes to which they are sensitive are called **stimuli** (singular = *stimulus*).

Sensory receptors are classified by type, location (internal or external), and complexity. For the purpose of the study of movement, we will focus on specific sensory receptors.

Some of the most significant receptors to movement are the **proprioceptors**. **Proprioception** is the perception of position in space. Proprioceptors are located in the muscles and joints and in connective tissues such as ligaments. Proprioceptors communicate the extent of movement to the brain by monitoring the stretch of the muscles during movement.

Pacinian corpuscles are found in the dermis and in the subcutaneous layer of the skin. They respond to pressure but accommodate to it quickly and feel it only when it is first applied.

Ruffini's corpuscles respond to continued deep pressure and are located in connective tissues. They are thought to monitor the stretch of tissue during movement.

The **muscle spindles** (also called neuromuscular spindles) are spindle-shaped receptors found in skeletal muscle. The **intrafusal fibers** contained within each muscle spindle responds to muscle stretch and initiates reflexive actions that control the amount of stretch in agonist and antagonist muscles.

Golgi tendon organs are proprioceptors that are found in the tendons of skeletal muscle near the point of muscle insertion. They work in concert with the muscle spindles. When a muscle contracts, the Golgi tendon organ is stimulated to inhibit the contracting muscle, causing it to relax at an appropriate time.

Joint kinesthetic receptors are located in the joint capsules and monitor the amount of stretch within the synovial joints. They provide information regarding joint position and movement, or the sense of **kinesthesia**.

Other sensory receptors include the **free dendritic endings**, which respond primarily to temperature and pain; **Meissner's corpuscles**, which transmit impulses related to discriminative touch; and **Merkel's disks**, which function in the perception of light touch.

Reflex Mechanisms of the Peripheral Nervous System

The proprioceptive receptors and reflexes of the PNS inform the CNS of the status of the muscles and maintain muscle tone that allows movement to occur. Muscle spindles and Golgi tendon organs are the sensory receptors that communicate with the brain. **Stretch reflexes** and **deep tendon reflexes** maintain tone in the muscles that allows functional movement.

The muscle spindle is made up of modified muscle cells with sensory neural fibers (receptors) wrapped around its center. These receptors are sensitive to excessive stretch; if a muscle stretches excessively, the receptors send a message to the spinal cord, which, in turn, sends return impulses that stimulate the muscle to contract to resume its optimal length. This is the stretch reflex. It maintains muscle tone and posture. The stretch reflex is constantly active, maintaining desired positions in space.

The Golgi tendon organs are located in the tendons of the muscles close to the point where the tendon joins the muscle and activate the deep tendon reflex. Stretch to the Golgi tendon organs, stimulated by contraction of the muscle, works opposite the stretch reflex. When stretched by muscle contraction, the Golgi tendon organ sends its message to the spinal cord, causing an impulse to be sent to the brain. In this case, the impulse goes on to the cerebellum, which responds by adjusting the muscle tension, causing the antagonist muscle to contract while the contracting muscle relaxes. This balances the muscle tone on both sides of the joint. The stretch reflex and deep tendon reflex work opposite one another continuously to maintain position and posture.

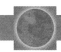 ## DISABILITY AND MOVEMENT

Neurological disorders and injuries impact an individual's function in many ways. As an OTA, you can use your knowledge of the nervous system to understand the background of your neurological patients' disabilities.

In general, certain deficits are expected with certain types of injuries. Some typical deficits are as follows:

■ When neural damage occurs to the pyramidal tracts above the spinal cord, the typical effect on movement is spastic (increased muscle tone) paralysis of the contralateral side of the body.

■ When damage occurs to motor nerves in the periphery, the typical response is flaccid (low muscle tone) on the ipsilateral side of the body.

■ Damage to a structure in the brain compromises the typical regulatory effect that the structure has on movement and on other brain structures with which it communicates. Deficits will be seen in movement and may include a lack of coordination, tremor, altered intensity of movement, disturbances in muscle tone, movement that is atypically slow or fast, and disturbances of the perception of position in space, to name a few.

■ Sensory disturbances will have an impact on movement becuase sensory input such as touch and proprioception play a major role in movement. Sensory stimuli provide the information to which the nervous system responds in regulating movement.

Functional movement are affected by many aspects of an injury or illness. Review your patients' diagnoses to learn as much as possible about the nature of their disability. First and foremost, remember that there are no hard and fast rules. Even though nervous system structures are the same in general terms, there are slight structural and chemical differences in all of them. Consequently, no two neurological cases are exactly the same and they will not necessarily be "textbook." Each patient is slightly different and even the same diagnosis or injury to the same part of the nervous system will show variations.

Ask yourself the following questions:

■ *Where is the location of the injury? What structures and functions might be affected?* Consider the location of the injury and the function typically carried out by the injured part. Knowing this, what deficits might you expect? For example, individuals who endure a CVA (stroke) in the left parietal lobe typically experience speech impairments. Individuals with head trauma in the area of the motor cortex may have deficits in voluntary movement. Taking into account the functions that might be affected will provide you with additional insight of your patient's injury.

■ *How is communication between structures affected?* If one of the association cortices is affected, familiar actions and movements may become unfamiliar.

■ *What are the psychological and emotional components?* These aspects should always be considered when physical dysfunction is of concern. Changes in the ability to carry out daily tasks and activities can result in a number of emotional responses, including, but certainly not limited to, depression, anger, frustration, and denial. The connections of the limbic system to other areas of the brain are significant and it is wise to consider their effect on movement.

■ *What are the cognitive components?* Recalling the functions of the frontal lobe, consider the impact that higher levels of thinking and executive functions can have on functional movement. Think about the role of judgment, decision making, planning, and problem solving in daily activities. How do these affect movement? Also, are there cognitive deficits, such as memory loss or inability to follow directions, that will affect your intervention with your patient.

■ *How are deficits reflected in the symptoms?* What behaviors and actions does your patient exhibit that reflect the disturbance in the nervous system?

There is much to know about the nervous system, and the information presented here is a brief overview. Challenge yourself to learn more as you need to in your practice. As an OTA, understanding the anatomy and physiology of the nervous system will guide you in understanding your patients' deficits.

KEY CONCEPTS

- The central nervous system (CNS) is comprised of the brain and spinal cord. Tracts are bundles of axons that conduct impulses between the brain and spinal cord.

- The peripheral nervous system (PNS) is comprised of nerves and neural structures outside the brain and spinal cord. The PNS is further divided into the voluntary system, which controls conscious, voluntary movement, and the autonomic system, which controls body functions over which we have no conscious control. The autonomic system is divided into the sympathetic and parasympathetic divisions, which have opposite effects on body organs.

- There are several types of neurons, or nerve cells in the body. The major structures of the neuron are the dendrites, the cell body, and the axon. Neurons are specialized to conduct electrical impulses, called action potentials, to other neurons or organs. The action potential causes a neurotransmitter to be released, which triggers a response or action in the postsynaptic neuron or organ.

- The brain has numerous landmarks, divisions, and structures. Each is specialized for a unique function. Each structure or division exerts its influence on other brain structures, on the spinal cord, and on the PNS. The various influences contribute to functional movement by regulating its timing, coordination, speed, and intensity. If one of the structures is damaged, movement deficits are likely to occur and other structures dependent on its influence will be affected.

- The spinal cord is encased in the vertebral column and is the structure from which the spinal nerves arise. The cord is divided into the cervical, thoracic, lumbar, and sacral regions. Thirty-one pairs of spinal nerves exit from the spinal cord through the intervertebral foramina of the vertebrae. Each nerve has a dorsal root consisting of sensory fibers and a ventral root consisting of motor fibers. Shortly after emerging from the spinal cord, the roots join together to form a mixed nerve. The nerve then splits into dorsal and ventral rami. The ventral rami form nerve plexuses in the cervical and lumbosacral regions, giving rise to the nerves that innervate the extremities and other areas of the body.

- Muscle tone is controlled by influences from the CNS, primarily by the basal nuclei of the cerebral hemispheres and the cerebellum. Muscle spindles and Golgi tendon organs, which are proprioceptive sensory receptors found in the muscles and tendons, react to the stretch of muscle and relay impulses to the spinal cord, which, in turn, sends impulses to the brain. The CNS responds by adjusting muscle contraction accordingly. This occurs continuously on an unconscious level and allows us to maintain posture and position and to move smoothly. Damage to the nervous system can affect this element of functional movement.

- The OTA or should consider the location of a patient's neurological injury, the structures and functions involved and how other structures might be affected, and how functional movement is affected. Psychological, emotional, and cognitive aspects must be considered.

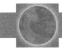

BIBLIOGRAPHY

Brown, D. R. (1980). *Neurosciences for the allied health therapies*. St. Louis, MO: C. V. Mosby.

Hole, J. W., Jr. (1993). *Human anatomy and physiology* (6th ed.). Dubuque, IA: W. C. Brown.

Marieb, E. N. (2003). *Human anatomy and physiology* (6th ed.). Menlo Park, CA: Addison Wesley Longman, Inc.

Rizzo, D. C. (2001). *Delmar's fundamentals of anatomy and physiology*. Clifton Park, NY: Thomson Delmar Learning.

Scott, A. S., & Fong, E. (2004). *Body structures and functions* (10th ed.). Clifton Park, NY: Thomson Delmar Learning.

WEB RESOURCES

- The Web site www.bbc.co.uk/science/humanbody// features an interactive site that examines the students' knowledge of the different systems found in the human body.
- For disorders of the nervous system, go to www.alm.nih.gov/medlineplus/brainandnervoussystem.html.
- Go to www.ama-assn.org/ama/pub/category/7172.html for clear examples of the nervous system. It also includes links to different major nervous system conditions and charts that explain the resulting neurological deficits according to the location of the nervous system injury.
- Go to www.acm.uiuc.edu/sigbio/project/nervous/ for illustrations and descriptions of major anatomical structures and functions of the nervous system.

(These Web addresses were current as of February 2004.)

REVIEW QUESTIONS

Fill in the Blanks

Provide the word(s) or phrase(s) that best completes the sentence.

1. The central nervous system consists of the _____ and _____.

2. The two divisions of the autonomic nervous system are the _____ and _____.

3. _____ impulses travel toward the brain from the body's periphery, and _____ impulses travel from the body's periphery to the brain.

4. An impulse traveling into a neuron enters at the _____, is processed in the _____, and moves onto the next neuron or organ through the _____.

5. The white, fatty coating on some neurons is called _____ and its main purpose is to _____.

6. The junction between two neurons or a neuron and an organ is called the _____. _____ is secreted from the neuron to allow the impulse to cross the _____ _____.

7. The four main divisions of the brain are the _____, the _____, the _____, and the _____.

8. The bundles of neural processes that transmit impulses between the brain and spinal cord are called _____. The processes that communicate within a hemisphere are called _____ and processes that communicate between hemispheres are called _____.

9. The part of the brain that controls voluntary movement is called the _____ _____ _____ and is located on the _____ _____. The tract that carries motor impulses is called the _____ _____.

10. The two structures of the brain most involved in the control of movement are the _____ _____ and the _____.

11. In the medulla, the _____ _____ crosses over, meaning that _____ is controlled by _____.

12. The structure that maintains general awareness and arousal is called the _____ _____ _____.

13. The _____ _____ provides buoyancy and protects the brain from being jostled. It is found in the _____ layer of the meninges.

14. The _____ _____ are found deep in cerebral hemispheres and play an important part in the control and regulation of movement.

15. Sensory neurons enter the spinal cord at the _____ horn, and motor neurons arise from the _____ horn.

16. Muscle tone is maintained by the _____ and _____ _____ reflexes.

17. An interlacing of the ventral aspects of the spinal nerves is called a _____.

18. Oculomotor, trochlear, and trigeminal are names of _____ nerves.

19. When working with patients, three things that you should keep in mind regarding their movements are _____, _____, and _____.

Multiple Choice

Select the best answer to complete the following statements.

1. Superiorly to inferiorly, the major divisions of the brain are the _____ .
   a. cerebellum, cerebrum, diencephalons, and brainstem
   b. cerebrum, cerebellum, diencephalons, and brainstem
   c. diencephalons, cerebrum, cerebellum, and brainstem
   d. cerebrum, diencephalons, cerebellum, and brainstem

2. The sympathetic and parasympathetic divisions of the nervous system _____ .
   a. regulate organ function
   b. are part of the peripheral nervous system
   c. exert complimentary influences on body structures
   d. are part of the central nervous system

3. The *primary* function of the central nervous system is _____ .
   a. controlling and integrating function
   b. regulating consciousness
   c. maintaining awareness
   d. interpreting stimuli
   e. executing thought

4. The statement that *best* describes the difference between neurons and other cells of the body is that _____ .
   a. neurons last a lifetime
   b. neurons use significantly more energy than other cells
   c. neurons are amitotic (they do not divide)
   d. neurons last a lifetime, they use significantly more energy, and they are amitotic

5. The part of the neuron that receives impulses is the _____ .
   a. axon
   b. cell body
   c. dendrite
   d. node of Ranvier

6. Myelin functions to _____ .
   a. protect the cell body
   b. facilitate the transmission of impulses and insulate the axon
   c. facilitate the transmission of impulses and insulate the dendrites
   d. protect the Schwann cells

7. In order, the steps of an action potential are _____ .
   a. opening of the sodium-potassium pump, depolarization, repolarization, release of neurotransmitter
   b. depolarization, opening of the sodium-potassium pump, repolarization, release of neurotransmitter
   c. depolarization, repolarization, opening of the sodium-potassium pump, release of neurotransmitter
   d. depolarization, release of neurotransmitter, opening of the sodium-potassium pump, repolarization

8. The most commonly used neurotransmitter in the human body is _____ .
   a. acetylcholine
   b. endorphins
   c. epinephrine
   d. serotonin

9. The mechanism that prevents unwanted and potentially harmful substances from entering the brain is the _____ .
   a. neuroglial network
   b. dopamine
   c. microglial network
   d. cerebrospinal fluid
   e. blood-brain barrier

10. Second-order neurons extend _____ .
   a. from the periphery of the body to the spinal cord
   b. from the spinal cord to the thalamus
   c. from the thalamus to the cerebral cortex
   d. between the hemispheres

11. The structure that separates the two hemispheres is the _____ .
   a. central sulcus
   b. corpus collosum
   c. lateral fissure
   d. longitudinal fissure

12. The lobe of the brain that is chiefly concerned with spatial perception is the _____ .
   a. frontal lobe
   b. parietal lobe
   c. temporal lobe
   d. occipital lobe

13. The system that identifies each function area of the brain by a series of 52 numbers is known as _____ .
   a. Broca's areas
   b. Brodmann's areas
   c. somatotrophic areas
   d. Wernicke's areas

14. The primary motor cortex is located in the _____ .
   a. postcentral gyrus
   b. precentral gyrus
   c. somatosensory gyrus
   d. frontal gyrus

15. Of the following, _____ is *not* a function of the basal nuclei.
   a. starting and stopping movement
   b. coordinating voluntary movement
   c. regulating the intensity of movement
   d. inhibiting unnecessary movement

16. The *main* function of the thalmus is to _____ .
   a. function as a sensory relay center
   b. sort information from sensory areas
   c. sort information from emotion areas
   d. control the function of the hypothalamus

17. The pyramidal tracts (also called the corticospinal tract) conduct _____ .
    a. impulses related to emotion
    b. impulses related to motor responses
    c. impulses related to sensory input
    d. impulses exerting control from the cerebellum

18. The neurotransmitter dopamine functions in conjunction with _____ .
    a. the basal nuclei
    b. the cerebellum
    c. the cerebral cortex
    d. the pons

19. The part of the brain that controls life-supporting functions (with influence from the thalmus) is _____ .
    a. the cerebral cortex
    b. the cerebellum
    c. the midbrain
    d. the brainstem

20. The cerebellum _____ .
    a. plays a role in memory
    b. regulates muscle contraction
    c. adjusts movements via the motor cortex
    d. is the center for the reticular activating system
    e. regulates muscle contraction and adjusts movements via the motor cortex

21. The amygdala and hippocampus are structures of the _____ .
    a. basal nuclei
    b. limbic system
    c. cerebellum
    d. thalamus

22. Cerebrospinal fluid is located inferior to the _____ .
    a. dura mater
    b. arachnoid mater
    c. pia mater
    d. periosteum of the skull

23. The spinal nerves exit the vertebral column via the _____ .
    a. cribiform plate
    b. foramen magnum
    c. intervertebral foramina
    d. orbital foramen

24. The spinal nerves that control motor function originate in the _____ .
    a. anterior or ventral horn of the gray matter of the spinal cord
    b. posterior or dorsal horn of the gray matter of the spinal cord
    c. anterior or ventral horn of the white matter of the spinal cord
    d. posterior or dorsal of the white matter of the spinal cord

25. The cutaneous sensory regions of the body are called _____ .
    a. dermazones
    b. dermatomes
    c. dermal regions
    d. dermaplexes

26. The *best* description of a plexus is that it is _____ .
    a. a group of spinal nerves
    b. a group of spinal nerve roots and fibers
    c. an interweaving of neural fibers
    d. an interweaving of neural fibers from several spinal segments

27. The advantage that a plexus provides is _____ .
   a. increased motor control
   b. increased discriminatory sensation
   c. supplementary innervation in the event of injury
   d. supplementary innervation to the sympathetic ganglia

28. The brachial plexus _____ .
   a. supplies cutaneous innervation to the neck region
   b. supplies the upper extremity
   c. supplies the lower extremity
   d. supplies the abdomen and perineal areas

29. The cranial nerves arise *primarily* from the _____ .
   a. cerebral cortex
   b. midbrain
   c. pons
   d. brainstem

30. The function of the stretch and deep tendon reflexes is *best* described as _____ .
   a. controlling coordination
   b. controlling voluntary movement
   c. maintaining muscle tone
   d. regulating extension and flexion

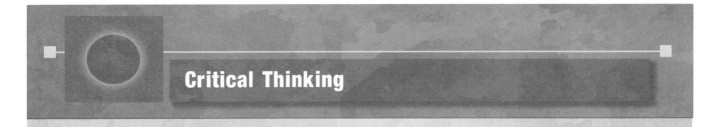

Critical Thinking

1. Draw and label the brain structures as you study them.

2. Create a schematic of the tracts, label each, and briefly describe their function in the role of movement.

3. Make a chart that lists the lobes of the brain and the primary and association cortices and their functions.

4. Study the effects of brain structures on movement by asking yourself what the expected effect might be if certain structures were damaged. Illustrate both the typical function and the affected function and present the comparison to the class.

5. To help you understand the effects of injury on movement, list as many effects on movement as you can, assuming injury to the midbrain (or other structure) and resulting interruption in its function. Create a game that challenges participants to do the same.

6. Compose a list of neurological diagnoses and injuries commonly seen in practice. Or use case studies of patients with neurological dysfunction. Research their symptoms and write a brief description of how the symptoms reflect the condition of the nervous system.

7. Pay close attention to your daily activities from the time you get up in the morning until you arrive to your first class. Make note of your actions and movements and the nervous system structures and functions that are regulating them. Write a paper on your observations or share in a class discussion.

8. Research and describe the clinical picture of a 65-year-old male patient who sustained a severe stroke 3 days before, resulting in a right hemiplegia. Describe the side of the body affected and how the patient will present physically at this time. Because the symptoms can vary, describe a patient with symptoms that you think would be consistent with his condition. Describe this same patient 3 weeks later when he has regained some function and has been moved to a rehabilitation facility. Describe the goals of OT at this time.

9. A 24-year-old male sustained a complete spinal cord lesion at the T4 level. Surgery was performed to stabilize the fracture. Describe the role of OT in the initial stages of bed rest and then research the functional ability of a patient with a lesion at this level. Describe how he would transfer and become independent.

10. Define the following terms: *spasticity, flaccidity, ataxia, dysarthria, dysphagia*

11. Impulsive behaviors, ineffective problem solving, impaired judgment, poor memory, and inaccurate interpretations of spatial perceptions are just a few of the resultant diminished capacities that may occur from brain damage. The natural healing process, medications and other medical interventions, and the effects of therapy all might influence the client's recovery. In the meantime, in the following scenario, the OTA needs techniques to successfully engage the client, who has sustained a head injury, in therapeutic interventions for improving fine motor coordination (motor skills within the performance skills domain), safe performance in areas of occupation such as instrumental activities of daily living (IADL) and the specific task of grocery shopping, and the functional mobility necessary for climbing a flight of stairs. In a treatment session, the client initiated climbing a flight of stairs—he needs to be able to do this, carrying a sack of groceries, in order to be able to return home—and he "missed" the second step, falling backward. What does the OTA *consider* and then *do* in order to determine the root of the problem? Was it a cognitive function of inattention? Was it a visual perceptual deficit of spatial relations or depth of field? Was it a sensory processing impairment such as a proprioception deficit? Was it caused by poor movement—lack of range of motion in the knee or ankle, or poor strength in the leg muscles? Or was the stairway cluttered, slippery, or poorly lit? What is the likelihood that a "misstep" will happen again while carrying a bag full of groceries? What information does the OTA gather and then share with the OTR in order to problem solve, and possibly change the treatment plan? These factors, and others, all influence the client's ability to move—to engage in purposeful and meaningful tasks—and in order for the OTA to provide quality therapy, numerous aspects within the domain of OT need to be addressed. Although it is imperative the OTA study kinesiology and the nervous system, these are just two areas that influence, and are influenced by, other contexts important to the client and to the field of OT.

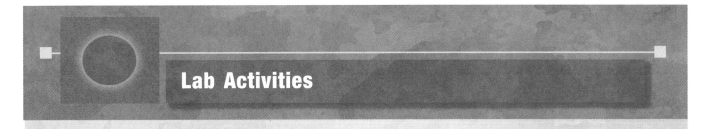

Lab Activities

Lab 4-1: Range of Motion (ROM)

Objective: To properly administer ROM exercises in the care of the patient with an injured spine.

Equipment Needed: A lab partner, pen/pencil, paper

Step 1. Using your partner perform passive ROM exercises for a patient who has sustained a complete spinal cord injury at C5.

Step 2. Describe the number of repetitions that should be performed and four benefits of passive ROM.

Lab 4-2: Stretching Techniques for the Patient with Hemiplegia

Objective: To properly provide stretching techniques in the care of the patient with hemiplegia.

Equipment Needed: A lab partner, pen/pencil, paper

Step 1. Your partner has a spastic hemiplegia of the left side of the body. Assuming he or she has a flexor spasticity of the upper extremity and an extensor spasticity of the lower extremity, have your partner correctly mimic the position that each joint would adopt.

Step 2. Perform passive stretches and techniques to reduce the tone.

Lab 4-3: Cranial Nerves

Objective: To identify cranial nerves and their basic functions.

Equipment Needed: Puzzle, pencil, paper, textbook, and a lab partner (if students are to create their own puzzle)

Step 1. Find the 12 cranial nerves in the "Word Find" puzzle on the next page (the words may be vertical, horizontal, diagonal, forward, or backward).

Step 2. Identify the basic function of each cranial nerve located on the puzzle.

Step 3. Choose two cranial nerves, and with your partner, discuss what the potential functional deficit would be if those nerves were damaged. Be prepared to discuss your impressions with the class.

Step 4. With a partner, create and solve a similar puzzle using other vocabulary words from this chapter e.g., terms that pertain to the CNS, the PNS, or the gross structure of the brain. As you create the puzzle, think about, discuss, and list their influences on movement and how those abilities or deficits might affect function.

Lab 4-4: Giving and Following Directions

Objective: To recognize the complexities of directions and how they impact treatment.

Equipment Needed: Pencil, paper, textbook, a lab partner, and access to an environment to carry out directions (if that is to be part of the lab activity)

Step 1. Participate in giving directions by giving and following an exercise suggested in the OTA Perspectives box. Give your partner a direction, paying attention to its complexity. How many steps were involved? Did you use hand or facial gestures to augment your verbal directions? Did you use any jargon or slang words in your language? Did your instructions rely on information you assumed your partner knew? Is the activity that you expect your partner to do something familiar or new to him or her? Is there any preparation involved? For example, if the direction involves going outside to perform a task, does the weather indicate that a coat be worn?) With your partner pick apart the direction given, and, if possible, relate different aspects of the direction to functions of the nervous system. An entry-level OTA will be expected to "grade" activities—essentially, to make the activity simpler or more complex. Do so with the direction you gave your partner. Be prepared to share your findings with the class.

(continues)

Lab Activities *(continued)*

K	I	N	E	S	S	T	U	D	Y	O	T	A
G	A	B	O	L	F	A	C	T	O	R	Y	V
L	O	A	C	V	D	S	T	U	R	O	C	E
O	O	C	R	A	N	I	A	L	W	C	R	S
S	P	C	U	F	N	E	R	V	E	H	A	T
S	T	E	C	L	A	Q	P	T	A	L	N	I
O	I	S	E	R	O	C	P	U	N	E	I	B
P	C	S	V	K	A	M	I	N	L	A	A	U
H	N	O	R	A	I	N	P	A	K	R	L	L
A	E	R	E	D	G	N	I	T	L	I	J	O
R	R	Y	N	B	C	U	E	A	O	H	G	C
Y	V	A	C	O	T	A	S	S	L	R	F	O
N	E	L	A	S	S	O	L	G	O	P	Y	H
G	T	R	I	G	E	M	I	N	A	L	D	L
E	C	R	A	N	I	A	L	N	E	R	V	E
A	C	C	E	S	S	O	R	Y	O	T	A	A
L	P	T	S	N	E	C	U	D	B	A	E	R

Lab 4-5: Sensory Testing

Objective: To recognize various aspects of sensory testing.

Equipment Needed: A lab partner, pencil, paper, textbook, OT sensation testing manuals and materials, OT textbooks and resources

Step 1.   Research OT sensory testing.

Step 2.   Match the ability of each of the following sensations to impact the spinal tract:

Discriminative touch:

Pain/temperature:

Crude touch/pressure:

Proprioception:

Chapter 5

BONE

Key Words

anatomical landmarks
appendicular skeleton
appositional growth
atlas
axial skeleton
axis
canaliculi
carpal bones
cervical vertebrae
clavicle
coccyx
compact bone
costae
diaphysis
epiphyseal structure
femur
fibula
flat bone
haversian canal

humerus
inferior appendicular skeleton
irregular bone
lacuna
lamella
long bone
lumbar
manubrium
medullary cavity
metacarpal bones
metatarsals
osseous tissue
osteoblast
osteoclast
osteocyte
osteon
patella
pelvic bone

periosteum
phalanges of the foot
radius
sacrum
scapula
short bone
spongy bone
sternal body
sternum
tarsals
thoracic
tibia
trabecular bone
ulna
vertebral
Volksmann's canal
xiphoid process

INTRODUCTION

Simple movements such as reaching for a glass of water, driving a car, walking around the block, or even moving our fingers would be impossible if bones did not provide a sound structure and base of support for the muscles to pull on. Without this structure and support, we would mimic "the blobs," rolling from one location to the next. Fortunately, however, the human body has 206 named bones, which provide a strong base of support for movement, and bony processes, which attach the muscle firmly to the skeleton. Movement of the various body segments through a full range of motion depends on these sound structures and the solid base of support that bones provide.

PURPOSE OF BONE

Although we often think the only purpose of bone is that of support, it has underlying systematic functions that extend past the realm of structure and support. Bones provide five totally separate functions: anatomical landmarks, hematopoesis, vitamin and mineral storage, protection, and support.

Anatomical Landmarks

Bones provide landmarks for muscle attachment. These **anatomical landmarks** are important because they increase the surface area provided by the various bones. This, in return, helps increase the mechanical efficiency of the contracting muscles that attach to these landmarks.

OTA Perspective

OT practitioners use clinical reasoning—sound professional judgment based on theory—to guide decision making that affects client treatments. In order to develop problem-solving skills used in clinical reasoning, one method might be to correlate a change in the body's skeletal system to the OT Practice Framework (further explored in the lab exercise).

When something "breaks" (e.g., bone), or does not function in its typical or expected manner, one must determine the what-where-when-why-how of the break or dysfunction in order to fix it and restore function—and for the OT practitioner, how this all affects OT function. That means employing the OT process: An evaluation includes the occupational profile and an analysis of occupational performance, intervention—planning, implementation, and review—and outcomes.

Simplistically, in kinesiology terms of bones—purpose, structure, location—determining what broke and where, along with how that affects function, is similar to performing an OT evaluation. Bone function, purpose, and location guide intervention. Prevention of future "breaks" depends on outcomes and education—"why" it originally occurred.

Hematopoesis

During the early years of life through puberty, blood cell formation occurs primarily in the medullary cavity of long bones. As we age, up through puberty, the blood cell formation duties shift toward the spinous processes of the vertebrae and the bones of the head. As the shift occurs, the red marrow, once found in the medullary cavity, turns into fatty yellow marrow.

Vitamin and Mineral Storage

Bone serves as a storing structure for many of the vitamins and minerals within the human body. Specifically, bones contain calcium, phosphate, and vitamin K. Throughout the day, the concentration of these minerals and vitamin in the bone fluctuate to ensure proper nourishment of the cells that use them.

Protection

One of the more important physiological roles of bone is its anatomical relationship to the vital organs. The close proximity of the bones to the vital organs allows for solid protection of the organs. Picture what would happen to the brain if the skull did not surround it or if the ribs and sternum did not protect the heart and lungs.

Support

The final purpose of bone, and the most important for kinesiological purposes, is support. The bones in the body provide a strong attachment site for the muscles to pull on. This chapter primarily focuses on the anatomical structures of bone.

 STRUCTURE OF BONE

Often it is thought that bone tissue is solid, nonpliable, and continuous and that the structure of bone resembles solid wood or dense concrete without pores and fibers. However, taking a cross section of any bone in the body would reveal that this solid, continuous arrangement is not present. Typically, depending on their type, bones are made up of a dense superficial layer and a series of bone fibers meshed together in a deep layer (Figure 5-1).

The superficial covering of bone is comprised of **compact bone**. Compact bone is smooth to the touch and provides the hard outercoat appearance that is commonly associated with bone. Immediately deep to the compact bone is **trabecular bone**, better known as **spongy bone**. Trabecular bone is made up of fibrous **osseous tissue** that forms pores, allowing blood vessels and nerves to pass through into deeper layers of bone. The term *trabecular* in Latin means "beams," and the

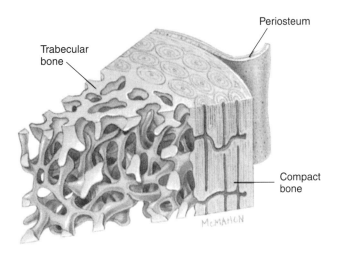

Figure 5-1 *Structure of Bone*

direction of the osseous fibers are laid down along lines of mechanical compression. This structural alignment maximizes the ability of the bone to withstand greater than normal forces occurring in that area.

When considering the difference between compact and trabecular bones, picture a high-rise building. Imagine that the trabeculae are the steel beams and the compact bone is the cement outercoat. In this situation, the beams provide the structural strength, whereas the cement increases the strength of the structure.

 TYPES OF BONES

There are four types of bone in the human body: short, irregular, flat, and long. The shape that each bone possesses, as their names indicate, help classify each of the bones in the body. For instance, the humerus (superior arm) would be classified as a long bone because of its long appearance. The surface area and length of the bones are crucial for the outcome of the muscular contraction in a specific region.

Short Bone

Short bones are cuboid shaped, meaning that they are three-dimensional, with the length of each side being of equal distance in a shape resembling a square or rectangle (Figure 5-2). The best examples of the short bones are the carpals of the hand and the tarsals of the foot. Unlike long bones, short bones provide a small amount of surface area for muscle attachment and mainly provide structural support for the body. Short bones consists of a thin superficial layer of compact bone with a large area of trabecular bone deep to the compact bone.

Irregular Bone

The bones in the body that do not have a definite identifiable shape are called **irregular bones** (see Figure 5-2). Examples of irregular bones are the vertebrae and the sphenoid bone in the skull. With many different shapes, irregular bones provide a large surface area for muscle attachments and are structurally sound bones. The structural makeup of irregular bones is similar to those of short bones. These bones are made up of a thin superficial layer of compact bone with a deep layer of trabecular bone.

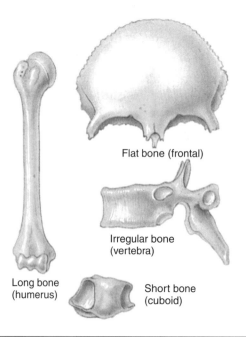

Flat bone (frontal)

Irregular bone
(vertebra)

Long bone
(humerus)

Short bone
(cuboid)

Figure 5-2 *Bone Shapes*

Flat Bone

As the name indicates, **flat bones** are thin, wide, and typically provide a large amount of surface area for muscle attachment (see Figure 5-2). Prime examples of flat bones include the scapula and pelvis. Flat bones are made up of a thin superficial layer of compact bone and a thick layer of trabecular bone found between the compact bone.

Long Bone

The most simple bone type to recognize is the **long bone**. As the name indicates, long bones are longer than they are wide. Examples of long bones found in the body include the humerus (arm), femur (thigh), metacarpals (hand), and metatarsals (foot).

Each long bone in the body has a similar anatomical structure. It has two rounded ends connected by a long shaft (Figure 5-3). The external connective tissue found on bone is the periosteum. Immediately deep to the periosteum are the Sharpey's fibers, which firmly attach the periosteum to the compact bone. A second osseous tissue, the endosteum, is found in the medullary cavity. This structure houses osteoblasts and osteoclasts and lines the haversian and Volksmann's canals.

Epiphysis At the proximal and distal ends of the long bone are two individual **epiphyseal structures**. These structures are primarily composed of trabecular bone, with a thin superficial layer covering of compact bone. The major makeup of each epiphysis is trabecular bone, which increases the strength of the region and helps with the mechanical stresses that often occur to bone. Lining the end of each epiphysis is articular cartilage, which helps provide a cushion where the bones come together. Another distinct feature to the epiphysis is the epiphyseal line, which can be found near the diaphysis. During the growing years, the bone grows lengthwise as new bone tissue spreads lengthwise from these centers.

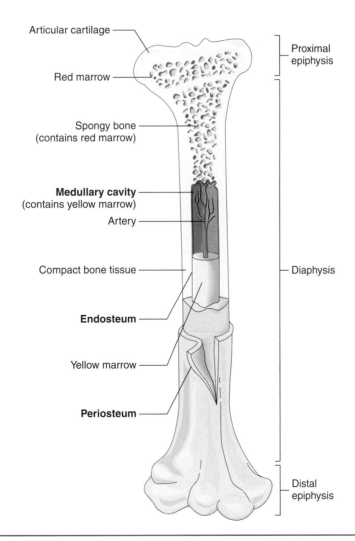

Figure 5-3 *Structure of Long Bones*

Diaphysis   The portion of the long bone that provides the most length is the **diaphysis**. The diaphysis is primarily composed of compact bone surrounded by the superficial **periosteum**. Found in the center of the diaphysis is the **medullary cavity**, which is primarily responsible for the formation of red blood cells in the early years of life. One important feature of the diaphysis to mechanical support is the thick middle region of the structure that provides much of the mechanical support. The thickness of the bones in this region prevents bones from buckling when mechanical forces increase.

MICROSCOPIC ANATOMY OF COMPACT BONE

Understanding the microscopic anatomical structures of compact bone is important to the study of the physiological and mechanical functions that bones provide. When studying these structures, realize that bone is a living tissue that constantly remodels itself to provide an optimally sound structure and strong base of support for the muscles to pull on.

Osseous Tissue

The osseous tissue of compact bone is organized into concentric rings that resemble the rings found in trees (Figure 5-4). Each ring grouping can be distinguished as the **osteon**, which is the structural unit of bone. Contained within each osteon are three distinct bone cells responsible for the formation and remodeling processes of bone. In the long bone, as new tissue is formed and old tissue is reabsorbed, the growth of new bone tissue occurs from the center and pushes outward. This growth is referred to as **appositional growth**.

    Found toward the center rings of bone are the **osteoblasts**, which lay down new bone tissue. The hormone calcitonin regulates the activity of the osteoblast cells by stimulating them to form new bone tissue through the use of calcium in the bloodstream. As a result, new osseous tissue is formed and pushes from the center outward. Mature osseous tissue is found in the middle of the osteon and is maintained by the **osteocytes**, which are the mature bone cells. These cells maintain the

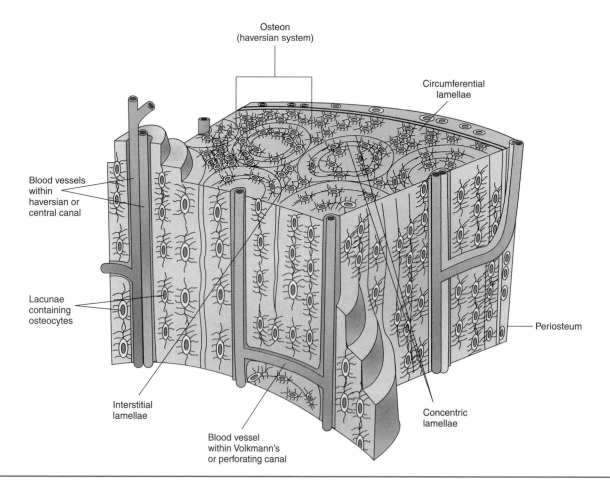

Figure 5-4   *Osseous Tissue*

bone's structural integrity by nourishing the osseous tissue and removing waste products. As osseous tissue matures, it further pushes outward from the center and over time becomes less structurally sound. Aging of the bone results in an increased activity of the **osteoclast** bone cells, which result in the reabsorption of the aging bone. The activity of the osteoclasts increases when the concentration of parathyroid hormone increases. The actions of each of these three cells ensure that the bones will maintain their structural integrity.

Haversian and Volksmann's Canals

The blood vessels and nervous tissues that extend from the superficial to deep layers of compact bone traverse through a series of hollow anatomical pathways that lie within the osteon. These hollow anatomical structures deliver blood and nutrients to the osteocyte and remove waste products from these structures. The first of these hollow canals are the **haversian canals** found in the center of the osteon running parallel to it. The second hollow canals are the **Volksmann's canals**, which run perpendicular to the osteon and allow the blood vessels to extend into the deeper osteon layers.

Osteon

Closer examination of the osteon will reveal that each individual ring is identified as a **lamella**. The structural makeup of the lamella is important to the mechanical support provided by bones because the osseous tissue is inlaid with collagen fibers that run parallel along the entire length of the lamella. The collagen fibers of one lamella are laid down in opposition to the direction of the fibers in the next lamella. The arrangement of these fibers provides support against the twisting mechanical forces that are often applied to bone, helping prevent fractures.

Found between each lamella is a series of microchannels and cavities that allows the osteocytes to communicate with one another. The first of these structures is a large cavity called the **lacuna** that houses the osteocytes. Running from one lacuna to the next are hairline canals called the **canaliculi**, which are built into the lamella and which allow extensions of the osteocytes to communicate with one another. The close proximity of the osteocytes ensures that nutrients and waste products can pass between the osteocytes of the internal to external lamellae. These processes maintain the bone tissues.

 THE AXIAL AND APPENDICULAR SKELETON

The 206 named bones that are found in the human body can be divided into two functional skeletons: the axial skeleton and the appendicular skeleton (Figure 5-5). To differentiate between the two skeletons, remember that the **axial skeleton** pro-

OTA Perspective

Fracture means a loss of continuity of a bone. Sometimes patients think that a fracture of a bone is different from a break; this, however, is incorrect. A fracture and a break are the exact same thing. Fractures are classified into many different groups. A *simple* or *closed* fracture is one where the skin remains intact. A *compound* or *open* fracture is one where there is soft tissue damage and an open wound. The wound may be from the fractured bone protruding out of the skin or from penetration to the bone from the outside. Healing time of a fracture depends on many different outside factors as well as the type of bone affected and the type of fracture. Fractures can result from a direct blow or from an indirect cause such as a twisting injury. *Pathological fractures* occur in already weakened bone, possibly due to a tumor. *Stress fractures* occur in areas where there is repeated stress, for example, a fracture found in the foot of a long-distance runner.

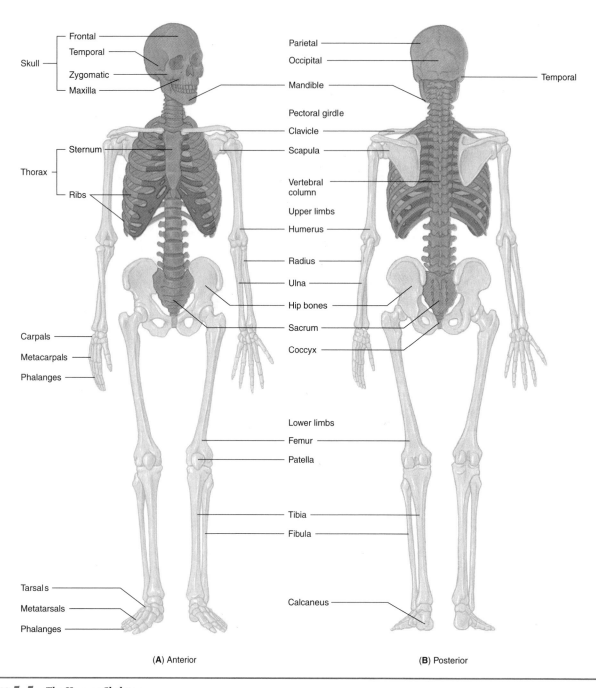

Skull
- Frontal
- Temporal
- Zygomatic
- Maxilla

Thorax
- Sternum
- Ribs

Carpals

Metacarpals

Phalanges

Tarsals

Metatarsals

Phalanges

(A) Anterior

Parietal

Occipital

Mandible

Pectoral girdle

Clavicle

Scapula

Vertebral column

Upper limbs

Humerus

Radius

Ulna

Hip bones

Sacrum

Coccyx

Lower limbs

Femur

Patella

Tibia

Fibula

Calcaneus

Temporal

(B) Posterior

Figure 5-5   *The Human Skeleton*

vides the base of support for the body, and the **appendicular skeleton** moves more freely through a full range of motion around the axial skeleton. Therefore, the axial skeleton often remains stable while the muscles of the appendicular skeleton pull from the axial skeleton to move the appendages.

THE AXIAL SKELETON

The axial skeleton can be subdivided into three regions based on the base of support that these regions provide for appendicular movement: vertebrae, sternum, and ribs.

Vertebrae   Located in the posterior region of the body are five separate **vertebral** sections: cervical, thoracic, lumbar, sacral, and coccygeal (Figure 5-6). When the bones of the vertebral regions are identified, the first letters of the region and number order of bones labeled from superior to inferior are used. For example, the second thoracic vertebra is the second vertebral bone in the thoracic region and is named T2.

OTA Perspective

The literal definition of *osteoporosis* is "soft bones." Medically, it is defined as a loss of bone mass, resulting in weak bones and a predisposition to fractures. According to the U.S. National Osteoporosis Foundation, this disease affects 28 million Americans, 80% of them women. After menopause, women lose bone mass at the most accelerated rate, a fact that often triggers hormone replacement therapy. Preventive measures include exercise (especially weight-bearing exercise), diet, adequate calcium intake, and sun exposure. In OT, the results of osteoporosis frequently present in the form of fractures, most commonly of the wrist and hip. A good knowledge of the disease process is therefore important.

Vertebral bones are important to the human body because it relies on the protection they provide for the spinal cord and the numerous anatomical landmarks that increase the surface area for muscle attachment.

On closer observation of the vertebrae, notice how the anatomical alignment of the bones forms several distinct curves. As one walks, runs, jumps, or even sits in a chair, the curves act as a spring and help to absorb the forces that are applied to these regions. Also note how the size of the vertebral bones change from smallest in the superior cervical region to largest in the lumbar region. This anatomical arrangement allows the vertebral column to absorb the weight of the body, which increases, as weight is applied in the inferior direction. Form follows function with a vertebral column; as it is tracked in the inferior direction, the bones get larger.

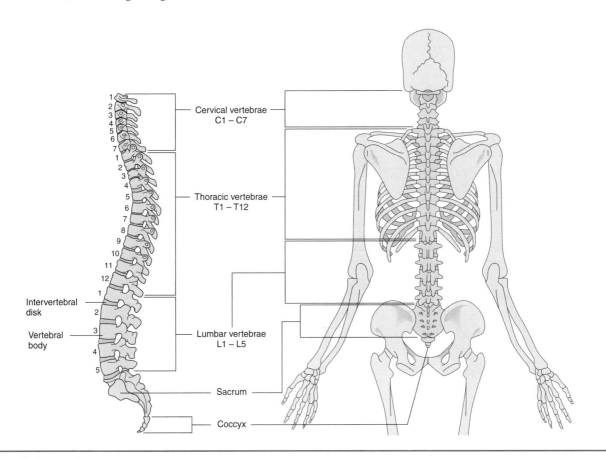

Figure 5-6   *Vertebrae*

Cervical Vertebrae. When observing the **cervical vertebrae**, note how the structure of the bones forms a concave curve located in the neck. The first two cervical bones have individual names: atlas (C1) and axis (C2). Remember from Greek mythology that Atlas held up the weight of the world with his hands. In this example, the **atlas** bone holds the weight of the head. The **axis**, on the other hand, has a point that projects through the anterior portion of the atlas. When the head moves, it pivots and moves around the axis point that projects through the atlas. The remaining cervical vertebrae are labeled C3–C7 and increase in size from superior to inferior.

Thoracic Vertebrae. Notice that the distinguishing factor identifying the **thoracic** region from the cervical and lumbar regions is that individual costal bones (ribs) originate from each of these vertebrae. Unlike the cervical vertebrae, the thoracic region has a convex curve comprised of 12 individual bones labeled T1–T12.

Lumbar Vertebrae. Five individual vertebrae make up the **lumbar** region and are identified as L1–L5. They form a concave curve and are the largest vertebral bones. The reason for this arrangement is that these bones absorb the large amounts of weight that are applied to the body by gravity.

Sacrum. The **sacrum** is located between the two pelvic bones of the inferior appendicular skeleton. The true form of the sacrum is convex and is comprised of five individual bones fused together and labeled S1–S5. The fusion of the five bones creates eight separate foramen, allowing the passage of nerve and blood vessels into the inferior appendicular skeleton. When studying human movement, the sacrum represents the final component of the axial skeleton that provides support. The location of the sacrum also differentiates the axial skeleton from the appendicular skeleton.

Coccyx. The final region of the vertebral column is the **coccyx**. This small tip of the vertebral column is made up of four individual bones. In terms of human movement, the coccyx serves little or no function.

Sternum The **sternum** is a dagger-shaped bone found in the anterosuperior region of the chest (Figure 5-7). Anatomically, the sternum is positioned directly in an area that protects the heart. When observing the sternum, note the three distinct portions that make up the structure. At the superior region of the sternum is the trapezoidal-shaped **manubrium**. The manubrium provides a base of support around which superior appendicular movements occur and is the attachment point for the first and second costal cartilage. Found in the middle of the sternum is the **sternal body**, which is the largest component. This bony structure provides a large surface area for the attachment of the pectoralis major muscle, which is an extremely strong muscle of the chest. Palpate your sternum and locate its inferior tip. This landmark is pointed and represents the **xiphoid process**. The importance of the xiphoid process to human movement stems from its attachment of the linea alba and from movements of the abdominal region. Also, the xiphoid process is an important landmark for the administration of cardiopulmonary resuscitation (CPR).

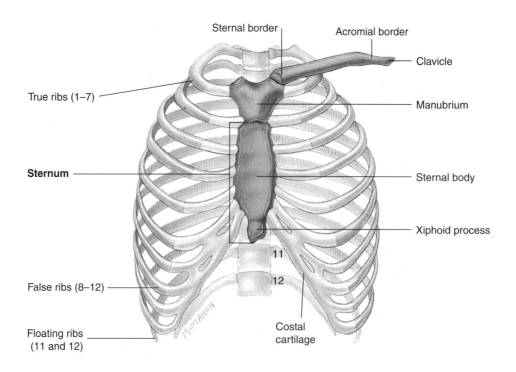

Figure 5-7 Sternum, Ribs, and Clavicle

The Ribs Twelve pairs of ribs (**costae**) are found in the thoracic cavity. They protect the vital organs of the cardiorespiratory system and provide increased surface area for muscle attachment. Of the 12 pairs of costae, 7 pairs are considered true costae and 5 pairs are false costae. Each of the seven true costal bones (ribs 1–7) originates from the corresponding thoracic vertebrae 1–7 and are attached to the manubrium and body of the sternum via costal cartilage.

The false costae, however, do not attach to the body of the sternum via their own individual costal cartilage; in some instances, they may not attach to the sternum at all. The costal bones, numbered 8–10, originate from T8 through T10 and attach to the body of the sternum via one common costal cartilage. The remaining two costae (ribs 11 and 12) originate from T11 and T12 and do not have a sternal attachment. Ribs 11 and 12 are known as floating ribs because they lack a sternal attachment and because they protect the kidneys.

THE APPENDICULAR SKELETON

The appendicular skeleton can be divided into two separate regions: superior and inferior. The superior appendicular skeleton consists of the shoulder, arms, wrists, and hands. In this region, there are 64 bones, or 32 bones per appendage. The inferior appendicular skeleton, on the other hand, is made up of 66 bones, or 33 per appendage, including the pelvis, thighs, legs, and feet. The bones located in the superior and inferior appendicular skeletons commonly provide support for lifting and carrying movements. They also extend body segments throughout a full range of motion to grasp, lift, and carry objects.

Superior Appendicular Skeleton The superior appendicular skeleton consists of 64 bones, including the clavicle, scapula, humerus, radius and ulna, carpals, metacarpals, and phalanges. These bones provide strong attachment points for the superior appendicular muscles.

Clavicle. When working with a skeleton, note the bones that make up the shoulder region. Moving from proximal to distal, the first bone is the **clavicle**. The clavicle is an S-shaped bone found on the anterosuperior surface of the shoulder joint. The clavicle is important to human movement because the medial portion connects the superior appendicular skeleton to the axial skeleton at the manubrium.

Scapula. Moving in the distal and posterior direction is the **scapula** (Figure 5-8). The scapula is an irregularly shaped triangular bone that is important to the muscles that move the shoulder joint and shoulder girdle. The numerous landmarks that extend off the scapula increase the surface area for muscular attachment of the shoulder region.

Humerus. The next region of the upper appendicular skeleton consists of the major long bones of the superior appendicular skeleton. Distal to and articulating with the scapula at the shoulder (glenohumoral) joint is the longest bone of the superior appendicular skeleton, the **humerus** (Figure 5-9). The area that the humerus takes up is called the arm.

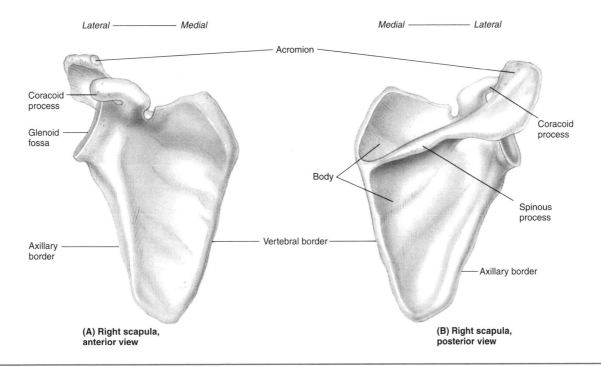

(A) Right scapula, anterior view

(B) Right scapula, posterior view

Figure 5-8 *Scapula*

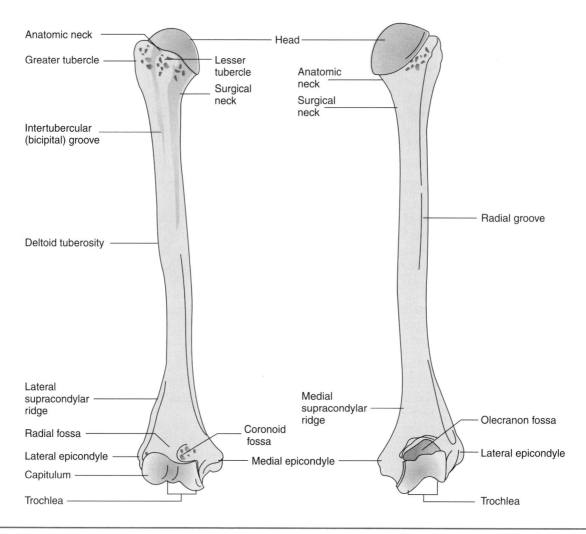

Figure 5-9 *Humerus*

Radius and Ulna. Moving from the humerus distally is the forearm, which includes the **radius** and **ulna** bones (Figure 5-10). When standing in the anatomical position, the radius is located on the lateral side of the forearm and the ulna is on the medial side. These bones have several other distinguishing factors, such as the radius is always connected to the thumb side of the wrist, whereas the ulna is always found on the pinky (digiti minimi) side. These positions allow for simple identification of bone location as the muscles of the wrist and forearm pull these bones through a full range of motion. Further in-depth study of these bones reveals that the ulna has a hook on its proximal segment and is longer than the radius.

Carpals. Distal to the forearm is the wrist (Figure 5-11). This region of the superior appendicular skeleton consists of eight complex **carpal bones**. The wrist contains two rows of carpal bones, with four carpal bones per row. When naming the carpal bones, move from a lateral (thumb side) to medial (digiti minimi side) position and proximal to distal direction (make sure to remember that when naming the bones, the body is in the anatomical position). Palpating the carpal bones while learning their names helps to identify them. The first row of carpals is proximal and, from lateral to medial, consists of the scaphoid, lunate, triquetrum, and pisiform bones. Moving distally from the first row, the second row of carpal bones include the trapezium, trapezoid, capitate, and hamate. When learning the names of the carpal bones, use a mnemonic device to help remember their names, such as "some" could stand for scaphoid or "play" could stand for pisiform.

> **Note:** *The scaphoid bone attaches to the metacarpal of the thumb. When palpating the scaphoid bone, look at the top of the hand and pull the thumb upward. When this movement occurs, the "anatomical snuffbox" is formed. Palpate the bone located in the snuffbox; this bone is the scaphoid. Until recently, the scaphoid bone was named the navicular and may still be identified as such in some old anatomy books. For identification purposes, the scaphoid name should be retained because there is a navicular bone in the foot.*

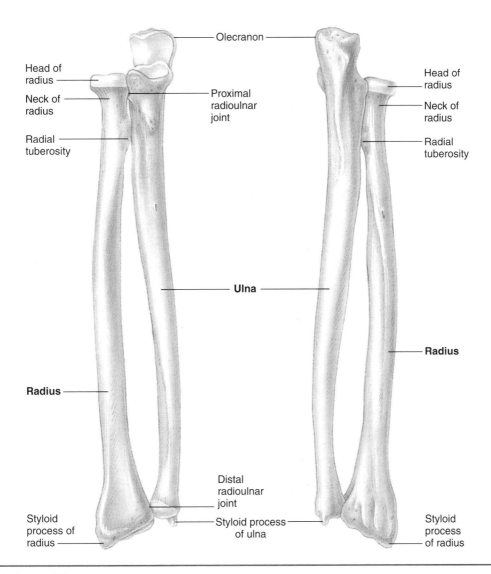

Figure 5-10 *Radius and Ulna*

Metacarpals. The **metacarpal bones** are immediately distal to the carpal bones. There are five metacarpals, which correspond with each digit. These bones are labeled with Roman numerals I–V and are identified from lateral (thumb side) to medial (pinky side). Therefore, metacarpal I articulates with the thumb, metacarpal V articulates with the digiti minimi, and so on.

Phalanges. Articulating with the metacarpals are the individual phalanges of the hand. When identifying the phalanges of the hand, move from lateral to medial beginning with the thumb. Like the metacarpals, these bones are labeled I–V. Unlike the metacarpals, however, several fingers have specific names. For instance, the thumb is identified as pollicis, the index finger is the indicis, and the little finger is the digiti minimi. When identifying the individual bones of the phalanges, realize that there are 14 individual phalanx bones. Each digit contains three individual phalanx bones except for the thumb, which contains two phalanx bones. These individual phalanx bones are identified as the proximal, intermediate, and distal phalanx bones in digits II – V and proximal and distal phalanx in digit I.

Inferior Appendicular Skeleton The **inferior appendicular skeleton** consists of 66 bones, including the pelvis, femur, tibia and fibula, tarsals, metatarsals, and phalanges. These bones provide strong attachment points for the inferior appendicular muscles.

Pelvis. The first bones of the inferior appendicular skeleton are the **pelvic bones** (Figure 5-12). The pelvic bones are important in kinesiology because in similar fashion to the clavicle, the pelvis attaches the inferior appendicular skeleton to the axial skeleton at the sacrum. The paired pelvic bones can be broken down into three specific regions: the ilium, located superior and lateral; the ischium, located inferior and posterior; and the pubic located anterior and inferior. Pelvic bones are

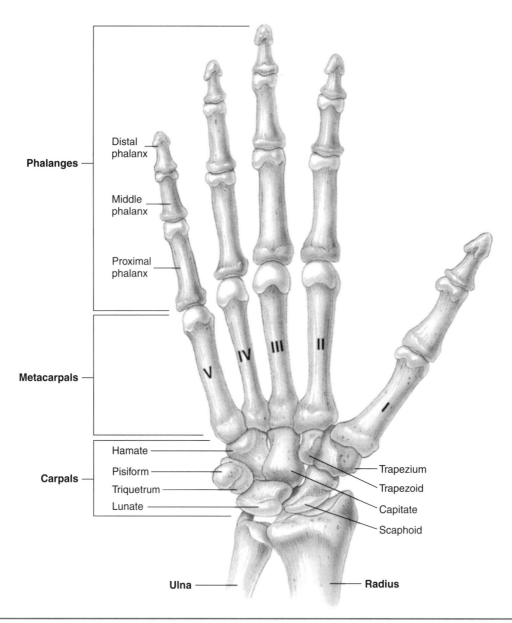

Phalanges —
  Distal phalanx
  Middle phalanx
  Proximal phalanx

Metacarpals —

V IV III II I

Carpals —
  Hamate
  Pisiform
  Triquetrum
  Lunate

  Trapezium
  Trapezoid
  Capitate
  Scaphoid

Ulna ———   ——— **Radius**

Figure 5-11 *Bones of the Hand*

classified as flat bones because of their shape. In terms of human movement, the pelvis provides a large amount of surface area for muscle attachment.

Femur. Moving distally from the pelvis is the longest bone in the body, the **femur** (Figure 5-13). The average length of a femur varies from 1 1/2 feet to 3 feet depending on the size of an individual. The long length of the femur makes it ideal for large muscle attachment.

Located at the distal end of the femur on the anterior surface is the **patella**. This sesamoid bone is important to human movement because it acts as a strong anatomical pulley that increases the contraction effects caused by the quadriceps muscles. When the patella is relaxed, one can move it by palpating the anterior surface of the knee. However, during muscle contractions, the patella tracks, locks, and provides the support necessary for the contracting quadriceps muscle and stabilizes the knee joint.

Tibia and Fibula. Located distally to the femur are two long bones that make up the lower leg region (Figure 5-14). In the anatomical position, the **tibia** is found on the medial side of the leg and the **fibula** is found on the lateral side. Several distinguishing factors are noticed when identifying the tibia and fibula. The most obvious is that the tibia is large and thick in comparison to the fibula, which has a much smaller diameter.

Tarsals. The final component of the inferior appendicular skeleton is the foot (Figure 5-15). Similar to the bony anatomy of the hand, the foot is made up of three distinct areas: the tarsals, metatarsals, and phalanges.

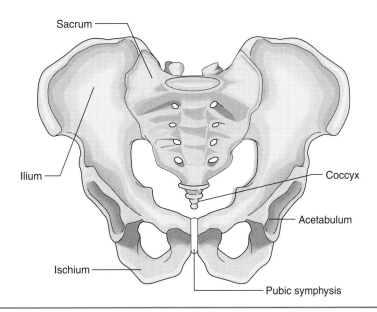

Figure 5-12 *Pelvis*

One difference between the hand and foot is the number of carpals versus **tarsals**. In the hand there are eight carpal bones that make up the wrist; in the foot there are seven tarsal bones. In addition, the metatarsals are arranged in a more parallel manner, allowing for a stronger base of support.

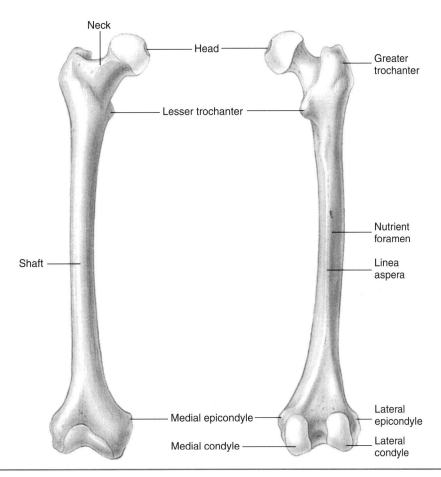

Figure 5-13 *Femur*

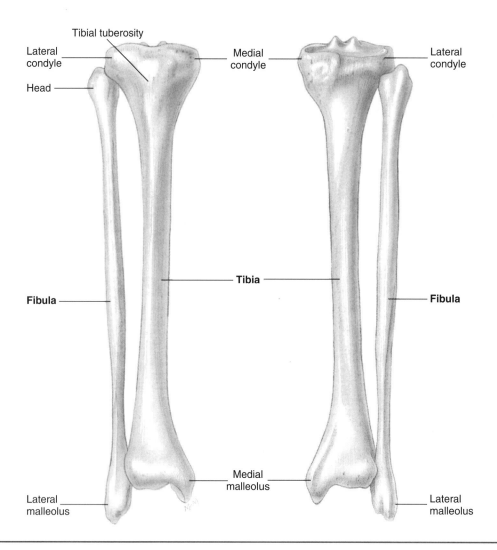

Lateral condyle
Tibial tuberosity
Head
Fibula
Lateral malleolus

Medial condyle
Tibia
Medial malleolus

Lateral condyle
Lateral condyle
Fibula
Lateral malleolus

Figure 5-14 *Tibia and Fibula*

OTA Perspective

Rather than restore function, the what-where-when-why-how of the break or dysfunction may indicate the necessity for compensation or adaptation to account for the change or loss of function within occupational performance.

Scientific knowledge, OT theory, and the client's goals are pieces of information that, along with clinical reasoning, guide treatment. For example, a young child with an incomplete fracture of the femur that resulted from a fall while playing in a tree house will receive therapy that focuses on restoration of function. On the other hand, an elderly woman with a medically complex diagnosis, including osteoporosis and post CVA with right-sided hemiparesis, who sustains a comminuted fracture of the right radius from a fall out of bed, might receive therapy that follows an occupational performance model with a focus on compensation and environmental adaptations.

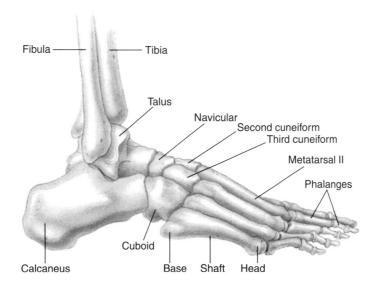

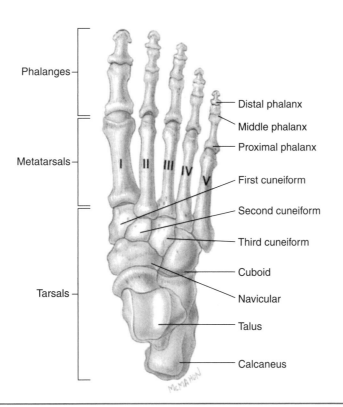

Figure 5-15 *Bones of the Foot*

Beginning at the posterior end of the foot and moving anteriorally is a large bone, the calcaneus, commonly known as the heel. Moving anteriorally and superiorly is the talus bone, which articulates with the tibia. The junction of the tibia and talus forms the talocrural joint and is significant to the movements of the ankle. Immediately anterior to the talus bone is the navicular bone. (Do not become confused when looking at older anatomy books when they make reference to the navicular in the hand and foot.) Anterolateral to the navicular is a short bone named the cuboid. The cuboid bone provides lateral support for the foot region. The final bones of the foot make up the arches and are named the cuneiforms. The cuneiforms are located medial to the cuboid bone and are labeled first, second, and third from medial to lateral. However, these bones may also be labeled as the medial, intermediate, and lateral cuneiforms in some books.

Metatarsals. Anteriorly to the tarsals are five long bones named the **metatarsals**. The metatarsals are labeled I–V, starting on the large toe side from medial to lateral. Note the difference between the structure of the metatarsals of the foot and the metacarpals of the hand.

Phalanges. Articulating with the metatarsals are the individual **phalanges of the foot**. In a similar manner to naming bones in the hand, the great and little toes have specific names. The great toe is known as hallicus, whereas the little toe is known as the digiti minimi. When identifying the individual bones of the phalanges note that there are 14 individual phalanx bones. Each digit contains three individual phalanx bones except for the hallicus, which contains two. These individual phalanx bones are identified as proximal, intermediate, and distal in digits II–V and proximal and distal in digit I.

BONE LANDMARKS

Bones provide attachment points for muscles. Structurally speaking, the landmarks found on the bones increase the surface area for muscle attachment and enhance the mechanical efficiency of muscle contraction. Various bone landmarks have simple names that identify their structure, such as an angle or line. Other bones, however, have difficult names to remember and offer no identifiable form, such as a tuberosity or meatus. Table 5-1 shows the common names associated with the bone landmarks.

WOLFF'S LAW

When observing bones, notice that some are thicker and wider in some areas and thinner in others. Wolff's law can further explain the optimal strength that a bone provides in relation to the thickness of the anatomical features. Wolff's law states that:

1. *Bones are thickest where muscles attach.* For example, look at the distal end of the humerus. Notice that the bone is much thicker than the bone of the shaft. When studying the muscles in the shoulder and elbow joints, notice that many of these bones have their attachments on the distal humerus.

2. *Long bones are thick in the middle of the shaft.* This arrangement prevents buckling of the bone during movement and increases the strength of the long bone. For example, what would happen to the femur during weight-bearing exercises if the bone tissue along the diaphysis was thin? Obviously, the structure provides mechanical support for the middle of the long bone.

3. *Curved bones are thickest in areas where they are most likely to break.* Take a look at the costal bones. Starting at the sternum and moving laterally, note that the costal bones are thickest in the middle. Remember that the costal bones protect the vital organs of the cardiovascular system and that these bones are thick where they are most likely to break.

4. *An area where trabecular bone is abundant is where mechanical forces are the greatest.* Where in the long bone do you find the greatest amount of trabecular bone? The answer is the epiphysis. The different muscles acting on a specific joint due to the mechanical forces that are applied to these regions during weight-bearing activities and the increased force are the reason for this.

KEY CONCEPTS

- The physiological properties of bone include five basic functions: mineral storage, protection, support, blood cell formation, and anatomical landmarks for muscles to attach to.

- All four types of bones are made up of a thin layer of compact bone surrounding a thicker layer of trabecular bone. The thick layer of trabecular bone resembles beams that provide strong support for the bone structures.

- There are four types of bones in the human body: long (e.g., humerus), short (e.g., carpals), irregular (e.g., sternum), and flat (e.g., skull).

- The bones in the human body consist of numerous microscopic structures that provide the physiological purposes of bones. Each structure is responsible for the integrity of bone.

Table 5-1 *Common Anatomical Landmarks*

Name	Description	Example and Location
Angle	Section of a bone that changes direction from anterior to posterior or medial to lateral	Inferior angle of the scapula Inferior scapula
Border	Process of a bone that defines the edge	Medial border of the scapula Medial scapula
Condyle	Projection of bone that increases the surface area	Medial and lateral condyle of the humerus Distal medial and lateral humerus
Crest	Semicircle-shaped projection on the superior region of a bone	Iliac crest Superior pelvis
Epicondyle	Projections that extend off a bone	Medial and lateral epicondlyle of the femur Posterior distal femur
Foramen	A large hole formed by several bones	Obturator foramen Pubic and ischium-pelvis
Fossa	A large, wide depression formed into a bone	Supraspinous fossa Superior to the spine of the scapula
Groove	A long, narrow depression formed between two landmarks	Bicipital (intertrubercular) groove Proximal humerus
Head	Proximal part of a bone that articulates with another socket	Head of the radius Proximal radius
Line	An elevation of a bone that forms an evident line	Linea aspera of the femur Posterior femur along the diaphysis
Meatus	A small hole that allows nerves or passages to run into a bone	External auditory meatus Base of the temporal bone
Notch	Indentation into a bone	Sciatic notch Distal ischium of the pelvis
Process	Extension of a bone in any direction	Acromion process of the scapula Posterolateral scapula
Spine	Process that forms a spine shape	Anterior superior iliac spine Anterior pelvis
Trochanter	Large projection that attaches to large muscles	Greater trochanter of the femur Lateral projection of the superior femur
Tubercle	Large projection that attaches to large muscles	Greater tubercle of the humerus Anterolateral humerus
Tuberosity	Small projection that attaches a large muscle group to a bone	Tibial tuberosity Proximal anterior surface of the tibia

■ The axial skeleton consists of those bones found along the spine and skull. These bones provide a sound structure around which movements occur. The appendicular skeleton consists of the bones that pull about the axial skeleton to cause movements.

■ There are four components of Wolff's law that explain the optimal strength that bone can provide. These are: bones are thickest where muscles attach, long bones are thick in the middle of the shaft, curved bones are thickest in areas where they are most likely to break, and an area where trabecular bone is abundant is where mechanical forces are the greatest.

BIBLIOGRAPHY

Guyton, A. C. (2000). *Textbook of medical physiology* (10th ed.). Philadelphia: W. B. Saunders.

Marieb, E. N. (2003). *Human anatomy and physiology* (6th ed.). Redwood City, CA: Benjamin/Cummings.

Stone, R. J. & Stone, J. A. (1999). *Atlas of skeletal muscle* (3rd ed.). Dubuque. IA: W. C. Brown.

Taber's cyclopedic medical dictionary (19th ed.). (2001). Philadelphia: F. A. Davis.

Thompson, C. W., & Floyd, R. T. (2001). *Manual of structural kinesiology* (14th ed.). St. Louis, MO: Mosby.

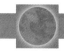

WEB RESOURCES

- Visit the Web site of the *Journal of Bone and Joint Surgery* at www.ejbjs.org/ for articles related to bone and joint injuries and surgical reports or injuries to specific joints.
- The Web site, www.innerbody.com, features some anatomical animations, including the skeleton, bone structure, and types of fractures.

(These Web addresses were current as of September 2003.)

REVIEW QUESTIONS

Fill in the Blank

Provide the word(s) or phrase(s) that best completes the sentence.

1. When you look at bone, _____ tissue makes up the superficial layer and _____ tissue lines the medullary cavity.

2. The _____ _____ is the growth center of bone and causes the bone to grow _____ _____.

3. _____ bones are made up of a thin layer of compact bone with a large layer of trabecular bone between them.

4. There are _____ bones in the human body.

5. The sphenoid bone in the skull is butterfly shaped and has a/an _____ shape.

6. Trabecular bone is known as _____ _____ and is laid down along lines of mechanical _____.

7. The type of bone cell that forms bone is known as a/an _____, whereas the bone that breaks down bone is known as a/an _____.

8. The other purposes of bone in addition to support include _____, _____, _____, and _____.

9. A hollow structure that runs parallel and down the center of an osteon is known as a _____ _____.

10. A hollow structure that runs perpendicular and connects one osteon to the next is known as a _____ _____.

Multiple Choice

Select the best answer to complete the following statements.

1. The structural unit of bone is known as the _____.
    a. osteocyte
    b. osteoclast
    c. osteoblast
    d. osteon

2. Cells that are responsible for the breakdown of bone that primarily exist in the lateral layers of the osteon are the _____ cells.
    a. osteocyte
    b. osteoclast
    c. osteoblast
    d. osteon

3. Mature bone cells are known as the _____ cells.
    a. osteocyte
    b. osteoclast
    c. osteoblast
    d. osteon

4. The second carpal bone of the first row is the _____.
    a. hamate
    b. triquetrum
    c. navicular
    d. scaphoid

5. The heel bone is also known as the _____.
    a. talus
    b. calcaneous
    c. anconeus
    d. tarsus

Matching

Match each of the following bones with the type of bone.

_____ **1.** Thoracic vertebrae 7	A.	Short
_____ **2.** 12th rib	B.	Long
_____ **3.** Radius	C.	Flat
_____ **4.** Frontal bone	D.	Irregular
_____ **5.** 4th metacarpal		
_____ **6.** Medial cuneiform		
_____ **7.** Triquetrum		
_____ **8.** Proximal phalange		
_____ **9.** Patella		
_____**10.** Occipital bone		
_____**11.** Pisiform		
_____**12.** 1st metatarsal		
_____**13.** Fibula		
_____**14.** Sacrum		
_____**15.** Body of the sternum		

Critical Thinking

1. Reflect on what you know about clinical reasoning to elaborate on the scenarios described in the perspective boxes, with a focus on bone function, purpose, and location, to plan a course of recovery. What other medical and therapy information would be beneficial to this plan?

2. Discuss the following with regard to the scenario of the child with the fractured femur: In what case would the child *not* need OT intervention? In what case might the child need a combination of OT and PT (be careful not to duplicate services)?

3. Your 55-year-old mother has been diagnosed with early-stage osteoporosis following a routine bone scan. She is concerned with the possible progression of the disease and seeks your advice. As a rehabilitation professional, describe the advice that you would give her and explain your reasons.

4. Review the different types of fractures listed below. For each one, draw a diagram of the fracture and give a possible cause of that type of fracture.

   ■ Greenstick

   ■ Spiral

   ■ Oblique

   ■ Comminuted

   ■ Transverse

   Which one of these fractures would heal the fastest and which would heal the slowest?

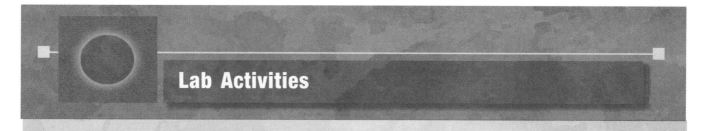

Lab Activities

Lab 5-1: Bones, Fractures, and Function

Objective: To relate the effects of a bone fracture to OT treatment and functional gains.

Equipment Needed: Skeleton or other mock-up of human skeletal system depending on the scenario

Step 1.   Choose a bone in the human body. Identify its location, type, and purpose and how it functions in relation to surrounding bones. For those who are interested in learning more, expand that identification to muscles, tendons, and ligaments.

Step 2.   Suppose that bone you have chosen breaks. Imagine its effect on function. List three possible changes in occupational performance.

Step 3.   Imagine how and why the bone broke (e.g., motor vehicle accident [MVA] versus a fall due to osteoarthritis). Create a client profile to determine possible interventions.

Step 4.   Name three possible OT treatments with a focus on addressing bone function.

Step 5.   Discuss outcomes in terms of restoring function or compensating for or adapting to loss of full functional return. Also discuss the necessary client education.

Lab 5-2: Review of Bones in the Human Skeleton

Objective: To identify all the bones in the human skeleton.

Equipment Needed: Skeleton or models of specific skeletal structures, a lab partner, self-stick notes, pen/pencil

Step 1.   Using the skeleton, label each bone of the appendicular skeleton with self-stick notes with your lab partner.

Step 2.   Using the skeleton, label each bone of the axial skeleton with self-stick notes with your lab partner.

Step 3:   Discuss the relationships of the bones in certain regions of the skeleton.

Lab 5-3: Identification of Bone Structure

Objective: To properly identify the structure of particular types of bone.

Equipment Needed: Models of a skeleton or parts of a skeleton, self-stick notes, pen/pencil

Step 1.   Choose an area of the skeleton, such as the shoulder girdle, spine, pelvic girdle, head, or chest.

Step 2.   Label the type of bones found in the area you chose as long, short, irregular, or flat.

Step 3.   Determine the function of the bone based on the structure.

Chapter 6

JOINT STRUCTURE

Key Words

amphiarthrosis joint
arthrosis
articular capsule
articular cartilage
biaxial joint
circumduction
condyloidal joint
diarthrosis, or synovial, joint

gomphosis
hinge joint
ligament
nonaxial joint
pivot joint
saddle joint
suture joint
symphysis joint
synarthrotic joint

synchondrosis joint
syndesmosis joint
synovial fluid
tendon
triaxial joint
uniaxial joint

INTRODUCTION

How would the segments of the body move if joint structures did not exist at the locations where two bones come together? We would be like trees in the forest with only the mountain breeze to make us sway from side to side. Movement of the various body segments through a full range of motion is dependent on the union of two bones and the joint structures that exist between these bones. In many cases, the joints provide an axis that allows the muscles to pull the bones in different directions. Other times, however, the joint structure in a given location fuses two bones together and provides additional support for human movement.

Joints are made up of several unique structural components that cushion the bones to absorb force, support the sides of a joint with strong fibrous tissues, and provide an axis around which the movements of the various segments occur. Although joints enhance movement, these structures are the weakest of all skeletal structures in the human body. As the demands for mobility increase, the joints sacrifice the sound structures that strengthen a given area, increasing the likelihood of injuries at a specific joint.

JOINT CLASSIFICATIONS

When studying the joint structures in the human body, observe the different bone shapes where they articulate (come together at a joint). The structure of the joint at this junction determines the amount of stability and mobility it provides for a given segment in the body. For instance, the cranial bones of adults articulate and form a union similar to fitting two pieces of a puzzle together. This close proximity enhances the structural strength of the cranium and helps protect the brain. Although this arrangement is beneficial for protection, however, the close proximity of the cranial bones limits their mobility. Some joints, on the other hand, have more space between the articulating ends of the bones. For example, observe a joint where two epiphyses are located. The increased space between the bones enhances mobility, yet their structural strength is compromised because they lack the structures that provide optimal support found in other joints. In-depth observations of the joints of the human body reveal three different joint classifications based on strength and mobility: fibrous (synarthrotic), cartilaginous (amphiarathrotic), and synovial (diarthrotic).

FIBROUS JOINTS

The immovable joints in the human body are classified as **synarthrotic joints**. When the term *synarthrotic* is broken down into its two components, the first part "syn" refers to "joined" or "together" and the second part **arthrosis** refers to the joints. The structural components of synarthrotic joints include a dense layer of fibrous connective tissue that firmly attaches the bones together, which limits the amount of movement around these joints. The three synarthrotic subclasses are called suture, gomphosis, and syndesmosis joints.

Suture Joints   **Suture joints** are found where two cranial bones come together (Figure 6-1A). Dense fibrous connective tissue holds the cranial bones firmly in place and prevents them from moving under any circumstance. The suture joint increases the support of the cranial region by providing a sound structure and inhibiting separation of these bones. At childbirth, however, the cranial bones are not fused, which allows the brain to grow and which results in a soft spot on the head to be formed. This soft spot is present from infant years through childhood, decreasing the cranial bones' capabilities to protect the brain during that peroid. Over time, the cranial bones grow and mesh together and form a suture at the union between them.

Gomphosis Joints   A fibrous joint, **gomphosis**, is not important to structural support or human movement. It occurs between the teeth and the underlying mandibular and maxillary bones. At this location, the teeth are cemented into place and only move when an external force is great enough to displace the fibrous tissue.

Syndesmosis Joints   The **syndesmosis joint** structure is important for supporting the nonmovable joints between the bones of the extremities such as the distal radioulnar and tibiofibular joints (Figure 6-1B). The joints found in these areas have long, fibrous connective tissues that firmly attach the ends of the bones together. The fibers support and enhance the movement of the segments and provide additional structural support for the two bones they attach.

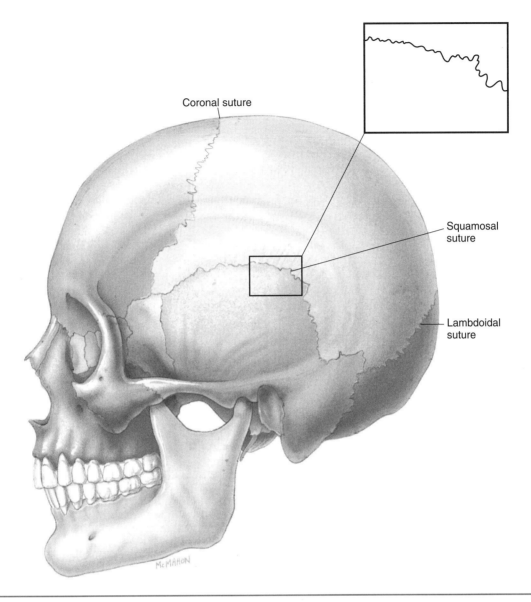

Figure 6-1A *Suture Joint*

CARTILAGINOUS JOINTS

The type of joints that primarily joins two bones together by cartilaginous connective tissue are classified as **amphiarthrosis joints**. Amphiarthrosis joints lack a specific joint cavity, are slightly movable, and function similarly to synarthrosis joints in that they limit the amount of movement that occurs in a specific region. The cartilage, however, promotes various movements that are essential to such important physiological functions as breathing, regional movement, and childbirth. Amphiarthrosis joints can be broken down into two subclasses: synchondrosis and symphysis joints.

Synchondrosis Joints **Synchondrosis joints** are located between bones where compression forces of gravity are increased and limited movements occur. The synchondrosis joint is found between the vertebrae and makes up much of the vertebral disk and spinal column. Synchondrosis joints also are found in the long cartilaginous extensions between the sternum and the ribs. The costal cartilage, in this case, allows the chest to rise and fall as we breathe on a continual basis.

Symphysis Joints The only location of a **symphysis joint** in the human body occurs at the symphysis pubis where the two pubic regions of the pelvic bones attach to one another (Figure 6-2). The symphysis joint provides structural strength for the inferior appendicular skeleton and provides a strong base of support around which the inferior appendicular skeletal muscles pull. The only occasion when movement occurs in this area is during childbirth as the baby moves through the birth canal. In this case, the symphysis expands, allowing the baby to be pushed forward into the world.

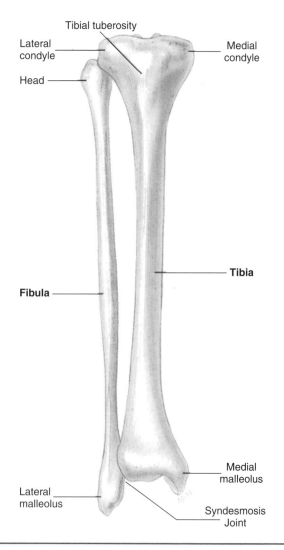

Figure 6-1B *Syndesmosis Joint*

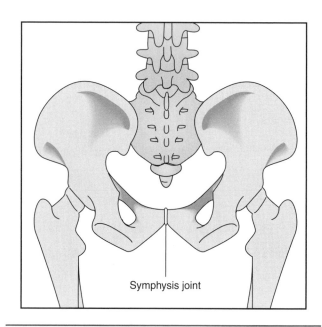

Figure 6-2 *Symphysis Joint*

SYNOVIAL JOINTS

The joint structures that are most important to human movement are those that possess a synovial joint capsule. They are classified as **diarthrosis, or synovial, joints**. The structures contained within the diarthrodial joints are common throughout and enhance the mobility of the joints through a wide array of complex movements. The need for enhanced mobility allowed by the synovial joints sacrifices the sound structural components of the synarthrosis and amphiarthrosis joints. As a result, diarthrosis joints are more susceptible to injuries following overextension of these structures. There are four classes of diarthrodial joints: nonaxial, uniaxial, biaxial, and triaxial joints.

Nonaxial Joints Synovial joints that do not provide movements in a specific plane or specific axis are called **nonaxial joints** (Figure 6-3A). Nonaxial joints have a joint cavity yet the bones in the region are in close proximity, which decreases their ability to move around a specific joint axis. Examples of nonaxial joints include the articulations between the carpal and tarsal bones, which provide sliding movements as these bones move past one another.

Uniaxial Joints The joints in the human body that allow for movement around one axis in one plane are called **uniaxial joints** (Figure 6-3B). Often, rigid bony structures and ligaments of uniaxial joints prevent movements from occurring in other planes of motion. For instance, the elbow joint (articulation between the ulna and humerus) is a uniaxial joint that is supported by the olecranon process of the ulna and various ligaments of the elbow region. The bony process of the olecranon prevents movements of the elbow in the frontal and transverse planes. Two types of uniaxial joints are found in the human body: the hinge and pivot joints.

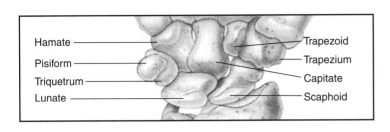

Hamate	Trapezoid
Pisiform	Trapezium
Triquetrum	Capitate
Lunate	Scaphoid

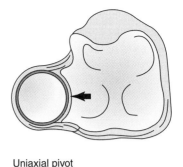

Uniaxial pivot

Figure 6-3A *Nonaxial Joint*

Figure 6-3B *Uniaxial Joint*

OTA Perspective

In terms of joint mobility, and specifically of the upper extremity (U/E), analyze the task of petting a cat within the role of pet owner (task or activity analysis of an occupation). Conduct a performance analysis of your classmate petting a cat. Compare and contrast the two. Did your classmate use the joint movements that you anticipated were necessary to accomplish the task of petting a cat? Review U/E joint movements and planes and axes as one would typically reach out for the cat's back and stroke it with the anterior hand surface, using elbow flexion and extension to provide most of the active movement, with the hand and wrist in relative stability.

Hinge Joints. The classic **hinge joints** of the human body are at the elbow, knee, and interphalangeal joints (Figure 6-3C). Based on the anatomical position, movements of the hinge joints occur in the sagittal plane around a frontal axis. For example, think of a weight lifter performing a biceps curl. Imagine a rigid bar through the elbow joint: the rigid bar would be located in the frontal plane. As the movement occurs, the arms move anterior to posterior, resulting in movement in the sagittal plane. Observations of the bony structures in these areas reveal that the bones prevent movements in other planes and axes.

Pivot Joints. The primary **pivot joint** in the human body is found at the radioulnar joint where the proximal head of the radius articulates with the radial notch of the ulna. Avoid confusing the elbow and radioulnar joint as one joint because they each are individually classified. The pivoting movement of the radius over the ulna provides for uniaxial movement in this location. An in-depth movement analysis reveals that the actions at the radioulnar joint occur around the vertical axis in the

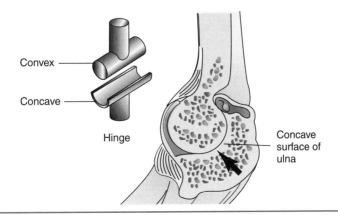

Convex

Concave

Hinge

Concave surface of ulna

Figure 6-3C *Hinge Joints*

transverse plane. For example, a jar that is sitting on a countertop rests in the transverse plane. If one was to place a hand on the jar and extend the arm vertically, the movement occurs in the transverse plane around a vertical axis.

Biaxial Joints

The name **biaxial** infers that movements of these joints occur in two planes around two different axes (Figure 6-4). Structural identification reveals that biaxial joints are supported on all sides by ligaments and tendons without additional bony support. The subclassifications for the biaxial joints include the condyloidal and saddle joints.

Condyloidal Joints. **Condyloidal joints** are found at the metacarpophalangeal joint (where the metacarpals articulate with the proximal phalanx of the phalange) of the hand and the metatarsophalangeal joint (where the metatarsals articulate with the proximal phalanx of the phalange) of the foot and allow movements in two planes around two separate axes. For example, observe the structures and movements that occur at the metacarpophalangeal joint of the hand. Are there additional bony landmarks that provide additional support? Can an individual rotate the fingers without manually forcing them to move in the transverse plane? The answer to both of these questions is no. The movements at the metacarpophalangeal joint occur in both the sagittal and frontal planes around a frontal and sagittal axis, respectively. If a rigid bar were extended from the lateral surface through the joints to the medial surface of the hand, movements would occur in the sagittal plane around a frontal axis. Similarly, if the same rigid bar were extended from the anterior surface through the joint and out through the posterior surface, the movement would occur in the frontal plane around a sagittal axis. Notice that the metacarpophalangeal joint does not allow actions to occur in the transverse plane.

Saddle Joints. The second type of biaxial joint is the **saddle joint**. Saddle joints are located only between the trapezium bone and the first metacarpal bone. Observe the saddle shape of the trapezium. Analyzing its movement shows that it is similar to that of the condyloidal joint, with movements occurring in both the sagittal and frontal planes around the frontal and sagittal axes, respectively. Again, if a rigid bar were extended from the lateral surface through the joint to the medial surface of the joint, the ensuing movements would occur in the sagittal plane around a frontal axis. Similarly, if a rigid bar were extended from the anterior surface through the joint and out through the posterior surface, the movement would occur in the frontal plane around a sagittal axis. Notice also that the trapeziometacarpal joint does not allow actions to occur in the transverse plane.

Triaxial Joints

The **triaxial joint** is commonly referred to as a ball-and-socket joint (Figure 6-5). The mobility of the triaxial joint is enhanced when compared to the sound structural support provided by stable joints in the human body, such as the synarthroses and amphiarthroses joints. As a result, triaxial joints are often the most injured joints when the joint structures pass their normal range of motion. Sound ligaments and numerous muscle tendons exist on all sides of the triaxial joint to help strengthen and reinforce the joint region.

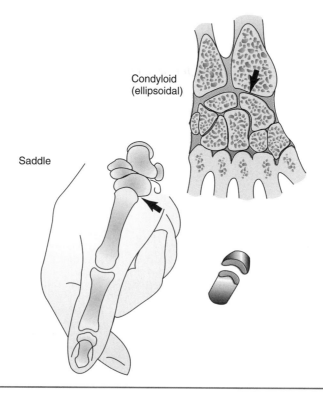

Condyloid
(ellipsoidal)

Saddle

Figure 6-4 *Biaxial Joint*

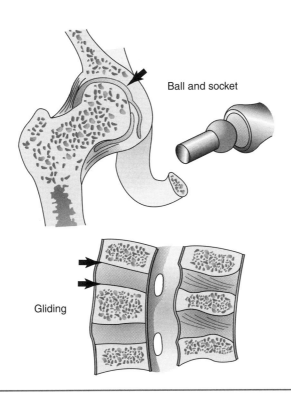

Figure 6-5 *Triaxial Joint*

The name "triaxial" refers to the ability of the joint to move in three planes around three axes. Observe the movements of either the shoulder (glenohumoral) or hip (acetabulofemoral) joint. Move these joints freely through a full range of motion and observe the different planes and axes in which the bones move. Extending a rigid bar from anterior to posterior and per-

OTA Perspective

Rheumatoid arthritis (RA) is a progressive inflammatory disease that affects joints in a symmetrical pattern. It is more common in women and the onset is usually before age 50. The disease affects the synovial lining of the joint capsule, and the joints become swollen, red, hot, and very painful. RA usually affects the hands and feet first, although characteristic deformities of all joints also occur and function can be severely limited. The cause of RA is unknown but may be an autoimmune factor. All patients have a positive rheumatoid factor present on a blood test. RA has systemic features that can also affect the rest of the body.

Osteoarthritis (OA) is the most common form of arthritis. It is a degenerative disease of the synovial joints. It affects the cartilage of the joints, resulting in deterioration, swelling, loss of ROM, and pain. It commonly affects the weight-bearing joints of the lower extremities, especially the hip and the knee, and has a nonsymmetrical presentation. Stiffness is severe, especially in the morning, and the most positive findings are seen on X-ray, where degeneration is seen. Causes of the disease are primarily wear and tear, and it most commonly affects people over age 65.

forming a jumping jack skill, the movement occurs in the frontal plane around a sagittal axis. Moving the bar through the medial and lateral surfaces causes anterior and posterior movement of the arm. Movement in the region would then occur in the sagittal plane around a frontal axis. The last movement at the shoulder joint occurs along a vertical axis. Using the jar-opening example from earlier in this chapter, extend your arm vertically and twist the jar at the shoulder. Notice that the movement occurs around a vertical axis in the transverse plane. The movement of the triaxial joint increases the ability of the superior and inferior appendicular skeletons to move through a full range of motion.

 ## STRUCTURE OF DIARTHRODIAL JOINTS

When observing the structures of the diarthrodial joints, remember that they are found among uniaxial, biaxial, triaxial, and nonaxial joints. Additionally, remember that when the need for mobility increases in a given area, the abundance of strong fibrous connective tissues is decreased.

Articular Cartilage

Located inferior and superior to the epiphysis of long bone is an area composed of **articular cartilage** (Figure 6-6) that is made of hyaline cartilage. Hyaline cartilage is important to human movement because of its ability to absorb the stresses caused by an increased gravitational influence on the joint. For instance, imagine the forces that are applied to the knee joint during running. As the compressional force increases, the hyaline cartilage absorbs the force and acts as a cushion to dissipate the force. When degeneration of the cartilage structure occurs, there is a marked increase in pain and dysfunction. The hyaline cartilage may be referred to as the meniscus, such as the medial or lateral meniscus of the knee.

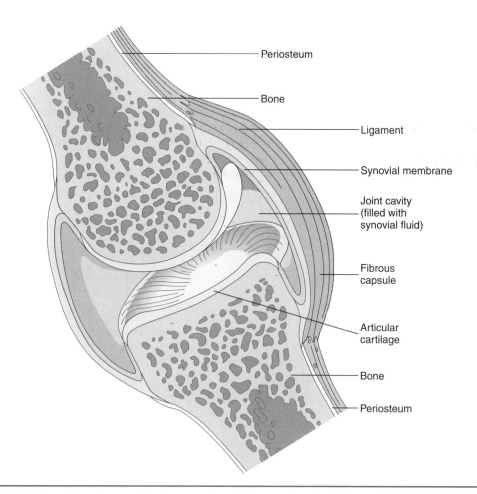

Figure 6-6 *Articular Cartilage*

Articular Capsule

A structure that is continuous with the periosteum and articular cartilage is the **articular capsule**. It is comprised of two structures that enhance the strength and pliability of the diarthrodial joint and are the fibrous capsule and the synovial membrane. The fibrous capsule is made of a distinct layer of fibrous connective tissue. This layer increases the flexibility and structural integrity of the joint. Immediately deep to the fibrous capsule is the synovial capsule. This structure lines the interior surface of the joint and aids in protecting the joint.

Synovial Fluid

The fluid that lubricates the inside of the articular capsule is called the **synovial fluid**. Much like the oil in the engine of a car, the synovial fluid is a low-viscous fluid that helps to decrease the frictional properties applied to the joint during human movement. During movements of the various segments, synovial fluid is released from the synovial membrane when the segment is compressed. Following the compression movement, the fluid is reabsorbed by the hyaline cartilage. Lack of synovial fluid results in decreased functions of the joint and increased pain associated with movements.

Ligaments

Much like the tendon of muscle, the origin of the **ligament** is continuous with the periosteum of bone. This fibrous connective tissue spans the joint and provides additional structural support for the joint during human movement. For example, picture the following two scenarios. In the first scenario, bones A and B form a joint and are connected by a rubber band on one side. When a force is applied to the opposite side of the rubber band, the joint buckles and the rubber band provides support for the joint. As the force is released from the joint formed by A and B, the rubber band contracts and returns this mock joint to its original position. In the second scenario, picture bones A and B without a rubber band crossing the joint. When an external force is applied to the joint and then released, the joint would not recoil and return to its prior shape. Replace the rubber band and imagine a ligament that spans the joint surface; notice that ligaments can be stretched to a given point. If a ligament is stretched beyond its normal limits, it will snap much like a rubber band that has been overstretched beyond its limit. Otherwise, the ligament supports the joint and prevents it from buckling.

Tendons

One final structure that provides additional support for the joint is the **tendon** of the muscle that crosses a particular joint. For instance, one of the more infamous regions where the tendons provide support for the joint is at the shoulder joint and includes the tendons of the shoulder cuff muscles. In this region, the tendons of the teres minor, infraspinatus, supraspinatus, and subscapularis muscles provide additional support for the shoulder. Depending on their location, the teres minor and infraspinatus muscles provide posterior support, the supraspinatus provides superior support, and the subscapularis provides anterior support for the shoulder joint. The tendons that cross the joints increase the strength of the shoulder joint during a muscle contraction and ensure that the joint is stable for all muscle actions.

 MUSCLE MOVEMENTS AROUND A PLANE OR AXIS

Understanding normal human movement is extremely important for analyzing the movements of clients during various modes of exercise. It is increasingly important to understand that the various movements occur in a specific plane (sagittal, frontal, and transverse) around a specific axis (sagittal, frontal, and vertical). Variations from these normal movements can often exacerbate a problem that occurs in a joint. For example, say you were an athletic trainer watching a videotape of an athlete who recently broke the humerus at the elbow. During the video you see that the athlete was hit from the side and the elbow joint moved in the frontal plane. An analysis of this movement would reveal that flexion and extension movements occur at this joint and that these movements occur in the sagittal, not the frontal, plane. In addition to observing the planes and axes around which the movement occurs, remember that there are four different diarthrodial joints, nonaxial, uniaxial, biaxial, and triaxial, that allow different movements at the different joints.

Recall the discussion in Chapter 1 about the breakdown of the different planes in the human body. These planes are the sagittal, frontal, and transverse planes. When further learning about human movement, observe that the actions of the muscles cause specific movements in these planes. For example, the muscles that allow us to perform a jumping jack cause an

OTA Perspective

Ligament injuries are called *sprains*. Clinically there are three grades of injuries. Grade I sprains involve minimal tissue damage, such as slight swelling and slight local tenderness. Function is only minimally affected in this type of injury. Grade II sprains involve more tearing of the fibers of the ligament, local pain is intense, and there is loss of function. Grade II tears constitute any amount of tearing between minimal and severe but without full rupture. Grade III sprains involve a total rupture of the ligament with loss of joint stability and substantial loss of function. These total ruptures may require surgery to repair them. Ligament sprains heal by fibrous tissue, and physical therapy may be needed to maximize the joint function.

action that occurs in the frontal plane. Recall that the frontal plane separates the body into two parts: anterior and posterior. Imagine that your arms are a pendulum when performing a jumping jack movement. The motion of the pendulum would separate the body into anterior and posterior halves.

A difficult concept to understand about human movement is the axis around which movements occur. An *axis* is defined as a rigid bar that runs through an object at its pivot point. For example, observe a pair of scissors. The axis is the point where the scissors attach and around which movements of the scissors occur.

When identifying human movements, realize that the axis around which movement occurs is perpendicular to the plane of motion (Table 6-1). For example, when observing the jumping jack skill, the segments have movement in the frontal plane around the sagittal axis. As a rigid bar is extended out from the shoulder and hip joints from anterior to posterior, observe that the sagittal axis is the only axis that corresponds with movement in the frontal plane.

Table 6-1 *Pairing of a Plane and its Perpendicular Axis*

Plane	Axis	Example
Sagittal	Frontal	Biceps curl
Frontal	Sagittal	Jumping jack
Transverse	Vertical	Spinning on ice skates

Joint Movements of the Sagittal Plane

Muscles that have their origin and insertion toward the anterior and posterior of the joint cause movements in the sagittal plane (Figure 6-7). Take, for instance, the tendons of the biceps brachii (biceps tendon—anterior) and triceps brachii (triceps tendon—posterior) at the elbow joint (Table 6-2). The movements in this location occur around the frontal axis in a sagittal plane. For example, isolate the elbow joint during performance of a biceps curl. When extending a rigid bar through the elbow joint from the medial surface through to the lateral surface and making the movement around the frontal axis, the movement would occur in the sagittal plane around a frontal axis.

Table 6-2 *Movements that Occur in the Sagittal Plane around a Frontal Axis*

Movement	Description of the Movement	Location of the Movement
Flexion	Decrease in the joint angle as the movement occurs in the sagittal plane	Elbow, knee, ankle, wrist, neck, trunk, shoulder, hip
Extension	Increase in the joint angle as the movement occurs in the sagittal plane	Elbow, knee, ankle, wrist, neck, trunk, shoulder, hip

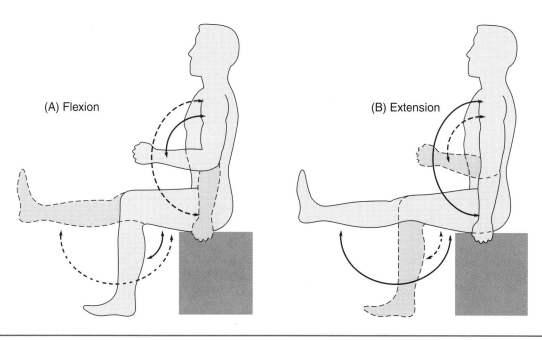

Figure 6-7 *Flexion and Extension*

OTA Perspective

To an OT practitioner, an activity analysis is an investigation of sorts, or a scrutiny, of a task. It is a process that contributes to clinical reasoning and is a basis for choosing and adapting or grading activities used in OT treatment. Its focus is on the task components in terms of activity demands—what needs to be done to the activity in order for it to be accomplished. A performance analysis is a skilled observation of what and how a person accomplishes a task, focusing on the performance skills and client factors; outcomes may be viewed in terms of independence, safety, effectiveness, and efficiency. The rest of the aspects of *The Framework* should be taken into consideration with both activity and performance analyses.

OT practitioners are uniquely skilled in analyzing the demands of both the activity and occupation and in analyzing the person's performance—ability to engage in occupation—and then determining the necessity for bridging the gap in any dissonance between the two. Using OT models of practice guide "what" is done to bridge that disparity.

Joint Movements of the Frontal Plane

Movements of the human body that occur in the frontal plane do so around a sagittal axis (Figure 6-8A–F). The existing tendons that cause movement in the frontal plane, in most cases, cross either the medial or lateral surface of the joint (Table 6-3). For example, the tendon of the supraspinatus muscle crosses on the superolateral surface, whereas the latissimus dorsi muscle crosses the inferomedial portion of the shoulder joint. The best example of a movement that occurs in the frontal axis is a jumping jack movement. While observing this movement, imagine a rigid bar that extends from the anterior surface through the posterior surface of the shoulder and hip joints. As the muscles contract to move the joint through a full range of motion, they cause movement in the frontal plane around the sagittal axis.

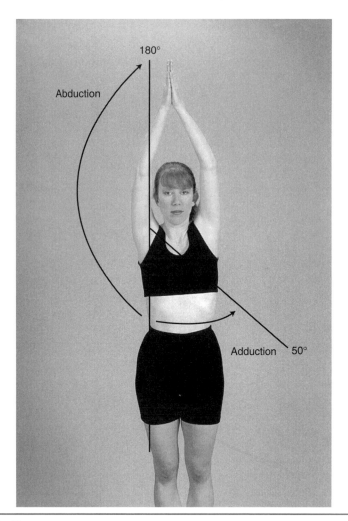

Figure 6-8A *Abduction and Adduction*

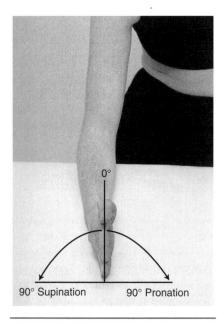

Figure 6-8B *Supination and Pronation*

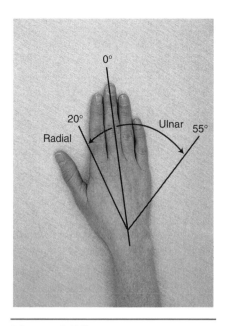

Figure 6-8C *Radial and Ulnar Deviation*

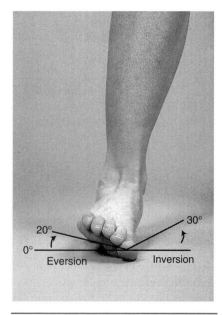

Figure 6-8D *Eversion and Inversion*

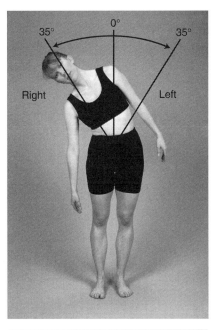

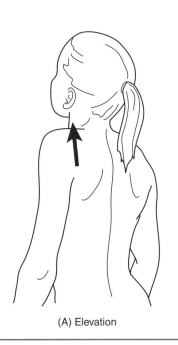

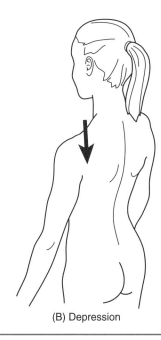

(A) Elevation

(B) Depression

Figure 6-8E *Lateral Bending*

Figure 6-8F *Elevation and Depression*

Table 6-3 *Movements that Occur in the Frontal Plane around a Sagittal Axis*

Movement	Description of the Movement	Location of the Movement	Figure
Abduction	Lateral and superior movements of a segment away from the midline	Shoulder and hip	6-8A
Adduction	Medial and inferior movements of a segment toward the midline	Shoulder and hip	6-8A
Elevation	Superior movement of the segment	Clavicle and scapula	6-8F
Depression	Inferior movement of the segment	Clavicle and scapula	6-8F
Inversion	Medial border of a segment moves in the superior direction	Medial border of the foot	6-8D
Eversion	Medial border of a segment moves in the inferior direction	Medial border of the foot	6-8D
Lateral Bending	Trunk moves toward either side	Trunk region	6-8E
Pronation	Elbow is flexed to 90 degrees and the palm is turned down toward the floor	Wrist	6-8B
Supination	Elbow is flexed to 90 degrees and the palm is turned up toward the ceiling	Wrist	6-8B
Radial Deviation	Thumb is moved toward the radius	Wrist	6-8C
Ulnar Deviation	Digiti minimi is moved toward the ulna	Wrist	6-8C

Joint Movements of the Transverse Plane

The third type of motion that occurs in various joints takes place around a vertical axis in the transverse plane (Figure 6-9A–D). The movements in this category are similar to those of an ice skater skating on a pond. The ice is the transverse plane, and the blade of the skate is in the vertical plane. As the skater makes a rotation, the movement occurs in the transverse plane around a vertical axis plane (Table 6-4). The tendons of the muscles that cause movements in the transverse plane often wrap around the muscle and insert into a large muscle groove that lies in the transverse plane. For example, the insertion of the latissimus dorsi muscle runs from the posterior portion of the humerus, around the lateral side, and inserts into the medial lip of the bicipital groove. The position of this tendon enhances the rotating movements that occur in the transverse plane.

Table 6-4   *Movements that Occur in the Transverse Plane around a Vertical Axis*

Movement	Description of the Movement	Location of the Movement	Figure
Internal Rotation	Digit is moved toward the midline around a vertical axis	Shoulder and hip	6-9B
External Rotation	Digit is moved away from the midline around a vertical axis	Shoulder and hip	6-9B
Horizontal Abduction	Joint is flexed to 90 degrees and the segment moves away from the midline	Shoulder and hip	6-9C
Horizontal Adduction	Joint is flexed to 90 degrees and the segment moves toward the midline	Shoulder and hip	6-9C
Protraction	The medial border of the scapula moves away from the midline	Scapulothoracic joint	6-9D
Retraction	The medial border of the scapula moves towards the midline	Scapulothoracic joint	6-9D

Circumduction

One movement that is often confused with a planar movement is **circumduction** (Figure 6-10). Circumduction is a movement that occurs when one is standing in the anatomical position and moves the arms or legs in a circular fashion. This movement does not occur in a specific plane around a specific axis. In fact, it is a combination of movements that occurs in the frontal and sagittal axes. As the arm moves in a circle, it does so with flexion and extension movements in the sagittal plane and abduction and adduction in the frontal plane. These movements are nonplanar and, therefore, are classified as a combination movement.

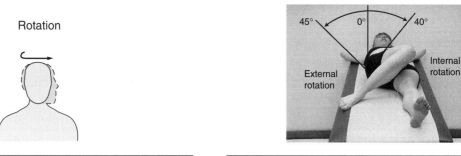

Figure 6-9A   *Rotation*

Figure 6-9B   *Internal and External Rotation*

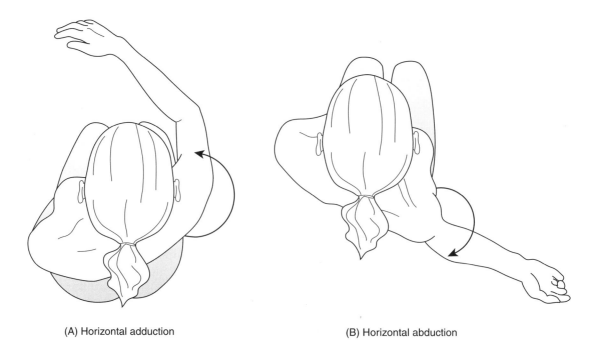

(A) Horizontal adduction

(B) Horizontal abduction

Figure 6-9C   *Horizontal Adduction and Horizontal Abduction*

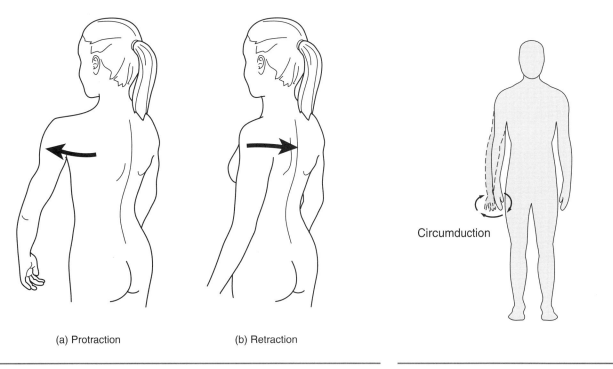

(a) Protraction   (b) Retraction

Figure 6-9D *Protraction and Retraction*   **Figure 6-10** *Circumduction*

KEY CONCEPTS

■ Movements occur in three different planes around three different axes.

■ The three major joint classifications are fibrous, cartilaginous, and synovial.

■ The four subclasses of diarthrodial joints are nonaxial, uniaxial, biaxial, and triaxial.

■ The common structures found in all synovial joints are articular cartilage, articular capsule, synovial fluid, ligaments, and tendons.

■ Ligaments play an important role in the structure of each joint and in human movement. They provide support for the joint, allowing the joint to move within a certain area while also allowing the joint to return to its normal state.

■ There are many movements that occur at the different joints. Review Tables 6-2 through 6-4 for a complete list.

BIBLIOGRAPHY

Green, D. P., & Roberts, S. L. (1999). *Kinesiology: Movement in the context of activity*. St. Louis, MO: Mosby.

Guyton, A. C. (2000). *Textbook of medical physiology* (10th ed.). Philadelphia: W. B. Saunders.

Konin, J. G. (1999). *Practical kinesiology for the physical therapy assistant*. Thorofare, NJ: Slack.

Marieb, E. N. (2003). *Human anatomy and physiology* (6th ed.). Menlo Park, CA: Addison Wesley Longman.

Taber's cyclopedic medical dictionary (19th ed.). (2001). Philadelphia: F. A. Davis.

WEB RESOURCES

- The Arthritis Foundation at www.arthritis.org features the many different facets of the Arthritis Foundation, such as current events and arthritis news.
- Arthritis.com at www.arthritis.com features facts about treatment of arthritis, pain management, assistive products, and more.
- Sports Injury Clinic.net at www.sportsinjuryclinic.net features links to fact sheets regarding many common types of sports injuries. This includes a description of the injury, common treatments, and what modalities a sports medical doctor would prescribe for treament of sports-related injuries.
- Joint Injury.com at www.jointinjury.com features visual representations of different common joint injuries. This includes force vectors and how injuries occur.

(These Web addresses were current as of September 2003.)

REVIEW QUESTIONS

Fill in the Blank

Provide the word(s) or phrase(s) that best completes the sentence.

1. Articular cartilage is made up of _____ cartilage.

2. Movement in the _____ plane occurs around a frontal axis.

3. Movement in the transverse plane occurs around a _____ axis.

4. The tendons of the muscles that make up the rotator cuff include the _____, _____, _____, and _____ .

5. The type of connective tissue that makes up a synarthrodial tissue is strong _____ connective tissue.

6. A jumping jack movement would occur in the _____ plane.

7. The articular capsule is made up of two components, including the _____ capsule and the _____ membrane.

8. Ligaments are similar to the tendons of muscles by the fact that they are continuous with the _____ of bone.

9. Synovial joints are different than amphiarthrodial and synarthrodial joints because they allow for greater _____.

10. The motion that occurs around the knee joint when kicking a soccer ball occurs in the _____ plane around a _____ axis.

Multiple Choice

Select the best answer to complete the following statements.

1. The _____ joint is a triaxial joint because it allows motion in three planes.
   a. elbow
   b. metacarpophalangeal
   c. saddle
   d. acetabulofemoral

2. The _____ joint is a biaxial joint because it allows motion in two planes.
   a. elbow
   b. metacarpophalangeal
   c. interphalangeal
   d. acetabulofemoral

3. The _____ joint is a uniaxial joint because it allows motion in one plane.
   a. glenohumoral
   b. metacarpophalangeal
   c. interphalangeal
   d. acetabulofemoral

4. An axis is referred to as a rigid bar. Another term that could also describe an axis is _____ .
   a. segment
   b. pivot point
   c. force
   d. area where a movement occurs

5. The fluid found within the joint capsule is known as _____ fluid.
   a. articular
   b. ligament
   c. cartilaginous
   d. synovial

6. The flexion movement occurs in a _____ plane around a _____ axis.
   a. frontal/sagittal
   b. sagittal/frontal
   c. transverse/vertical
   d. vertical/transverse

7. The adduction movement occurs in a _____ plane around a _____ axis.
   a. frontal/sagittal
   b. sagittal/frontal
   c. transverse/vertical
   d. vertical/transverse

8. The rotation movement occurs in a _____ plane around a _____ axis.
   a. frontal/sagittal
   b. sagittal/frontal
   c. transverse/vertical
   d. vertical/transverse

9. The inversion movement occurs in a _____ plane around a _____ axis.
   a. frontal/sagittal
   b. sagittal/frontal
   c. transverse/vertical
   d. vertical/transverse

10. The _____ movement does not occur in a specific given plane, yet it occurs in two different planes.
   a. horizontal adduction
   b. circumduction
   c. lateral bending
   d. elevation

Matching

Match the following joints with the proper joint classification. A term may be used more than once.

_____ **1.** Pubic joint		A. Syndesmoses
_____ **2.** Glenohumoral joint		B. Gomphoses
_____ **3.** Vertebral disks		C. Synchondroses
_____ **4.** Found at the distal tibia and fibula		D. Suture
_____ **5.** Cranial joint		E. Uniaxial
_____ **6.** Radioulnar joint		F. Biaxial
_____ **7.** Metatarsophalangeal joint		G. Triaxial
_____ **8.** Found in the teeth		H. Symphysis
_____ **9.** Intertarsal joint		I. Nonaxial
_____**10.** Sacroiliac joint		

Critical Thinking

1. Draw a table showing the differences and similarities of osteoarthritis and rheumatoid arthritis. Include the following:

   ■ Age of onset

   ■ Gender ratio

   ■ Joints affected

   ■ Etiology

   ■ Pathology of the joints

   ■ Diagnostic tests

2. Define the following terms and describe a clinical situation in which they would occur. Name the specific joint and the pathology that would be occurring.

   ■ Joint effusion

   ■ Laxity

   ■ Hypomobility

   ■ Instability

3. Give examples of how the following factors may influence range of motion in synovial joints during goniometric assessment: psychological, environmental, skeletal.

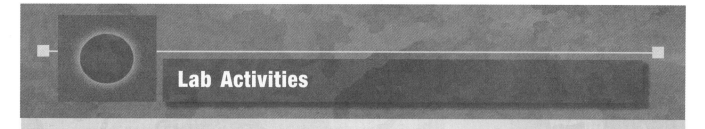

Lab Activities

Lab 6-1: Movement of Joints in Planes and Axes

Objective: To identify the planes and axes wherein different movements occur.

Equipment Needed: A lab partner, pen/pencil, paper

Step 1.   Starting in the anatomical position, instruct your partner in the following movements at the specific joints:
- Shoulder abduction
- Ankle dorsiflexion
- Elbow extension
- Foot eversion
- Forearm pronation
- Lumbar spine side bending
- Wrist flexion
- Cervical spine flexion
- Hip internal rotation

Step 2.   Document the planes and the axes wherein the movements take place.

Step 3.   Analyze whether these movements are a concentric, an eccentric, or a gravity counterbalanced activity.

Step 4.   Switch roles with your partner and repeat the steps above.

Lab 6-2: Petting a Cat Activity Analysis

Objective: To analyze the multiple functional components of a simple activity in terms of joint structure.

Equipment Needed: Group setting, cat, goniometer, pencils, paper

Step 1.   Observe the movements necessary for petting a cat.

Step 2.   Document the joints used and the planes and axes where the movements occur.

Step 3.   Consider how this activity would be altered in a person suffering from joint disease or an injury such as juvenile rheumatoid arthritis (JRA), a subluxed shoulder, or flexion contractures of the metacarpophalangeal (MCP) joints of the dominant hand. How does this joint condition affect the movement of petting the cat? Address the probable impairment in terms of (1) planes and axis of movement; (2) joint classification and corresponding subclassification; and (3) subsequent effects to common structures (e.g., ligaments).

Step 4.   As a means of developing clinical reasoning, move from the identifications mentioned in Step 3 to the *OT Framework* and to OT models of practice—in general, occupational performance based and impairment or deficit based. Discuss OT treatment from both perspectives.

Chapter 7

MUSCLE MECHANICS AND ARTHROKINEMATICS

Key Words

active insufficiency	force arm	osteokinematics
anatomical pulley	fulcrum	passive insufficiency
arthrokinematics	glide motion	resistance
closed kinetic chain	kinetic chain	resistance arm
closed-packed position	lever	roll motion
concave	lever classes	second-class lever
convex	leverage	spin motion
excursion	mechanical advantage	third-class lever
first-class lever	open kinetic chain	
force	open-packed position	

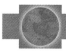

INTRODUCTION

Because you have chosen to explore the field of kinesiology, you are probably gaining an appreciation for the strategic design of the human body. For example, the fibrous suture joints of the skull allow a minute amount of movement for very good reason. Excessive movement at the suture joints of the skull could be detrimental to the protection of the brain. Now imagine some of the complex athletic movements or even the activities of daily living that the body and its segments allow. The wide range of human movements performed by the body and its segments are directly attributed to the various joints and joint structures that comprise the human body. Furthermore, the shape of the bones that comprise the joints determines the function of each specific joint in the body. This chapter explores the specific interaction between the bones and muscles, and the resulting movement that occurs.

The ability of a joint to move is directly related to the **arthrokinematics** that occur at a joint. The term *arthrokinematic* is taken from the Greek roots "arthro," meaning joint, and "kines," meaning movement. Arthrokinematics describes the interaction between the articular, or joint, surfaces of two bones, causing movement. In particular, the specific shape of each articulating bone in a joint has an impact on the type of motion that can occur at the joint. Contrast arthrokinematics with the term **osteokinematics**. Osteokinematics describes the specific joint motion occurring at a joint, such as flexion, abduction, and so on. In a sense, osteokinematics determines the "big picture" of joint movement, whereas arthrokinematics describes the more detailed relationship of bony segments moving with one another.

LEVER CLASSES

When an individual studies the distinct physical mechanics of the human body, one of the most important factors to understand is the complex mechanics through which the **lever classes** enhance human movements. A **lever** is a rigid bar around which a movement occurs around an axis. In human movement, the rigid bar is the bone segment and the pivot point, or fulcrum, is the joint around which the movements occur. Levers are also specifically designed to provide **leverage** to increase the amount of work that occurs during a muscle contraction. In addition to understanding lever principles, it is important to know that levers provide mechanical advantage to the movements that occur in a given region. The exact location of a muscle in the human body, in relation to the position of the joint where the muscle moves around, provides this advantage to human movement.

OTA Perspective

Consider the pediatric practice of not "labeling" or diagnosing children with physical disabilities that limit their ability to function "normally" or that is considered typical for their expected development. Rather, major symptoms that impede function are grouped as (1) muscle weakness, (2) limited joint range of motion (ROM), and (3) uncoordination. When an infant or very young child receives the diagnosis cerebral palsy (CP), the health care providers will associate functional abilities and disabilities; adaptive equipment and durable medical equipment (DME) for now and the predictable future; and even management of social, financial, and emotional issues to the diagnosis, sometimes without first considering who the child is. The danger is in "wearing blinders" that focus on the treatment, but do not readily allow for variations of each child's unique situations.

Reflect on what you consider the pros and cons of labeling very young children, both in the big picture and in terms of muscle mechanics.

The lever has three components that have to be present in order to function in an optimal manner. The first component of the lever is the **fulcrum** (Δ) around which movements in the body occur. In the human body, the fulcrum is a joint around which the muscles pull to move the different bone segments through a full range of motion. The second component to the lever system is the **force** (F) that moves the lever around a specific fulcrum. The force can be the force of a contracting muscle or the vertical force of gravity; for example, when performing a biceps curl, the force of the biceps' contraction causes the radius and ulna to move around the elbow joint. The third component of the lever is the **resistance** (R) that is applied to the lever, or what the force is moving against. Taking the biceps curl example once again, the resistance is the weight that is being moved. Both the force and resistance occur in opposite directions from one another in the vertical plane.

Mechanical Advantage

The **mechanical advantage** that a lever provides is directly related to the distance that the force and resistance are applied from the fulcrum of a given joint structure. The distance of the force to the fulcrum is called the **force arm**, and the distance of the resistance to the axis is called the **resistance arm**. To better understand this relationship, imagine one child weighing 100 pounds (Child A) and another child weighing 50 pounds (Child B) playing on a teeter-totter. In this scenario, if both children sat on the bar at the same time, Child B would be elevated off the ground because the force arm provided by Child B would be less than the resistance arm of Child A (Figure 7-1A). If Child B asked Child A to move closer to the axis around which the movement occurs, the lever arms would equal out and the two children would be able to proceed with the teeter-totter game (Figure 7-1B). This scenario is also an example of mechanical efficiency in that as Child A moves closer to the fulcrum of the teeter-totter, the weight distributes evenly, resulting in mechanical advantage for Child B. The equation for finding the mechanical advantage is as follows:

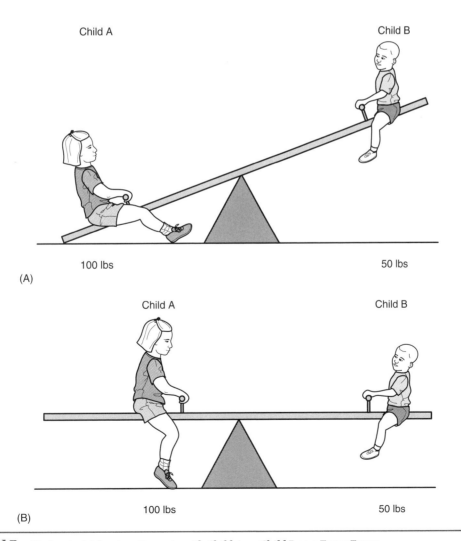

Figure 7-1A and B *Mechanical Advantage Scenario with Child A vs. Child B on a Teeter Totter*

$$MA = \frac{\text{The length of the force arm}}{\text{The length of the resistance arm}}$$

First-Class Levers

A **first-class lever** is found in situations where the fulcrum lies between the force and the resistance (Figure 7-2). The first-class lever is present when a segment of the body requires balance for optimal performance. For example, the head sits on the atlantooccipital joint (OA joint) where the base of the occipital bone articulates with the atlas bone. In this scenario, the OA joint is the fulcrum, and the force and resistance are applied lateral to the joint (Figure 7-3). Another example would be of an individual performing the lateral flexion activity of the neck where the head is displaced to the right. The sternocleidomastoid muscle of the right side would provide the force for the lateral bending movement, and the sternocleidomastoid muscle on the left combined with gravity would provide the resistance. Two other examples in which first-class levers are found are in teeter-totters and scissors.

Second-Class Levers

The **second-class lever** is found in locations where large weights can be moved by smaller amounts of force. They are defined by situations where the resistance lies closer to the fulcrum than the force (Figure 7-4). Figure 7-5 depicts a man moving a wheelbarrow full of dirt. In this example, the fulcrum is the tire, the barrel and load of dirt being moved are the resistance, and the force is located at the handlebars that are used to move the wheelbarrow. The mechanical advantage in this scenario is provided by the smaller forces applied to the heavy loads in the wheelbarrow.

Second-class levers are arguably the least common lever class in the human body. The main example of a second-class lever that can be applied to the human body occurs at the tibiotalar joint in which an individual moves from the standing to tiptoe position (however, this example is debatable). In the example shown in Figure 7-6, the fulcrum is found at the metatarsophalangeal joint in the foot, the resistance is the body weight, and the force is applied at the calcaneal tuberosity. As such, a smaller force is produced by the muscle contraction of the gastrocnemius muscle (calf) pulling on the calcaneal tuberosity, which results in moving the entire weight of the human body.

Third-Class Levers

The universal lever class in the human body is defined as the **third-class lever**. In this lever class, the force is applied closer to the fulcrum than to the resistance (Figure 7-7). The mechanical advantage provided by the third-class lever is opposite that of the second-class lever. In third-class levers, smaller amounts of resistance are moved by larger amounts of force. This arrangement allows the body to move an object for a greater amount of time over a greater distance.

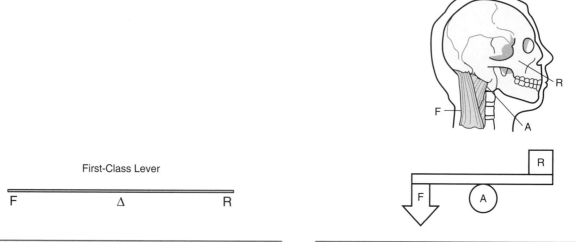

First-Class Lever

F   Δ   R

Figure 7-2 *Schematic Drawing of a First-Class Lever*

Figure 7-3 *Example of a First-Class Lever*

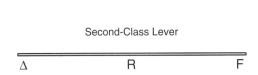

Second-Class Lever

Δ   R   F

Figure 7-4   *Schematic Drawing of a Second-Class Lever*

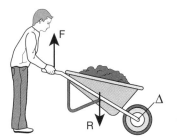

Figure 7-5   *Example of a Second-Class Lever*

The third-class lever is located around many joints in the human body where the muscle inserts proximal to where the resistance is moved during concentric exercise. The insertion directly enhances the amount of force produced at the joint. A great example of a third-class lever is that of the rectus femoris muscle of the quadriceps muscle group inserting into the tibial tuberosity of the tibia and performing a concentric movement (Figure 7-8). At this location, the knee acts as the fulcrum around which the movements occur. Proximal to the resistance on the leg is the insertion of the rectus femoris into the tibial tuberosity, which provides the force to move the resistance. Learning the muscles in the human body helps in identifying the third-class levers by observing the insertion of the muscle and where the resistance occurs when the muscle moves.

A difficult concept for students to understand is the "trade-off" of lever classes as the muscle action changes from concentric to eccentric. As the need for stability during a muscle contraction changes from concentric to eccentric, the lever class also changes from third class to second class. In the previous example, it has been well defined that during the concentric exercise, the force is produced by the contraction of the rectus femoris muscle that moves the resistance occurring at the leg and foot. During eccentric contractions, however, force becomes the force of gravity exerting a force in the inferior vertical direction on the extremities, whereas the eccentric movement of the rectus femoris causes the resistance acting in the superior direction. This trade-off scenario is true in most cases and allows for the mechanical efficiency involved in the muscle contraction to shift during concentric and eccentric muscle contractions.

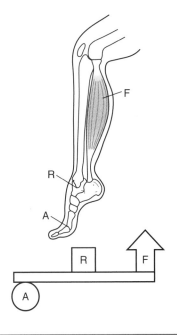

Figure 7-6   *Calf Raise Exercise as a Second-Class Lever*

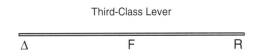

Third-Class Lever

Δ   F   R

Figure 7-7   *Schematic Drawing of a Third-Class Lever*

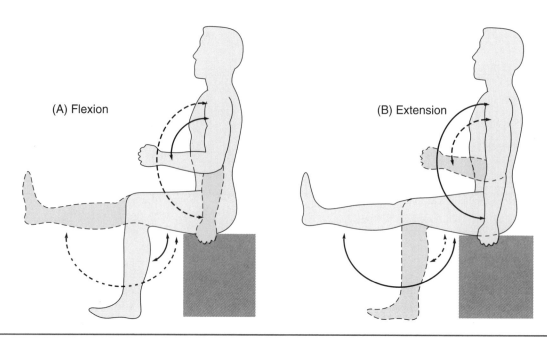

Figure 7-8 *Example of a Third-Class Lever*

ANATOMICAL PULLEYS

When people think of a pulley system, they often visualize numerous ropes threaded through devices that cause rotation. The purpose of the pulley is to produce equilibrium between the force arm and resistance arm by increasing the number of rotation axes. The action of the rope through the pulley system causes an increase in the force, which creates a situation wherein the application of force is maximized by the distance through which an object can be moved. Although the body is not made up of ropes, there are several instances where a bone is formed within a muscle, mimicking this pulley relationship. This anatomical arrangement causes an increase in the amount of force applied to an object during a muscle contraction, producing a more powerful contraction.

The classic example of an **anatomical pulley** in the human body is located at the knee joint (Figure 7-9). In this location, the patella lies within the tendon of the quadriceps muscle group. Through this arrangement, the patella increases the amount of force (force arm) produced by the quadriceps muscle group contractions by providing a larger surface area that the muscle can pull on. Therefore, the contractions of the quadriceps muscles are often the most powerful contractions that occur in the human body. Another location is where two sesamoid bones form an anatomical pulley on the inferior surface of the first metatarsal. These two bones are formed within the tendon of the flexor hallicus longus muscle and increase the force arm, which translates to a powerful muscle contraction of the foot. Another example is where tendons of various muscles wrap around bony processes and anatomical grooves. For instance, take the medial and lateral malleolus located at the distal end of the tibia and fibula. In these locations the muscles that cause movements of the ankle wrap posterior to these structures. This increases the force arm, resulting in a greater force production during muscle contractions of these muscles.

LENGTH AND TENSION RELATIONSHIPS

When performing muscle contractions during weight lifting or other physical activity, one may notice that when a given muscle is at variable lengths, different amounts of tension are produced. What is the cause of this phenomenon and how are these states overcome? To understand the change of force production during a muscle contraction, the physical events of the myofibrils and the events that occur when a muscle crosses more than one joint must be understood first.

When a muscle contracts or extends, it does so up to half of the length of the resting length, which is known as the muscle excursion. A muscle will also have enough **excursion** for it to move through a full range of motion. For example, the resting length of the rectus femoris muscle (quadriceps muscle) is 1 1/2 feet to 2 feet. When the rectus femoris muscle contracts and extends its excursion, its length becomes between 1 foot and 3 feet.

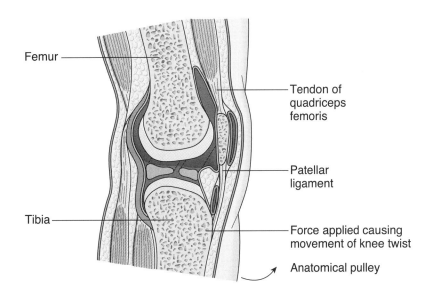

Femur

Tendon of quadriceps femoris

Patellar ligament

Tibia

Force applied causing movement of knee twist

Anatomical pulley

Figure 7-9 *Anatomical Pulley: Patella of the Knee Joint*

The different lengths that a muscle can be stretched or contracted often dictate the range of motion and the amount of force during its contraction. During the muscle contraction, the muscle also produces varied forces at different times.

The length-tension relationship of a muscle is a vital concept. Most of the work leading to the understanding of the relationship between the stretch on a muscle and the tension it is capable of producing was obtained in a laboratory through experiments with isolated single muscle fibers. Data were obtained by experimentally stretching a muscle to different lengths and stimulating it to contract.

The length-tension relationship of a muscle fiber describes the connection between the tension generation capability of a muscle and the overlap of the myofilaments of the contracting sarcomere. It is difficult to imagine that the actions of the microscopic myofilaments can have such a profound effect on the entire muscle. The optimal length-tension relationship occurs when the muscle is slightly stretched and the actin and myosin filaments slightly overlap. This slight overlap allows the myosin filaments to slide along the entire length of the actin, thus producing a great amount of tension. In other words, a muscle is strongest if it is slightly stretched before contracting. Think of instances in which this concept can be applied. Imagine a baseball player throwing a ball to first base. The pectoralis major, anterior deltoid, and internal rotators (to name a few) are all muscles that have to stretch before they can contract to create the greatest amount of force produced. What happens to a soccer player who kicks a ball? During the backswing, the rectus femoris and iliopsoas muscles are stretched before they shorten, or contract, thus producing more tension (Figure 7-10).

But what happens if a muscle is not in its ideal stretched condition before it contracts? If a muscle is stretched so far that there is no overlap of myofilaments before contraction, no tension can be generated because the cross-bridges have nothing to attach to. Imagine a baseball player attempting to throw a baseball if the shoulder joint and surrounding muscles are stretched much farther than normal. In addition to injury, those muscles will not be able to contract with a large amount of force because of the lack of overlap between actin and myosin filaments. On the other hand, imagine the myofilaments being so overlapped that the Z lines merge with the myosin filaments and very little shortening can occur.

One other factor regarding muscle function and the amount of excursion provided by a muscle is the relationship between the muscle and the number of joints that a muscle crosses. The amount of excursion provided by muscles that cross single joints is much greater than the amount of excursion provided for multijoint muscles. In multiple-joint muscles, one region of a contracting muscle produces a movement at one joint, whereas at the other joint the muscle produces a force that stabilizes the muscle contraction. For example, observe the differences between the biceps brachii and brachioradialis muscles that cause movements of the elbow joint. During elbow flexion, the brachioradialis (single joint) muscle shortens to one half of its resting length and has more than enough excursion ability to move the elbow through a full range of motion. The biceps brachii however, is a two-joint muscle. During contractions that involve the biceps, the origin on the scapula must stabilize the shoulder joint and produce the forces that cause the movement of the elbow through a full range of motion. The multifunctions of these muscles inhibit the action of the muscle and limit its ability to contract around two different joints.

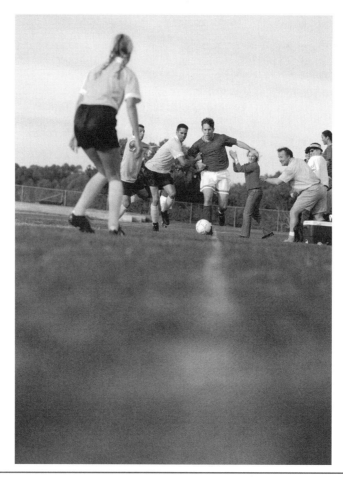

Figure 7-10 *Soccer Kick (Courtesy of Photodisc)*

Active Insufficiency

During a muscle contraction, the myofilaments pull both Z discs to the center of the sarcomere. In single-joint movements, the excursion of the muscle is large enough to ensure that the two actin strands of two adjacent sarcomeres never meet. This creates a situation where force and tension is maintained to work against resistance that occurs during human movement. In two-joint muscles, however, the excursion is less than the single-joint muscle and the distal ends of two adjacent actin myofilaments meet at the center of the sarcomere. Therefore, when the actin myofilaments join together in the center of the sarcomere, the contraction stops and the muscle is in a state of **active insufficiency**. When a two-joint muscle is in a state of active insufficiency, it loses its ability to shorten any further. Active insufficiency results in the termination of force production because of the termination of the contractile excursion. A muscle that crosses two joints has the potential for causing movements at two joints but can only perform one action efficiently.

When studying the concept of active insufficiency, try the following two examples with a partner. In the first example, shake your partner's hand with the elbow flexed and the hand in the same plane as the forearm. In this situation you will be able to give a firm handshake because you have not exceeded the excursion of the muscles that cause actions of the hand and fingers. In the second example, shake your partner's hand with the elbow and hand both in flexed positions. In these positions, the cross-bridges are complete and no further forces can be produced to adequately squeeze the hand of your partner. In the second example, the muscles that cause actions of the hand and fingers are at the point where the actin myofilaments have come together in the middle of the sarcomere and cannot contract any further.

Passive Insufficiency

Active insufficiency refers to the contractile excursion movements caused by the agonist muscle. In similar fashion, **passive insufficiency** is directly related to the full stretch of the antagonist muscle when the agonist is in a state of active insufficiency. During stretching movements, the actin myofilaments move away from the center of the sarcomere while stabilizing the muscle contraction. Much like active insufficiency, passive insufficiency directly relates the point at which the antagonist muscle can no longer be stretched.

The same handshaking example can be applied to passive insufficiency. In the first example, the single-joint muscles that act on the hand can be stretched to a point where the excursion is not sacrificed. However, in the second example where the elbow and wrist are both flexed, the antagonist muscles to the agonist are stretched to a point that they will not extend further. When you perform this movement for a second time, realize that the pain comes from the antagonist muscles located on the opposite side of the muscles that cause flexion of the elbow, wrist, and fingers.

FORCE–VELOCITY RELATIONSHIP

Another common concept or principle that is crucial to completely understand in muscle function is the relationship between the velocity of a contraction and the amount of force produced. Simply stated, the force generated in a muscle contraction is directly related to the velocity of a muscle contraction and vice versa. See Figure 7-11 to assist in understanding this concept.

At any certain point, the force generated in a muscle contraction depends on the number of cross-bridges attached. As muscle-shortening velocity is slowed, as in area A in Figure 7-11, more cross-bridges have time to attach, thereby increasing force. Conversely, if the myofilaments slide past each other at a rapid rate, force decreases owing to a lower number of attached cross-bridges. As you can see, the force drops off sharply when the shortening velocity switches from negative (eccentric) to positive (concentric).

As shown in Figure 7-11, a muscle can generate a great amount of tension during an eccentric contraction. Many activities of daily living, as well as athletic movements, require concentric-eccentric muscle patterns. In addition, eccentric muscle actions are used as a form of resistance training, so proper understanding of these actions is imperative for the fitness specialist or rehabilitation coordinator.

KINETIC CHAINS

As you probably know by now, the human body is comprised of a series of bones or rigid links held together by an array of musculature, ligaments, tendons, and cartilage. Simply stated, muscles contract and a force is exerted on the rigid links (bones), which cause movement of the bone or body segment. Many times movement is not restricted to just one body segment but on multiple joints or a series of body segments. The concept of the kinetic chain can be used to describe movement of a series of body segments that are connected to one another.

The **kinetic chain** of a given region refers to the ability of multiple joints to move together through a full range of motion. The farther the muscle is away from the axial skeleton results in a greater free range of movement, because the more proximal bones provide the sound base of support for human movements. The concept of a kinetic chain can be described in terms of open or closed kinetic chains.

Open Kinetic Chains

During contractions of the various muscle groups, the insertion of a muscle often moves freely through a full range of motion in the direction of its origin. For example, when performing a biceps curl, the forearm segment moves toward the upper arm or, more specifically, the radial tuberosity, and the forearm moves toward the supraglenoid tubercle and coracoid

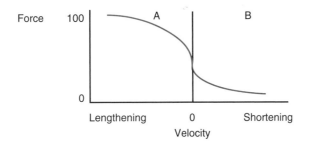

Figure 7-11 *Force-velocity Curve*

process of the scapula. The ability of the elbow to move in this sequence is known as an **open kinetic chain**. In most open chain circumstances the more distally located muscles pull on the more stable proximal bones, resulting in their greater ability to move freely through a full range of motion. Other examples of open kinetic chain movements include seated leg extensions and lateral shoulder raises.

Closed Kinetic Chain

Closed kinetic chain movements occur when a proximal bone is fixed in place and the origin moves toward the insertion. For example, in the classic pull-up exercise the hands are fixed about a bar. During the muscle contraction, the biceps brachii muscles contract to move the body in the superior direction toward the hands. As a result the origin of the biceps brachii muscle, located at the supraglenoid tubercle and coracoid process, move toward the fixed radial tuberosity or insertion. Other examples of closed kinetic chain movements include squatting and push-ups.

When studying movements in greater depth, observe the relationships between open and closed kinetic chains that occur throughout the body.

CONVEX AND CONCAVE RELATIONSHIPS

The specific design of the diarthrodial joints gives rise to the various movements that occur on the joint surfaces (Figure 7-12). Recall from a previous discussion that arthrokinematics describes the interaction of the articulating surfaces of the bones in a joint. Each of the diarthrodial joints has one projection that has a **convex** shape that articulates with a **concave** structure. However, the extent to the concavity and convexity is different between the different joints. For example, observe the relationship between the convex head of the femur and the concave acetabulum of the hip joint compared to the joint articulations that exist between the phalanges. In the first example, the head is extremely convex versus the concave acetabulum of the pelvis. In fact, the junction here is so close that when the head of the femur is displaced from the acetabulum during surgery, the close proximity creates a suction noise. In the second example, the articulations between the phalangeal joints are almost flat and do not complete a tight fit.

The shape of the diarthrodial joint allows for specific movements to occur when the two articulations of the joint move around one another, such as glide, spin, and roll motions (Figure 7-13). The importance of these motions ensures that a joint will move through a full range of motion around a small surface area when the muscles contract.

Glide Motions

During **glide motions**, the two bones of a region move past each other, much like the parts of the continents moving by one another in plate tectonics. For example, when the wrist performs ulnar and radial deviation, the carpal bones glide past one another. If this relationship were not present, the close relationship between the carpal bones would prevent movement of the wrist in any direction.

Spin Motions

Spin motions exist when the articulation of one joint rotates around a single axis of the second articulation similarly to a top spinning on the surface of a table. During this motion, the top spins around a central axis and prevents movements in other directions. In the human body, spin motions occur mainly in areas composed of triaxial joints; only a few biaxial joints permit spin motions. The shoulder joint and hip joint are the simplest joints in which to observe the spin motion. As the joint moves through internal and external rotations, the heads of the humerus and femur spin on one central point.

Roll Motions

The most common motion that exists between two joints occurs when a surface of a joint rolls over the surface of a second joint. **Roll motions** exist when one point of a moving articulation is in contact with the joint surface of a fixed joint. The uniaxial, biaxial, and triaxial joints allow for roll motion. Take, for instance, the interphalangeal joints in the phalanges. As the muscles that cause movement contract, the distal phalanx roll over the proximal phalanx with one point maintaining contact throughout the movement.

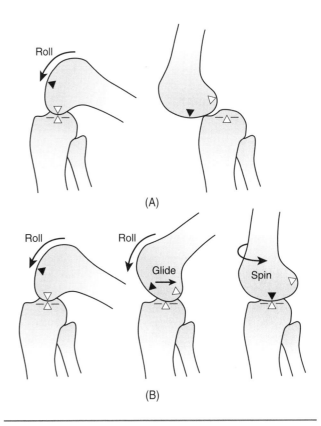

(A)

(B)

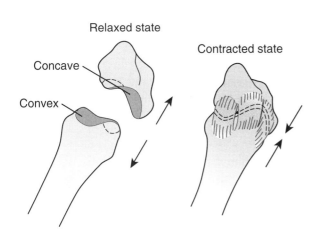

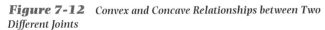

Figure 7-12 *Convex and Concave Relationships between Two Different Joints*

Figure 7-13 *Schematic Drawing of a Glide, Spin, and Roll Movement*

To help you understand the concept of glide, spin, and roll, use the skeletons in the classroom to help in your learning process. Observe each of the joints as they move through a full range of motion and determine what type of motion exists at the specific joint. Notice the importance of these movements in terms of surface area and range of motion.

Closed-Packed and Open-Packed Positions

The stability that the joint provides during a muscle contraction is based on what occurs to the structural support components and the convexity and concavity of a specific joint. As you observe the joints in the human body, you will notice that the convex and concave surfaces allow the bones to fit together much like two pieces of a puzzle. This close relationship enhances the stability and structural support of the joint. During the contraction and relaxation states, the joints maintain two totally different positions: closed and open packed.

Closed-Packed Position When the muscles that act around the major joints of the body contract, they cause the joints to fit together in a snug manner much like the two pieces of a puzzle as mentioned earlier. This action places the joint in the immovable position known as the **closed-packed position**. As the contraction occurs, it forces the two articulating concave and convex surfaces to make a sound immovable fit together. At this point the tendons that cross the joint also become taut, preventing movement of the joint. The combination of these events compresses the joint and limits the amount of movement that can exist in the given area.

A good example of the closed-packed position is at the knee joint when the muscles that act on it are contracted. Once the muscles around the knee joint contract, they force the medial and lateral condyles of the femur to compress into the medial and lateral meniscus of the tibia. As this action occurs, the tendons of the muscles that cause movement of the knee joint contract and prohibit movement of the knee joint.

Open-Packed Position Following a muscle contraction the joint moves back to the relaxed position. This is known as the **open-packed position**. The joint structures that were formerly compressed and the ligaments that pulled on the joint become relaxed. As a result of the relaxation process, the joints become pliable and more palpable.

Compared to the closed-packed position of the knee, in the open-packed position as the knee relaxes, the structures that were once compressed together and taut become relaxed. The joint can then be moved manually through a full range of motion.

Closed- and open-packed positions are important because of the support they give to the joints. Imagine what would happen to the structures of the joints if they did not lock into place or relax at different times. The amount of movement would be severely limited and the incidence of injury would be largely increased.

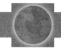 KEY CONCEPTS

■ Levers are found all around us. They assist us in moving and lifting tasks. Levers are also found in the human body. Various types of levers are designed for different functions.

■ There are three classes of levers; first, second, third. A first-class lever is designed for balance and is defined by the force and the resistance located on opposite sides of the fulcrum. A teeter-totter would be an example of a first-class lever. A second-class lever is defined by the resistance and force located on one side of the fulcrum, with the resistance closer to the fulcrum than the force. Second-class levers are designed for power. A wheelbarrow is an example of a second-class lever. Third-class levers are designed for range of motion. They are defined by the fulcrum at one end and the force and resistance on the same side, with the force located closer to the fulcrum than the resistance. An example would be the rectus femoris muscle attaching to the tibial tuberosity of the tibia and performing a knee extension exercise.

■ Active insufficiency describes a situation wherein a multijoint or two-joint muscle cannot shorten any further and thus incurs a loss of force production. Passive insufficiency occurs at the antagonist muscle and results in a decreased range of motion owing to the actin filaments moving away from the sarcomere.

■ Interactions between two-joint surfaces can give rise to various forms of movement, specifically, glide, spin, and roll motions. Glide motions can be described as two-joint surfaces gliding or sliding across one another during movement. Spin motions are described as one articulation rotating around a single axis during joint movement. Roll motions are described as various areas of one bone being in contact with a second bone throughout the range of joint motion. A conceptual understanding of these interactions is crucial to a practical understanding of joint movement and range of motion at various joints.

■ The convex-concave relationship of bones can provide further insight into the type of motion available at a specific joint. The convex portion of one bone comfortably "fits" into a concave portion of the articulating bone.

OTA Perspective

Be creative in designing your own "analogies" and methods for learning difficult concepts, for memorizing words and their meanings, and for drawing OTA conclusions from the study of kinesiology. Write a sing-song; make up a rhyme; create a memory/matching card game; make flash cards using symbols; highlight reading material in various colors; make a puzzle with items that have similar shapes or colors; bake cookies, cutting the dough into shapes that match bone structures; create a poem or limerick; make up a dance or a hand-clapping game to a specific sequence of words; or tell a far-fetched story illustrating related concepts. Using your "right brain" to learn concrete, linear, scientific concepts and "left brain" thinking really does assist one to become skilled in this tangible study of kinesiology.

BIBLIOGRAPHY

Luttgens, K. (2000). *Kinesiology: Scientific basis of human motion* (9th ed.). Madison, WI: McGraw-Hill.

Smith, L. K., Weiss, E. L., & Lehmkuhl, D. L. (1996). *Brunnstrom's clinical kinesiology* (5th ed.). Philadelphia: F. A. Davis.

Tipens, P. E. (1994). *Basic technical physics* (2nd ed.). New York: Glencoe.

WEB RESOURCES

Visit these Web sites for additional information on kinesiology:
- The Kinesiology Network at www.kinesiology.net/
- The International College of Applied Kinesiology at www.icak.com/
- The American Academy of Kinesiology and Physical Education at www.aakpe.org/

(These Web addresses were current as of September 2003.)

REVIEW QUESTIONS

Fill in the Blank

Provide the word(s) or phrase(s) that best completes the sentence.

1. A type of lever in which the resistance lies closer to the fulcrum than the force is referred to as a _____ class lever.

2. The part of a joint that has a sunken structure that articulates with another structure that protrudes outward is called a _____ structure.

3. A type of lever in which the fulcrum lies between the force and resistance is referred to as a _____ class lever.

4. The point at which two-joint muscles can no longer be stretched is referred to as _____ _____.

5. During _____ motion, one point of the humerus will articulate with the glenoid fossa, causing internal and external rotations.

Multiple Choice

Select the best answer to complete the following statements.

1. The movement that occurs when the origin moves toward the insertion is better known as a/an _____ .
   a. open kinetic chain
   b. open-packed position
   c. closed kinetic chain
   d. closed-packed position

2. A condition in which the two articulating bones of a joint are compressed and the tendons around a joint are taut is referred to as a/an _____.
   a. open kinetic chain
   b. open-packed position
   c. closed kinetic chain
   d. closed-packed position

3. During a/an _____ the insertion moves toward the origin.
   a. open kinetic chain
   b. open-packed position
   c. closed kinetic chain
   d. closed-packed position

4. When the joint is relaxed and is most pliable, it is referred to as a/an _____.
   a. open kinetic chain
   b. open-packed position
   c. closed kinetic chain
   d. closed-packed position

5. A/an _____ exists during a situation in which the insertion is fixed and a muscle contraction occurs.
   a. open kinetic chain
   b. open-packed position
   c. closed kinetic chain
   d. closed-packed position

Matching

Match each of the following examples with the appropriate lever class.

_____ **1.** Atlanto-occipital joint

_____ **2.** Biceps brachii muscle

_____ **3.** Rectus femoris muscle

_____ **4.** A pair of scissors

_____ **5.** A wheelbarrow

_____ **6.** Pectoralis major

_____ **7.** A door working around a hinge

_____ **8.** A tire jack

_____ **9.** A crowbar

_____ **10.** The gastrocnemius muscle working around the calcaneal tuberosity

A. First-class lever

B. Second-class lever

C. Third-class lever

Critical Thinking

1. Choose 5 of the 10 examples from the Matching exercise section and draw a picture of the scenario. For each example, label the fulcrum, resistance, and force.

2. Currently, strength training literature supports the notion that eccentric resistance training exercises are extremely beneficial in strengthening musculature. Why might this be? Recalling your knowledge of physiology, what might be a negative aspect to training eccentrically all of the time?

3. All OTA students study kinesiology. Which areas of practice will use this knowledge—muscle mechanics, bone and joint structures, muscle characteristics —the most? What is it about those areas of practice and treatment settings that intrigue you the most? Because you will be working with a variety of clients, what diagnoses do you expect to treat? Which will be more familiar and which will be less common? Sometimes keeping the big picture in mind and the reasons you are studying OT and, subsequently kinesiology, helps in maintaining interest, motivation, and thirst for knowledge.

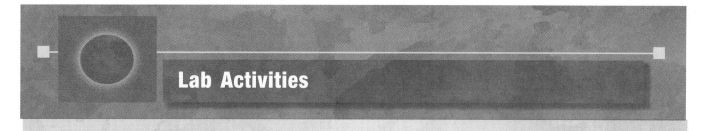

Lab Activities

Lab 7-1: Open and Closed Kinetic Chain

Objective: To identify and delineate between open and closed kinetic chain exercises.

Equipment needed: A lab partner, pen, paper, open fitness area

Step 1.   Choose a lower extremity conditioning exercise (walking, squatting, leg press, etc.) and perform this activity.

Step 2.   Your lab partner should record the name of the exercise and determine whether it is an open or closed kinetic chain exercise.

Step 3.   Have your lab partner choose an upper extremity conditioning exercise (push-up, dumbbell bench press, wall push-up, etc.) and perform this activity.

Step 4.   You should record the name of the exercise and determine whether it is an open or closed kinetic chain exercise.

Step 5.   Together discuss the benefits and drawbacks to open and closed kinetic chain exercises in a rehabilitation setting (remember to discuss the functionality of exercises and progression of rehabilitation exercises).

Lab 7-2: Arthrokinematics

Objective: To describe the various arthrokinematic motions that occur at various joints.

Equipment Needed: A skeleton

Step 1.   Locate the elbow joint on the skeleton. Manually move the elbow in a flexion/extension motion. Describe the type of motion (roll, spin, glide) occurring at the joint.

Step 2.   Locate the hip joint on the skeleton. Manually move the femur through internal and external rotation motions. Describe the type of motion (roll, spin, glide) occurring at the joint.

Step 3.   Locate the carpometacarpal joint of the thumb. Manually move the bones through motions. Describe the type of motion (roll, spin, glide) occurring at the joint.

Step 4.   Locate the wrist joint. Manually move the wrist through various motions (flexion, extension, radial and ulnar deviation). Describe the type of motion (glide, spin, roll) occurring at the joint.

Lab 7-3: Muscle Mechanics

Objective: To relate muscle mechanics to the growth and development of a child and then to OT interventions, including parent education.

Equipment Needed: Resource books and AOTA documents, child skeleton, group setting for role-play

Step 1.   Recall what you know about typical growth and development. Review the *OT Practice Framework*. Research or review OT in the school system and then reflect on the steps that follow in terms of mechanics of the musculoskeletal system. As an OTA, you are collaborating with the supervising OT about treatment ideas for a 5-year-old child you are treating in an academic (school) setting. This particular discussion concerns parent education and training of activities that can be incorporated into the family's home life and that augment the child's OT (education) goals. For the sake of reflection and discussion, assume a positive supervisory relationship, sufficient resources, an adequate comprehension of growth and development, and an appropriate level of confidence in your OTA skills and the ability to relate this knowledge to caregivers.

Step 2.   In terms of kinesiology concepts, specifically muscle mechanics, identify an activity that makes use of (1) third-class levers, (2) roll, spin, and glide motions, (3) open and closed kinetic chains, and (4) active and passive insufficiency. Identify one activity for each of the three symptom categories listed in the OTA perspectives boxes in this chapter. Incorporate the muscle mechanics into the identified activities, matching the major symptoms addressed.

(continues)

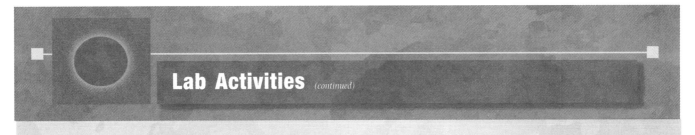

Lab Activities *(continued)*

Step 3. To expand on this scenario, and the activities you have identified with the incorporated muscle mechanics, role-play a discussion between the OT and the OTA regarding education treatment goals and subsequent home activities. Role-play an education session, with the OTA training the parent on specific goals and home treatment, involving the child in the training session. Does either of these role-plays seem realistic? Do OT practitioners really talk in terms of muscle mechanics? Do they talk that way to parents? If not, why study kinesiology to this depth? How does this study and ensuing knowledge impact clinical reasoning? Where does it fit within OT models of practice? It may be beneficial to observe an OT practitioner treat a child in a school setting and ask questions accordingly.

Part II
Muscles of the Axial
Skeleton & Respiration

Chapters 8-12

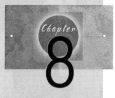
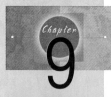
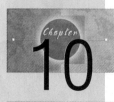
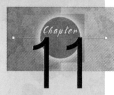

THE HEAD AND NECK

Objectives

Upon completion of this chapter, the reader should be able to:

- Describe the movements of the head and neck.

- Describe the various structures associated with the head and neck, including the bones and bony landmarks of the spinal column.

- Name the major muscles involved in the head and neck.

- Locate the origin, insertion, action, and innervation of each major muscle of the head and neck.

Key Words

longissimus capitis	occipital protuberance	splenius capitis
mandible	scalenes	splenius cervicis
masseter	semispinalis capitis	sternocleidomastoid
mastoid process	semispinalis cervicis	temporalis
nuchal ligamentum	spinous process	transverse process

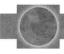

INTRODUCTION

The head and neck are obviously very vulnerable regions of the human body. Consider the injury potential to this region through athletics and unfortunate accidents. Regrettably, you may work with clients who have life-altering injuries to this region of the body. Your comprehension of this complex, but ever so important, area of the human body is essential. The learning process for the core region of the body starts in this chapter. Specifically, this chapter focuses on the regional area known as the head and neck. New structures and terms are introduced in this chapter, such as the erector spinae muscle group, specific areas of the spinal column (i.e., spinous and transverse processes), and various movements that are generally specific to this region of the body.

The muscles of the head and neck are defined as those that either originate or insert on any landmark of the head or cervical vertebrae. Generally, these muscles are responsible for strong contractions that produce flexion, extension, lateral flexion, and rotation movements of the neck.

MAJOR LANDMARKS OF THE HEAD AND NECK

As we begin our discussion of this region, you must realize that this section introduces muscles that have not yet been described. There are also several important bony landmarks on the skull and spine that provide attachment points for the muscles of the head and neck that are important to understand before the muscles are introduced. Once you gain an understanding for the muscles involved in this area, you are encouraged to refer back to the ligaments and structures involved to increase your comprehension.

Skull

The bones of the skull serve as attachment points for various muscles of the head and neck (Figure 8-1).

Mandible The **mandible** is the strong bone that makes up the lower jaw.

Zygomatic Bone The zygomatic bone forms the "cheek" bones and part of the orbital area.

Temporal Bone The temporal bone is located on the lateral side of the head. The temporal bones make up the inferolateral aspect of the skull as well as part of the underside of the cranium. In addition, they contain the bony landmark called the mastoid process, which is an anchor site for the sternocleidomastoid muscle.

Parietal Bone The top part of the lateral aspect of the skull is made up of the parietal bones.

Occipital Bone The base of the skull and the posterior area of the skull are made of the occipital bone. The occipital protuberance is also part of the occipital bone.

Mastoid Process The **mastoid process** is a round prominence located on the lateral side of the skull on the parietal cranial bones just behind the ear (see Figure 8-1). It provides an attachment point for the sternocleidomastoid, splenius capitis, and longissimus capitis muscles.

Occipital Protuberance The **occipital protuberance** is a large projection located on the posterior and inferior portions of the occipital bone of the skull (Figure 8-2). The occipital protuberance can be located by identifying the round prominence on the occipital bone that provides the attachment point for the nuchal ligament. In addition to providing an attachment point for the nuchal ligament, the occipital protuberance is a landmark for the muscles of the head and neck.

Vertebral Column (Spinal Column)

From the functional design perspective of the vertebral column, it is an amazing structure. The vertebral column and the adjoining structures perform a multitude of functions, such as support and stability, shock absorption, dispersion of weight, and protection of the spinal cord. It also serves as an attachment site for the many muscles of the neck and trunk. The vertebral column accomplishes all of these amazing functions while allowing movement in all directions.

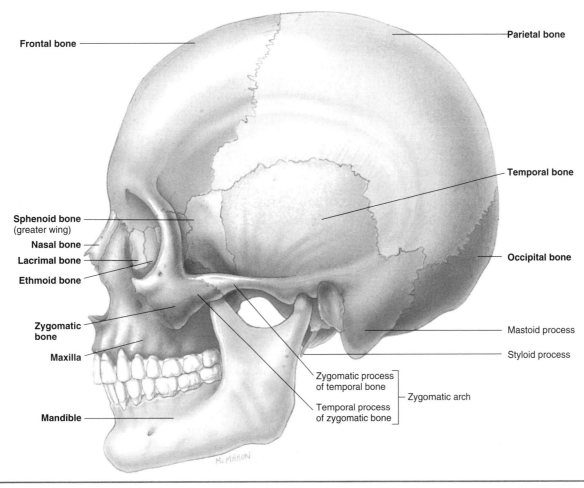

Figure 8-1 *Bones of the Skull*

The spinal column consists of 7 cervical, 12 thoracic, and 5 lumbar vertebrae, a sacrum (consisting of 5 fused vertebrae), and the coccyx (consisting of 4 fused vertebrae) (Figure 8-3). Each of the vertebrae has specific bony landmarks that are important to the discussion of the head and neck.

Because of the intense and important weight-bearing role of the vertebral column, the first through the fifth lumbar vertebrae become increasing larger in size. This allows for effective body weight distribution and dispersion to the lower body. Between each of these vertebrae lie specific structures called intervertebral disks, which are discussed in detail in Chapter 9.

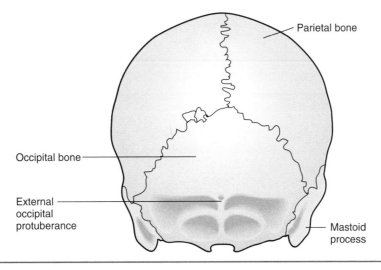

Figure 8-2 *Occipital Protuberance*

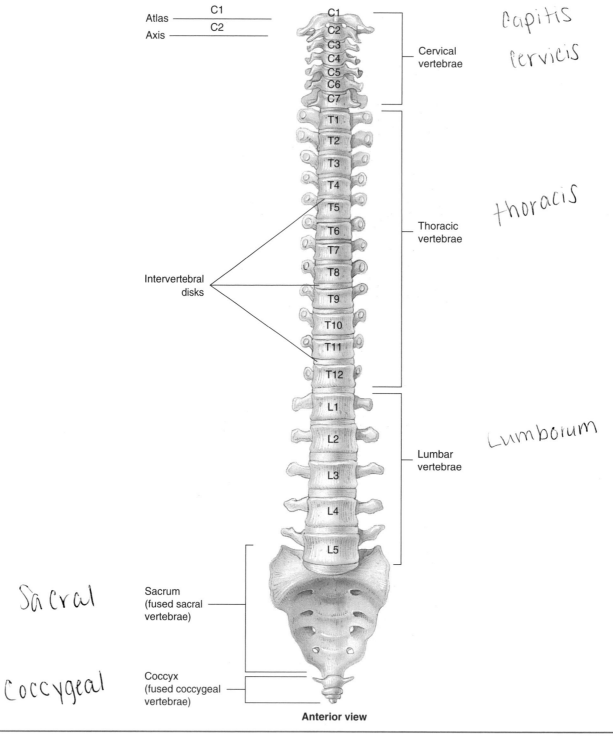

Figure 8-3 *Vertebral Column*

The following landmarks are crucial to the understanding of muscle attachment.

Spinous Process The **spinous processes** of the vertebra are the posterior projections along the midline of the vertebrae (Figure 8-4). These processes vary in shape from one section of the vertebral column to the next as the spine tracks from superior to inferior. The spinous processes provide attachment points for the splenius cervicis, semispinalis cervicis, and splenius capitis muscles.

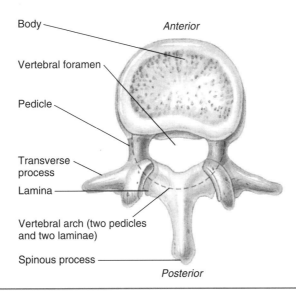

Figure 8-4   *Transverse and Spinal Processes of Vertebrae*

Transverse Process   The **transverse processes** of the vertebra are the lateral projections of the vertebrae (Figure 8-4). These processes provide attachment points for the semispinalis capitis, semispinalis cervicis, and longissimus capitis muscles. In addition, the transverse processes provide a sound, large surface area for the muscles of the lumbar, thoracic, and cervical regions.

 NERVOUS INNERVATION

The nerves that innervate the muscles of the head and neck originate from branches of the cervical spinal nerves and cranial nerves (Figure 8-5). These nerves further branch into distal cervical, trigeminal, accessory, and spinal nerve branches. The 12 pairs of cranial nerves are traditionally numbered using Roman numerals. Generally, the name of the cranial nerve reveals the primary function of the nerve or the area it affects. For our brief discussion of this region, only the trigeminal and accessory cranial nerves are discussed.

Trigeminal Nerve

When learning about the trigeminal nerve, realize that it is one of only several cranial nerves that innervate skeletal muscles. The trigeminal nerve is cranial nerve number V and originates at the inferior surface of the brain and tracks from an inferior to posterior direction to the sphenoid bone of the skull. From this location the nerve branches and innervates the masseter and temporalis muscles of the head.

Accessory Nerve

The accessory nerve is cranial nerve XI and originates at the inferior surface of the brain. The nerve tracks from an anterior to posterior direction following the curve of the spine. The accessory nerve can be found deep to the digastric muscle and posterior to the sternocleidomastoid. As the nerve continues posteriorly, it runs deep to the trapezius muscle. Becuase of its location, the accessory nerve innervates two muscles: the sternocleidomastoid and the trapezius muscle of the shoulder girdle.

Spinal Nerve Branches

Emerging from the spinal cord are 31 pairs of spinal nerves. These nerves supply all parts of the body except the head and some areas of the neck. Each of them is named for its point of origin from the spinal cord. Table 8-1 summarizes the nerves in the head and neck.

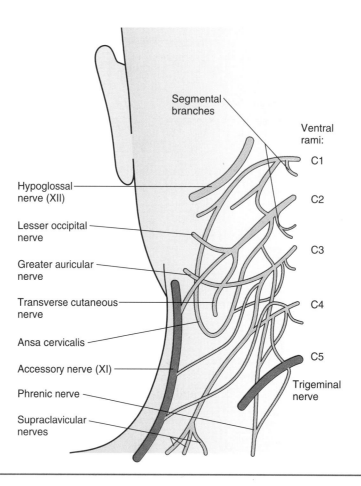

Figure 8-5 *Cervical Nerves*

Table 8-1 *Nerves of the Head and Neck*

Nerve	Affected Anterior Muscles	Affected Lateral Muscles	Affected Posterior Muscles
Cervical	None	None	Longissimus capitis Scalenes
Trigeminal	None	Masseter Temporalis	None
Accessory	Sternocleidomastoid	None	None
Spinal	None	None	Semispinalis cervicis Semispinalis capitis Splenius capitis Splenius cervicis

MOVEMENT OF THE HEAD AND NECK

The muscles of the head and neck create actions that cause movement of the head and cervical spine in the frontal, sagittal, and transverse planes. Flexion and extension movements both occur in the sagittal plane around a frontal axis. Lateral bending movements occur in the frontal plane around a sagittal axis. Lateral bending in the cervical region of the spinal column allows the most movement (relative to the thoracic or lumbar region). The final movement of the head and neck occurs as the muscles cause rotation of the cervical spine. These movements occur in the transverse plane around a vertical axis. Rotation in the cervical region of the spinal column provides the most movement relative to the rest of the spinal column. Perform the different movements referenced in Table 8-2 to help you better understand their actions.

Table 8-2 *Movements of the Head and Neck*

Movement	Plane	Axis	Description
Flexion	Sagittal	Frontal	The chin moves toward the sternum.
Extension	Sagittal	Frontal	The forehead moves up and back.
Lateral Flexion	Frontal	Sagittal	The ear moves toward the shoulder.
Rotation	Transverse	Vertical	The chin moves over the shoulder.

OTA Perspective

The treatment of a burn injury to the head, face, and neck is highly complicated and specialized. The skin is the largest organ, and it acts as a protective cover to all underlying structures. The epidermis (thin, outer layer that does not contain blood vessels) and the dermis (contains blood vessels, nerves, hair follicles, and sweat glands) are the two basic layers of normal skin. Classification of burn depth is determined by which anatomical structures have been damaged or destroyed. Superficial and deep partial-thickness burns were formally known as first- and second-degree burns. Full-thickness burns (the full thickness of the skin has been destroyed) were previously referred to as third-degree burns. Classic electrical burns (fourth-degree) require extensive surgical excision of necrotic tissue followed by skin grafting or possible amputation because deep soft tissue damage to fat, muscle, and bone does not allow for epithelialization (elements in the dermis from which skin regenerates).

The skin is "elastic." As a full-thickness burn heals, scar tissue is formed, which is not elastic. If the client is not properly treated, unmanaged growth of that scar tissue can result in disfigurement and deformity, which causes significant limitations in performance in areas of occupation, performance skills (namely, motor skills), and client factors (body functions and body structures, including ROM and strength). Think about this: if the skin is not malleable, muscle movement is compromised as is joint movement. Splinting, positioning, and exercise can assist in counteracting scar formation and enhancing participation in occupational performance.

The preceeding is a very simplified overview of burns. Treating a burn client, especially one who has sustained burns to the head or neck, is a complicated and lengthy process. (Skin maturation can occur up to 2 years post burn; a child may be involved in treatment through puberty.) To assist the OTA in relating a burn diagnosis to the study of kinesiology, further research is recommended. A visit to a burn unit and observing inpatient and outpatient OT treatment would be beneficial. Refer to the *Occupational Therapy Practice Framework* to link aspects of the OT domain together.

STABILITY OF THE HEAD AND NECK

A thick, strong ligament and many tendon attachments on the spine create the stability of the head and neck.

Nuchal Ligamentum

The **nuchal ligamentum** is located superficially between C7 (cervical vertebrae number 7) and the base of the skull and the occipital protuberance. This very strong ligament prevents extreme neck flexion. The functional purpose of the nuchal ligament, however, is not only for stability and support for the posterior neck region. This broad ligament also serves as an origin for the muscles of the shoulder girdle and shoulder joint.

MUSCLES OF THE HEAD AND NECK

At times studying the muscles of the head and neck can seem like a daunting task, but with the proper study time and techniques, you will find yourself gaining a proper understanding of these delicate muscles. The muscles of the head and neck are important to the stability of the head and neck and to the wide range of movements allowed in this area. The anterior and posterior locations of these muscles provide the movements required for the head and neck.

Masseter

The **masseter** muscle is a rhomboid-shaped muscle located on the lateral skull (Figure 8-6). When this muscle contracts, it provides movement of the jaw and clenches the teeth. It originates on the zygomatic process of the maxilla and the zygomatic arch and inserts on the lateral surface of the mandible. The masseter can be palpated on the lateral mandible.

Name:	Masseter
O:	Zygomatic process of the maxilla and zygomatic arch
I:	Lateral mandible
N:	Mandibular division of the trigeminal nerve
A:	Closes lower jaw
P:	Lateral mandible

Temporalis

The **temporalis** muscle is a triangular-shaped muscle located on the lateral skull (Figure 8-7). When this muscle contracts, it provides movements of the jaw and clenches the teeth. It originates on the temporal fossa of the frontal, parietal, and temporal bone and inserts on the lateral surface of the mandible. The temporalis can be palpated on the lateral aspect of the skull.

Name:	Temporalis
O:	Temporal fossa
I:	Coronoid process
N:	Mandibular division of the trigeminal nerve
A:	Closes lower jaw
P:	Temporal region

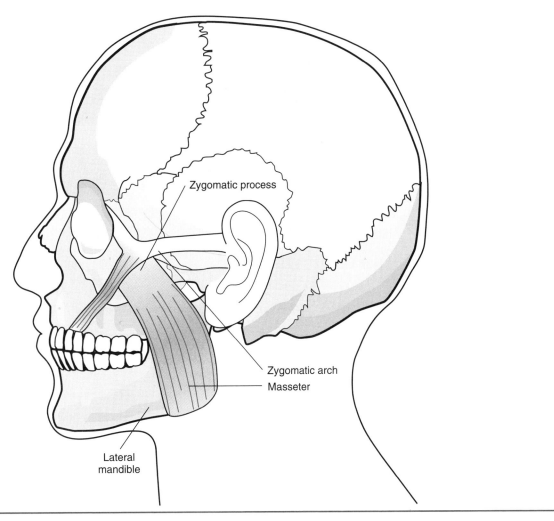

Zygomatic process

Zygomatic arch

Masseter

Lateral mandible

Figure 8-6 *Masseter*

Sternocleidomastoid

The **sternocleidomastoid** muscle is a strap muscle located superficially on the lateral and anterior neck (Figure 8-8). When both sides contract, the muscle produces cervical flexion; when one side contracts, it produces lateral bending to the same side and rotation to the opposite side. The sternocleidomastoid originates on the manubrium of the sternum and the medial clavicle and inserts on the mastoid process of the skull. The sternocleidomastoid is the large protruding neck muscle located on the anterior surface of the neck. Therefore, palpate the muscle as it tracks from superior to inferior.

Name: Sternocleidomastoid

O: Sternum and medial clavicle

I: Mastoid process

N: Accessory

A: Cervical flexion, rotation, and lateral flexion

P: Anterolateral neck

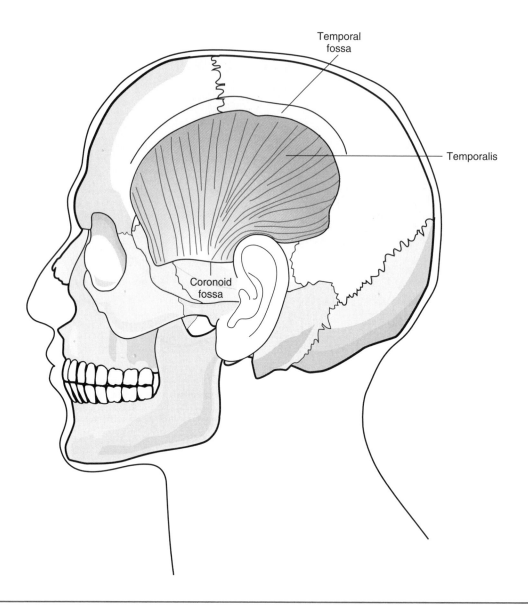

Figure 8-7   *Temporalis*

OTA Perspective

Torticollis is also called wryneck and is caused by either spasm or shortening of the sternocleidomastoid muscle. Contraction of the sternocleidomastoid will put the head in the characteristic side bent and rotated position.

It can occur in infants and in children and may develop from trauma to the neck during delivery. Usually, stretching of the muscle will correct the problem, although, occasionally, surgery is necessary. It can occur acutely in adults, with patients complaining of pain when they wake up in the morning and not having the ability to bring their head back to the neutral position. It is common in people who sleep on their stomachs.

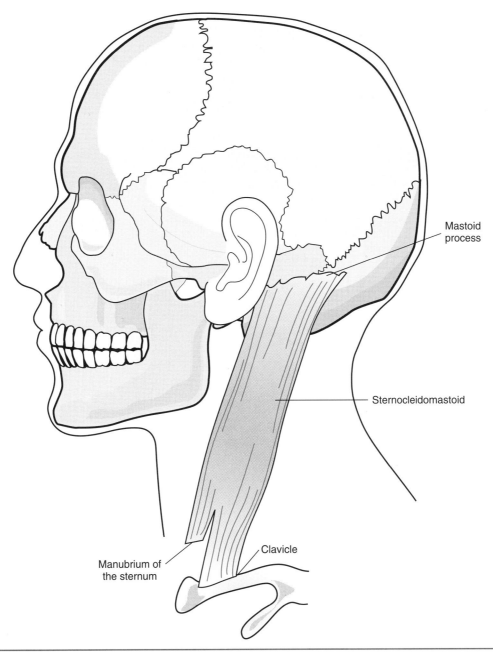

Figure 8-8 *Sternocleidomastoid*

Semispinalis Capitis

The **semispinalis capitis** is a multipennate-shaped muscle located on the posterior cervical and thoracic spine (Figure 8-9). When this muscle contracts, it produces cervical extension and head rotation. Because of its shape, this muscle has multiple origins. These are on the transverse processes of the lower four cervical vertebrae and the upper two thoracic vertebrae. The semispinalis capitis muscle inserts on the occipital bone. Palpation is only possible just below the occipital bone.

Name:	Semispinalis Capitis
O:	Transverse processes of C4–C7 and T1–T2
I:	Occipital bone
N:	Spinal nerve
A:	Extends and rotates the head
P:	Distal to the occipital bone

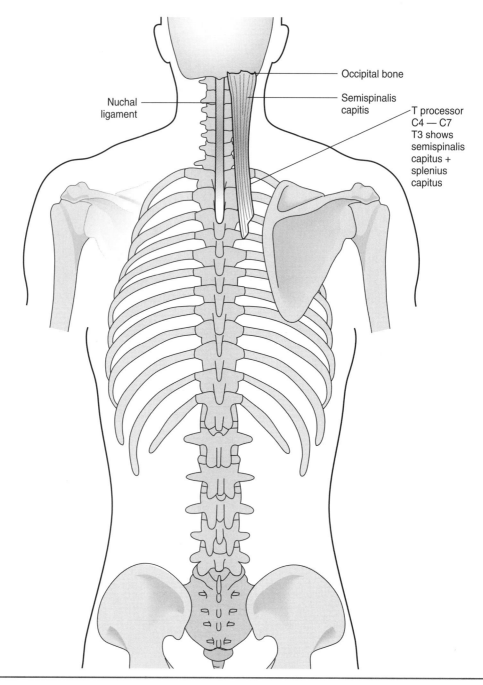

Nuchal
ligament

Occipital bone

Semispinalis
capitis

T processor
C4 — C7
T3 shows
semispinalis
capitus +
splenius
capitus

Figure 8-9 *Semispinalis Capitis*

Semispinalis Cervicis

The **semispinalis cervicis** is a multipennate-shaped muscle located on the posterior cervical and thoracic spine (Figure 8-10). When this muscle contracts, it produces cervical extension and head rotation. Because of its shape, this muscle has multiple origins. These are on the transverse processes of the upper five cervical vertebrae. The semispinalis cervicis inserts on the spinous processes of the lower six cervical vertebrae. Palpation is not possible because it is too deep.

Name:	Semispinalis Cervicis
O:	Transverse processes of T1–T5
I:	Spinous processes of C2–C7
N:	Spinal nerves
A:	Extends and rotates the head
P:	Cannot be palpated

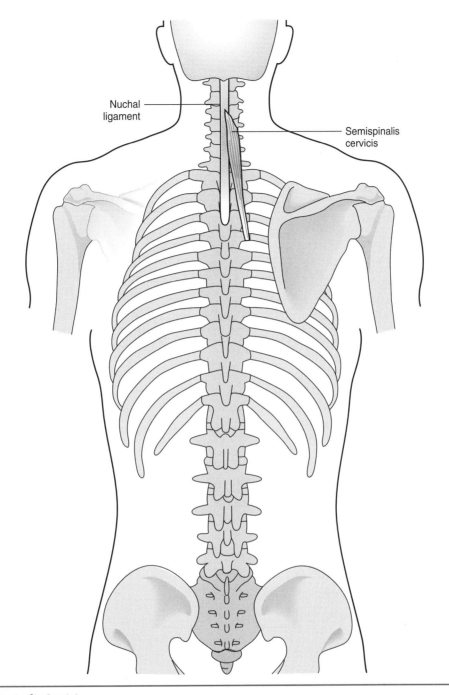

Figure 8-10 *Semispinalis Cervicis*

Splenius Capitis

The **splenius capitis** is a multipennate-shaped muscle located on the posterior cervical and thoracic spine (Figure 8-11). When this muscle contracts, it produces cervical extension and head rotation. Because of its shape, this muscle has multiple origins. These are on the lower half of the nuchal ligament and the spinous processes of the seventh cervical vertebrae and the spinous processes of the upper three thoracic vertebrae. The splenius capitis inserts on the mastoid process and the occipital bone. Palpation is possible on the posterolateral neck.

    Name: Splenius Capitis

    O: Lower half of nuchal ligament and spinous processes of C7–T3

    I: Mastoid process and occipital bone

    N: Spinal nerve

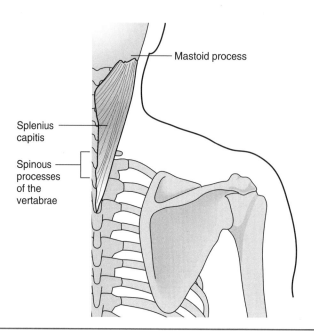

Mastoid process

Splenius
capitis

Spinous
processes
of the
vertabrae

Figure 8-11   *Splenius Capitis*

A: Bilateral: extends the head

            Unilateral: rotates the head to the same side

P: Posterolateral neck

Splenius Cervicis

The **splenius cervicis** is a multipennate-shaped muscle located on the posterior cervical and thoracic spine (Figure 8-12). When this muscle contracts, it produces cervical extension and head rotation. Because of its shape, this muscle has multiple origins. These are on the nuchal ligament and the spinous processes of the seventh cervical vertebrae. The splenius cervicis inserts on the spinous process of the second cervical vertebrae. Palpation is possible on the posterolateral neck.

    Name: Splenius Cervicis
    O: Nuchal ligamentum and spinous process of C7
    I: Spinous process of axis (C2)
    N: Spinal nerves
    A: Extends the cervial vertebrae
    P: Posterolateral neck

Longissimus Capitis

The **longissimus capitis** is a multipennate-shaped muscle located on the posterior cervical and thoracic spine (Figure 8-13). When this muscle contracts, it produces cervical extension and head rotation. Because of its shape, this muscle has multiple origins. These are on the transverse processes of the first five thoracic vertebrae and the articular processes of the lower three cervical vertebrae. The longissimus capitis inserts on the mastoid process. Palpation is not possible because it is too deep.

    Name: Longissimus Capitis
    O: Transverse processes of T1–T5 and articular processes of C5–C7
    I: Posterior mastoid process
    N: Cervical nerves
    A: Extends and rotates the head
    P: Cannot be palpated

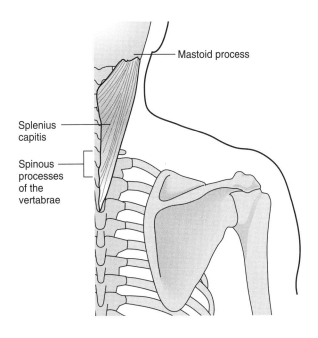

Figure 8-12 *Splenius Cervicis*

Scalenes

The **scalenes** muscle group is composed of three regional muscles: the anterior, middle, and posterior scalenes (Figure 8-14). For our discussion, it is not necessary to differentiate between the three muscles. They are only assistive at best in neck flexion and work unilaterally to produce lateral bending of the neck.

Name:	Scalene
O:	Cervical vertebrae and transverse processes
I:	First and second ribs
N:	Lower cervical nerve
A:	Assists in neck flexion and lateral bending
P:	Cannot be palpated

 KEY CONCEPTS

■ The muscles of the head and neck allow for motion in all three planes. These motions include flexion/extension, lateral flexion, and rotation,

■ The major landmarks of the head and neck are all important for the origin and insertion of the muscles that cause movements of the head and neck.

■ When learning the major muscles of the head and neck, group them together by anatomical location. Remember that the masseter and temporalis both act on the mandible and chewing. The sternocleidomastoid is located in the anterior and lateral regions of the neck and provides rotation, neck flexion, and lateral flexion. All four of the posterior muscles provide neck extension and rotation movements of the head and vertebrae and include the semispinalis capitis, semispinalis cervicis, splenius capitis, and longissimus capitis.

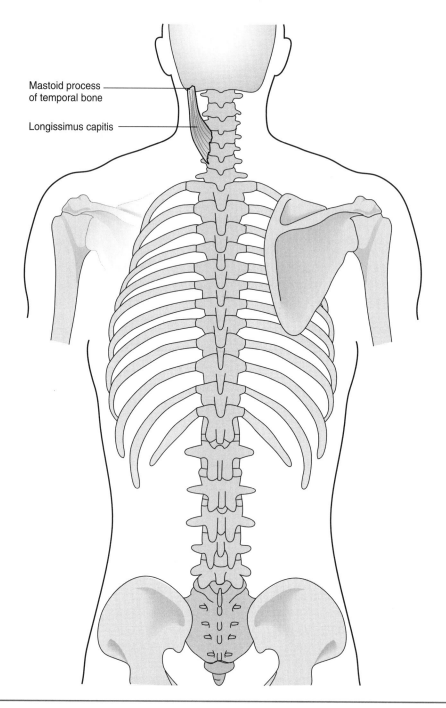

Figure 8-13 *Longissimus Capitis*

 BIBLIOGRAPHY

Luttgens, K. (2000). *Kinesiology: Scientific basis of human motion* (9th ed.). Madison, WI: McGraw-Hill.

Marieb, E. (2003). *Human anatomy & physiology* (6th ed.). Menlo Park, CA: Addison Wesley Longman.

Minor, M. (1998). *Kinesiology laboratory manual for physical therapist assistants.* Philadelphia: F. A. Davis.

Stone, R. (1990). *Atlas of the skeletal muscles.* Dubuque, IA: Wm. C. Brown.

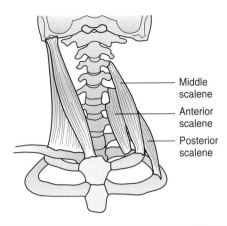

Figure 8-14   *Scalenes*

 REVIEW QUESTIONS

Multiple Choice

Select the best answer to complete the following statements.

1. The _____ muscle inserts on the mastoid process.
   a. splenius cervicis
   b. masseter
   c. temporalis
   d. longissimus capitis

2. The _____ process extends to the dorsal side of the body.
   a. mastoid
   b. spinous
   c. transverse
   d. occipital

3. The _____ muscle does not cause extension and rotation of the cervical spine.
   a. semispinalis cervicis
   b. splenius cervicis
   c. semispinalis capitis
   d. sternocleidomastoid

4. The _____ muscle produces unilateral movement on the opposite side.
   a. semispinalis cervicis
   b. splenius cervicis
   c. semispinalis capitis
   d. sternocleidomastoid

5. The _____ muscle is easily visible from the anterior side of the body.
   a. semispinalis cervicis
   b. splenius cervicis
   c. semispinalis capitis
   d. sternocleidomastoid

Matching

Match each of the following descriptions with the approproiate term.

_____ **1.** Lower jaw

_____ **2.** Lateral process on the vertebrae

_____ **3.** Lateral skull

_____ **4.** Posterior skull

_____ **5.** Posterolateral skull

_____ **6.** Strong support structure for the head

_____ **7.** Posterior process on the vertebrae

A. Temporal fossa

B. Nuchal ligamentum

C. Mastoid process

D. Spinous process

E. Transverse process

F. Mandible

G. Occipital protuberance

Critical Thinking

1. Many athletes, such as football players and wrestlers, benefit from strengthening the muscles of the neck to prevent injury. If you had unlimited weight training and strengthening equipment, describe three ways you could strengthen the neck muscles.

2. Imagine you were very limited on strength-training equipment. How could you strengthen the muscles of the neck using only your own body or body resistance? Identify and practice some techniques or exercises using only your body or body resistance. Then do the same thing with a towel or similar item. Write these exercises down and add them to your repertoire of strengthening exercises.

3. Pain from cervical nerve root compression is referred in dermatomal patterns. Review the pain referral of C1–C7 and draw a diagram. Also review the reflex loss associated with nerve root problems at C5, C6, and C7.

4. Your client is a 2-month-old baby with a torticollis resulting from delivery. The client was sent to you by the pediatrician. Describe the advice that you would give the mother regarding the condition. The mother is anxious and wants to know the prognosis. Research all you can on infant torticollis.

5. A 43-year-old client has undergone a surgical fusion of C4 and C5. She has been immobilized for 8 weeks and is now 4 weeks post immobilization. Record an exercise program that is applicable now that she can progress to within the next 4 weeks.

6. Regardless of the diagnosis, the OT practitioner must design and implement treatment that is age appropriate—one of the aspects of individualized and client-centered care. Read the brief case study in Lab 8-4. How might your treatment be different if your client was a 6-month-old child? If your client was an elderly gentleman who lived in the nursing home? Besides developmental reflexes for the infant, what other developmental factors might influence your treatment? What environmental factors might you consider when assisting the occuaptional therapist with the initial evaluation? What would you do if you suspect that the situation that led to the burn was not an accident but possible abuse? What would you do if your client is either purposefully noncompliant with your treatment (e.g., angry, acting-out teenager) or cognitively (e.g., early senile dementia) unable to independently comply with it, and with certainty you can predict life-long negative outcomes if the therapy regime is not consistently adhered to? What would you say to the client? The primary caregivers? The supervising occupational therapist, the physician, the treatment team? How would you document this? How much of client compliance is your responsibility?

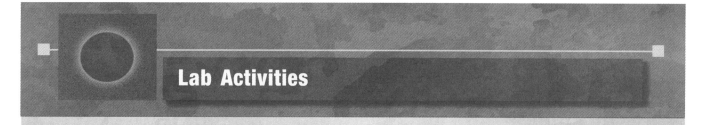

Lab Activities

Lab 8-1: Stretching Activities

Objective: To identify and plan stretching activities for particular muscles of the head and neck.

Equipment Needed: A lab partner

Step 1. Teach your partner a stretch for the following muscles:

    a. Anterior and middle scalenes

    b. Posterior scalenes

    c. Levator scapula

    d. Sternocleidomastoid

Step 2. Switch roles with your partner and repeat step 1.

Lab 8-2: Palpation of Landmarks

Objective: To properly identify and palpate the landmarks of the head and neck.

Equipment Needed: A lab partner

Step 1. With your partner in the supine position, palpate the following bony landmarks in the cervical spine:

    a. Spinous process of C1–C7

    b. Mastoid process

    c. Sternocleidomastoid process

    d. Scalenes

    e. Clavicle

Step 2. Switch roles with your partner and repeat step 1.

Lab 8-3: Assessment of Range of Motion

Objective: To identify and assess ROM of the head and neck.

Equipment Needed: A lab partner, measuring tools

Step 1. Assess the full ROM of the cervical spine of your partner. Have your partner play the role of a patient with neck pain and reduced ROM. Discuss how you would record the loss and use any measuring tools at your disposal.

Step 2. Switch roles with your partner and repeat step 1.

Lab 8-4: Facial Exercises for the Burn Client

Objective: To identify and link together muscles, movements, and activities indicated for normal facial movement.

Equipment Needed: Resource materials on burns, mirror, pen, and paper for writing answers

As you answer the following questions, keep this scenario in mind: A 10-year-old boy was experimenting with smoking a cigarette and sustained deep partial-thickness and full-thickness burns to his lower face, neck, and fingers of his right hand when the whole matchbook burned. No open burn areas; he has been wearing a thermoplastic neck conforming splint as ordered and thus far has been compliant with current outpatient OT treatment.

Step 1. Identify the muscles primarily used to open the mouth.

Step 2. Look in a mirror and see how wide you can open your mouth. What other mouth movements can you make?

Step 3. List several tasks in which you need to open your mouth as wide as possible.

Step 4. List as many activities and exercises that you can think of that promote this musculoskeletal movement and increase skin elasticity and movement.

Step 5. What other facial muscle movements are you concerned that this boy should be able to perform?

Chapter 9

THE LOWER BACK

Key Words

annulus fibrosus	longissimus muscle group	rotatores
anterior longitudinal ligament	multifidus	spinalis muscle group
erector spinae	nucleus pulposus	transversospinalis group
iliocostalis muscle group	posterior longitudinal ligament	
interspinales	quadratus lumborum	

INTRODUCTION

From a functional and human performance perspective, the trunk is the core structure around which everything else is built. Similar to a building, without a strong core, the bodily structures will not be strong and long lasting. The spinal column and lower back are the core structures of the human body. This chapter focuses on the ever-so-important lower back muscles.

Many muscles of the lower back are small and mainly contribute to posture, whereas others are larger and more powerful. The purpose of this textbook is to make learning muscles and their movements as simple as possible. We have attempted to simplify many of the origins and insertions of these muscles to facilitate the learning and studying process.

MAJOR LANDMARKS OF THE LOWER BACK

The vertebrae and spinal column were introduced in Chapter 8 and are, therefore, not discussed in great detail here. The important bones and landmarks to review for the muscles discussed in this chapter are the spinous and transverse processes of the vertebrae and the iliac crest of the pelvis. In addition, you may want to review the attachment of the spine and ribs because many of these lower back muscles have attachments to these structures as well.

NERVOUS INNERVATION

The multitude of muscles providing movement for the lower back are all innervated by the spinal nerves.

MOVEMENT OF THE LOWER BACK

Although the spinal column consists of individual adjoining vertebrae, the movements of two adjacent vertebrae are very minimal. When the individual movements of each adjoining vertebra are accumulated, the spinal column exhibits a much greater range of motion. As you learned in Chapter 8, much of the spinal column movement occurs in the cervical and lumbar regions, with limited motion occurring at the thoracic region.

There are four movements that occur in the spinal column, and the area of the spinal column where they are found specifies most of them. For example, extension of the spinal column can occur either at the cervical region or the lumbar region. However, it is important to specify which movement you are describing. The movements of the lower back that are important are flexion, extension, lateral bending/flexion, left or right spinal rotation, and reduction. Each of these movements is explained in Table 9-1.

As you learn the different movements referenced in Table 9-1, perform them to help you better understand their actions.

Table 9-1 *Movement of the Lower Back*

Movement	Description
Flexion	Movement of the torso toward the inferior skeleton
Spinal Extension	Return from flexion; posterior movement of the spine
Lateral Flexion/Bending	Lateral movement of the thorax toward the pelvis
Reduction	The return from lateral flexion/bending
Rotation	Rotary movement of the spine in horizontal plane

STABILITY OF THE LOWER BACK

The stability of the lower back is crucial to proper functioning, alignment, and pain-free living. The main ligaments and structures that are discussed here are the anterior and posterior longitudinal ligaments and the intervertebral disks.

Intervertebral Disks

The vertebral column allows a fair amount of motion, with the majority of the structure providing support for the axial skeleton. Some of the flexibility of the spinal column is due to the intervertebral disks located between adjoining vertebrae. These disks are composed of round fibrous and gel-like materials (Figure 9-1). The outer portion of the disk, the **annulus fibrosus**, is composed of concentric rings of fibrocartilage. This portion can be thought of as the rings of a tree when it is cut in half. The inner portion or core, the **nucleus pulposus**, is a soft gel-like substance mainly composed of water. These intervertebral disks serve several functions. First, they act as shock absorbers by absorbing and transmitting forces placed on the spinal column. Next, as each vertebra sits on another, these disks allow the vertebra to "rock" back and forth and rotate on one another. Lastly, these disks maintain the flexibility of the vertebral column.

Longitudinal Ligaments

The vertebrae are held together by two ligaments that run superior to inferior along the length of the spinal column. The ligament on the anterior side of the spinal column is termed the **anterior longitudinal ligament**, and the ligament on the posterior side is termed the **posterior longitudinal ligament**.

The anterior longitudinal ligament is a broad ligamentous structure that attaches on the anterior surfaces of the vertebral bodies and disks and inserts to the sacrum (Figure 9-2). Because of its location, its main job is to prevent excessive hyperextension of the spinal column.

The posterior longitudinal ligament runs along the posterior inside of the vertebral foramen (see Figure 9-2). It is thick toward the skull and tends to narrow in the lumbar region. This narrowing may contribute to increased injury to the lumbar region.

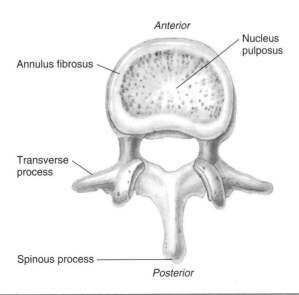

Figure 9-1 *Intervertebral Disk*

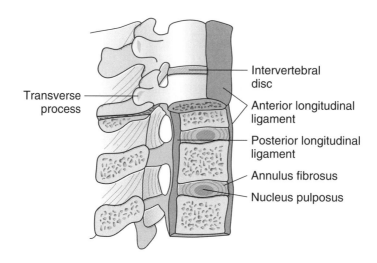

Figure 9-2 *Anterior Longitudinal Ligament and Posterior Longitudinal Ligament*

OTA Perspective

Low back pain (LBP) would be treated best via prevention techniques. These might include a diet adequate in calcium and vitamin D to support bone metabolism; use of proper body mechanics when moving or lifting objects; and maintaining an active vs. sedentary lifestyle to promote healthy bones, joints, muscles, and general well-being. LBP may result from a work-related injury or loss of spinal flexibility from degenerative disk changes as a result of the aging process; prevention education may reduce or delay those incidences.

The muscles of the spine function primarily to move the vertebral column, rather than to keep it erect. (That is accomplished more so by the hip and thigh muscles, primarily through strong ligamentous support of the spine.) Sustained static posture or lifting, or both, while twisting place an increased strain on the lower back structures and can result in soft tissue strain or compression fractures of the vertebral disks.

Understanding the functions of the lower back and postural assessments (see Chapter 11), not only provides a basis for preventing back injuries and illnesses, but also serves as a basis for treatments of those back ailments. The OTA student studying kinesiology may want to research LBP, compression fractures, and other diseases such as osteoporosis, along with body mechanics and work simplification concepts to appreciate the relationship between kinesiology and OT.

OTA Perspective

Disk pathology in the lumbar spine is more common than in any other area of the spine. It is more common in the lower two segments, and it frequently occurs in the third and fourth decade. The cause can be repetitive lifting, or one heavy lifting incident, and there is now some indication that genetics may play a part in it. Disk derangement can vary from a small protrusion to a large herniation that compresses the spinal nerve and causes referred pain into the lower extremity.

Symptoms arising from the disk are worse in the morning because of increased disk height, and worse with sitting, bending, and lifting. Pain can be relieved with therapy, including traction, joint mobilization, and exercises. In very severe cases when the pain does not resolve, surgery may be indicated. Symptoms that require urgent surgery include loss of bladder or bowel control.

MUSCLES OF THE LOWER BACK

The discussion of the lower back muscles is divided into three general sections based on the anatomical location of the muscles. We begin with the intermediate muscle layer—mainly the erector spinae muscle group. The deep muscles of the lower back—rotatores, multifidus, and interspinales—are discussed next. The last discussion is of the muscles that do not quite fit into one these groups but yet are important to lower back movement. Notice that our discussion begins with the intermediate back muscles and not the superficial muscles. This is because the main roles of the superficial muscles—latissimus dorsi, trapezius, and others— is not to exert an influence over the lower back or spinal column.

Erector Spinae Muscle Group

The intermediate layer of lower back muscles is called the **erector spinae** (Figure 9-3). This muscle group is difficult to define through dissection. Some people claim that individual actions cannot be assigned to one specific muscle group, but many of these muscles work synergistically to cause movement. We can make a few assumptions to make the learning process a bit easier. First, there are three main muscles that belong to this muscle group. From lateral to medial, these include the iliocostalis, longissimus, and spinalis (Table 9-2). Second, we also know that many of these muscles span many vertebrae and ribs. Therefore, each of these muscle groups actually contains three distinct muscles based on their location on the thorax. In addition, each of these erector muscles lies on both sides of the spine, which has implications for their actions.

Table 9-2 *Erector Spinae Muscle Group*

Iliocostalis	Longissimus	Spinalis
Iliocostalis Cervicis	Longissimus Cervicis	Spinalis Cervicis
Iliocostalis Thoracis	Longissimus Capitis	ISpinalis Capitis
Iliocostalis Lumborum	Longissimus Thoracis	Spinalis Thoracis

Iliocostalis The **iliocostalis muscle group** is the most lateral of the erectors (Figure 9-3). These are small long muscles that span the vertebrae. As with all of the erector muscles, the bilateral action extends the spine and the unilateral action provides lateral bending. They are innervated by the spinal nerves.

Name:	Iliocostalis
O:	Sacrum, vertebral spines of lumbar vertebra, posterior iliac crest
I:	Posterior ribs and cervical transverse processes
N:	Spinal nerves
A:	Bilateral: extension of spine
	Unilateral: lateral bending
P:	Either side of the spine at the lower lumbar region

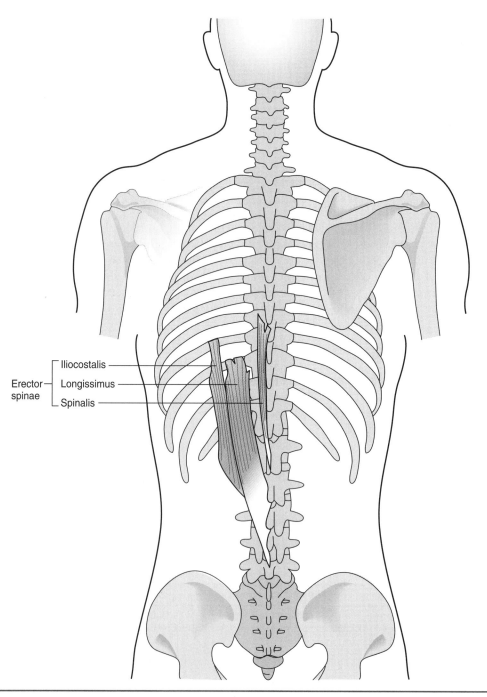

Figure 9-3 *Erector Spinae Muscle Group (Iliocostalis, Longissimus, Spinalis)*

OTA Perspective

When treating a client with a low back injury or illness, the OT practitioner might take the top-down treatment approach, utilizing occupational performance models of practice. The *Occupational Therapy Intervention Process Model* (OTIPM) might be a framework used for guiding assessment and intervention. Treatment would include a performance analysis, client and caregiver education, environmental changes as necessary, and a focus on occupational performance. Effectiveness, efficiency, safety, and independence of occupation (task) performance would be assessed, with adaptations or compensatory methods recommended to assist the client in his or her goals of continuing successful occupational performance with respect to the low back injury or illness issues.

The bottom-up approach, using a biomechanical framework, for example, might be the model of practice employed for assessment and treatment of a client with low back injuries or illnesses. In this approach, the OT practitioner would assess ROM, strength, endurance, balance, and the like, and then design treatment to restore those physical capacities back to the client's "norm." The OT and PT might share initial evaluation results, to avoid duplication of services, with the OT then focus on treatment and goals that would affect PADL/IADL tasks, such as education, strengthening exercises, and restoring function, for example.

The client's goals, prior medical history and functional status, the individual OT practitioner's experience with various models of practice, and facility procedures might dictate which approach is best—the top-down or bottom-up approach. The OTA student may want to review various OT frameworks to assist in guiding client-focused assessment and treatment. Considering many aspects of "the big picture"—kinesiology, OT models of practice, specific diseases of the human body, and the like—contribute to developing clinical reasoning skills.

Longissimus The **longissimus muscle group** is the intermediate muscle group when working from lateral to medial (see Figure 9-3). This is a small muscle group that spans multiple vertebrae. The actions are similar to that of iliocostalis where, bilaterally, they assist in extension of the spine, and, unilaterally, they cause lateral bending. The longissimus muscle group is innervated by the spinal nerves.

Name:	Longissimus
O:	Thoracolumbar fascia from the sacrum, transverse processes of the lumbar and thoracic vertebrae
I:	Mastoid process; transverse and cervical transverse processes
N:	Spinal Nerves
A:	Bilateral: extension of the spine
	Unilateral: lateral bending
P:	Either side of the spine at the lower lumbar region

Spinalis The **spinalis muscle group** is the most medial of the three erectors (see Figure 9-3). It is a small muscle group that spans multiple vertebrae. Unilaterally it acts to perform lateral bending, and bilaterally it acts to perform extension of the spine. The spinalis muscle group is innervated by the spinal nerves.

Name:	Spinalis
O:	Ligamentum nuchae, cervical and thoracic spinal processes
I:	Occipital bone and the cervical and thoracic spinal processes

N: Spinal nerves

A: Bilateral: extension of the spine

Unilateral: lateral bending

P: Either side of the spine at the lower lumbar region

Transversospinalis Muscle Group

Working from superficial to deep, the deep layer of muscles consists of **interspinales**, **multifidus**, and **rotatores** (Figure 9-4). Collectively, these muscles are termed the **transversospinalis muscle group**. Typically, these muscles span the distance from one to five vertebrae, thus they are quite small. Do not let their size fool you, however, because they play a large role in maintaining posture. Each of these muscles aids in rotating the trunk when unilaterally contracting and contributing to spinal extension when bilaterally contracting. Because these muscles work synergistically they are discussed as one muscle group. This muscle group is innervated by the spinal nerves.

Quadratus Lumborum

The **quadratus lumborum** is a deep muscle that lies on the lateral side of the trunk (Figure 9-5). It is a small muscle running vertically from the iliac crest to the 12th rib and the transverse processes of L2–L5. Because of its vertical direction, the quadratus lumborum acts to laterally bend the trunk. This muscle is generally too deep to palpate.

Name: Quadratus Lumborum

O: Iliac crest

I: Rib 12; transverse process of L2–L5

N: 1st lumbar nerve; 12th thoracic nerve

A: Lateral flexion

P: Cannot be palpated

 KEY CONCEPTS

■ There are four movements that occur in the spinal column: flexion and extension, lateral bending/flexion, left or right spinal rotation, and reduction.

■ The major ligaments associated with the lower back are the anterior longitudinal ligament and the posterior longitudinal ligament.

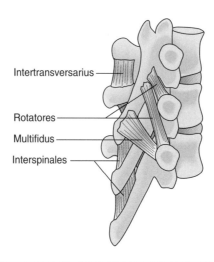

Intertransversarius

Rotatores

Multifidus

Interspinales

Figure 9-4 *Transversospinalis Muscle Group (Interspinales, Multifidus, Rotatores)*

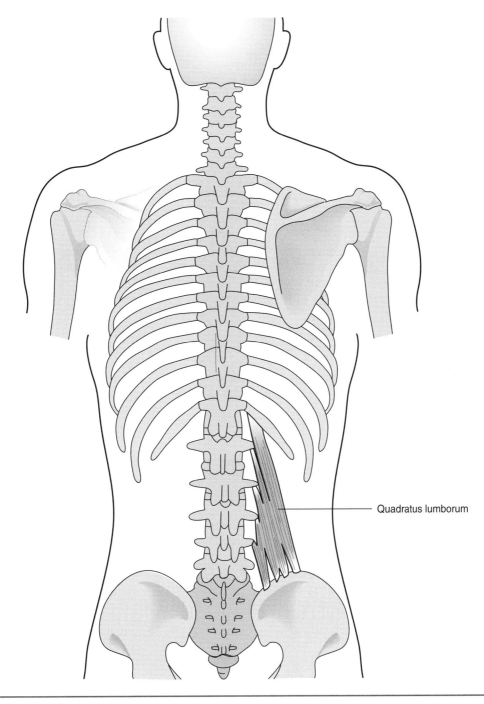

Quadratus lumborum

Figure 9-5 *Quadratus Lumborum*

■ The ligaments serve as support for the structures of the lower back and to prevent excessive hyperextension.

■ The major muscles of the erector spinae group are the iliocostalis, longissimus, and spinalis muscles. The major muscles of the transversospinalis muscle group are the interspinales, multifidus, and rotatores.

■ The erector spinae muscle group allows extension of the spine and lateral bending.

■ The transversospinalis muscle group allows rotating the trunk and spinal extension.

BIBLIOGRAPHY

Luttgens, K. (2000). *Kinesiology: Scientific basis of human motion* (9th ed.). Madison, WI: McGraw-Hill.

Marieb, E. (2003). *Human anatomy & physiology* (6th ed.). Menlo Park, CA: Addison Wesley Longman.

Minor, M. (1998). *Kinesiology laboratory manual for physical therapist assistants*. Philadelphia: F. A. Davis.

Stone, R. (1990). *Atlas of the skeletal muscles*. Dubuque, IA: Wm. C. Brown.

WEB RESOURCES

- The site www.fitness-advantage.com/injuries/lower-back.html features signs and symptoms, modalities, and correction of lower back pain issues.
- Go to www.spineuniverse.com/displayarticle.php/article399.html for features of the scope, studies, and related articles to lower back pain issues.

(These Web addresses were current as of February 2004.)

REVIEW QUESTIONS

Fill in the Blank

Provide the word(s) or phrase(s) that best completes the sentence.

1. From medial to lateral, the erector spinae muscles are _____, _____, _____.

2. Rotation of the trunk occurs in the _____ plane.

3. _____ is an example of reduction.

4. _____, _____, _____ are all part of the transversospinalis muscle group.

5. The quadratus lumborum muscle originates on the _____ of the pelvis.

Multiple Choice

Select the best answer to complete the following statements.

1. The _____ muscle group mainly contributes to posture.
   a. iliopsoas
   b. transversospinalis
   c erector spinae
   d. spinalis

2. Of the following activities, _____ would involve trunk rotation.
   a. performing a biceps curl with a dumbbell
   b. swinging a baseball bat
   c. pushing a gurney
   d. driving a golf ball

e. swinging a baseball bat and pushing a gurney

3. The posterior longitudinal ligament prevents excessive _____ .
a. hip flexion
b. trunk extension
c. trunk flexion
d. rotation

4. Two functions of the intervertebral disks are _____ and _____ .
a. to maintain posture of vertebral column
b. to absorb compressive forces
c. to provide nutrients to the vertebra
d. to produce synovial fluid

5. Of the following muscles, _____ is not a member of the erector spinae muscle group.
a. splenius capitus
b. spinalis
c. iliocostalis
d. longissimus

Matching

Match each of the following descriptions with the appropriate term.

_____ **1.** Erector spinae

_____ **2.** Transversospinalis

_____ **3.** Trunk rotation

_____ **4.** Lateral flexion

_____ **5.** Reduction

A. Movement of the trunk away from the midline

B. Rotatores, multifidus, interspinales

C. Movement of the trunk in the horizontal plane

D. Return of the trunk from lateral position to anatomic position

E. Iliocostalis, longissimus, spinalis

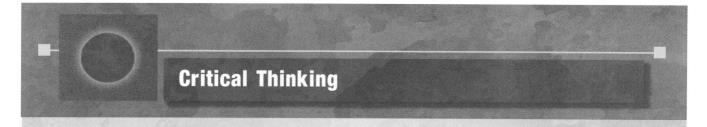

Critical Thinking

1. Describe ways to strengthen the muscles of the lower back without using any contraindicated exercises.

2. Draw the deep rotator muscles (transversospinalis muscle group) from origin to insertion.

3. On the figures provided, draw the major muscles of the lower back, including:

   ■ Iliocostalis muscles   ■ Multifidus

   ■ Longissimus muscles   ■ Rotatores

   ■ Spinalis muscles   ■ Quadratus Lumborum

4. On the drawings from number 3, label the origin, insertion, action and innervation for each of the above muscles.

5. Public education regarding prevention of back injuries is prevalent. Work injuries contribute to economic loss; falls and fractures in the elderly population contribute to decreased independence and, therefore, a possible increased burden on society. Think of prevention education ideas you have seen implemented (e.g., Certified Nursing Assistants [CNAs]) who wear low back support binders while lifting nursing home residents, or posters in the workplace aimed at safety while moving heavy objects). Debate the pros and cons of their effectiveness. How many times have you "moved wrong" and "pulled a muscle" in your back? Did you change your behavior to prevent a future incident? "Prevention" and "wellness" are buzzwords in the business of health care. But we continue to be more focused on rehabilitation "after the fact." Why do you suppose that is?

6. Define *spondylitis* and *spondylosis*. Describe how a patient with spondylosis would present, including age, pain distribution, aggravating and easing factors, and limitations. What advice would you give this patient in terms of managing his or her pain?

7. Research the following surgeries, then describe briefly their procedures and indications.

   a. Laminectomy

   b. Discectomy

   c. Spinal fusion

8. Patients with referred pain from the nerve root will present with pain in dermatomal patterns. Draw a picture reflecting the pain distribution of each dermatome from L1 to L5.

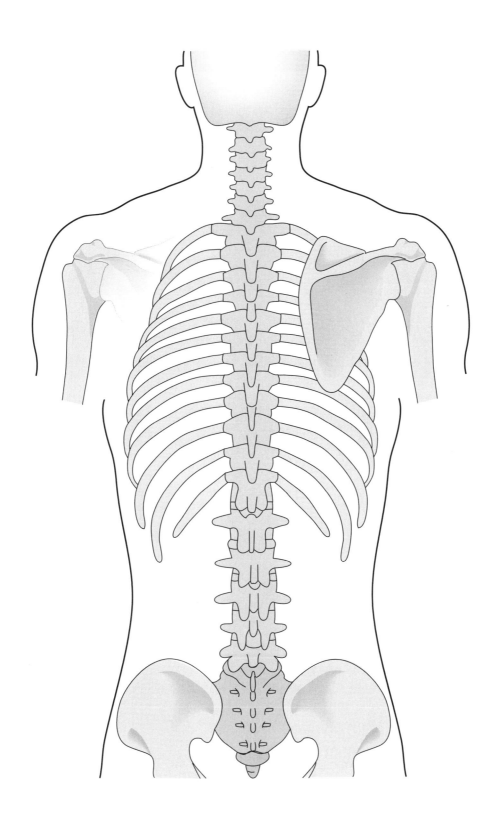

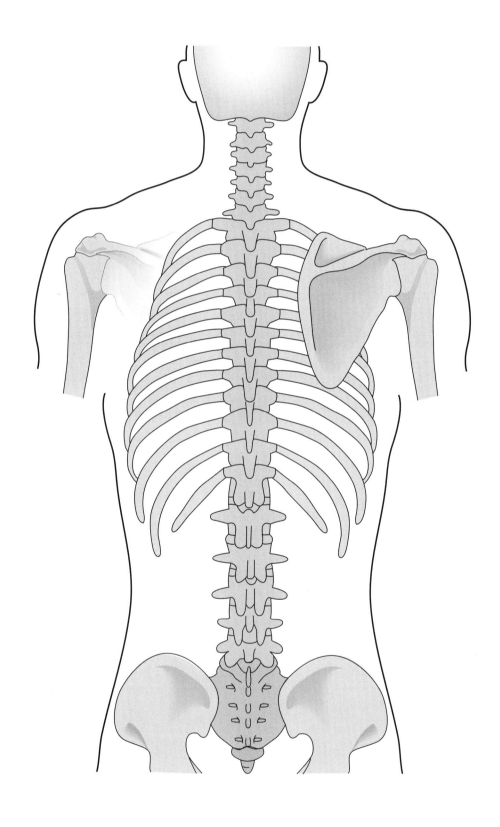

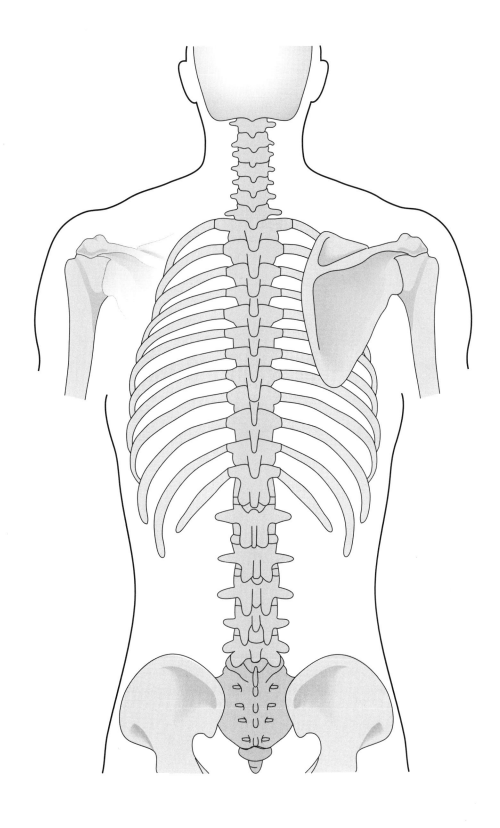

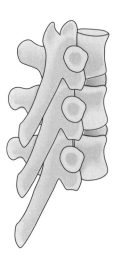

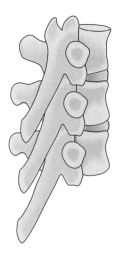

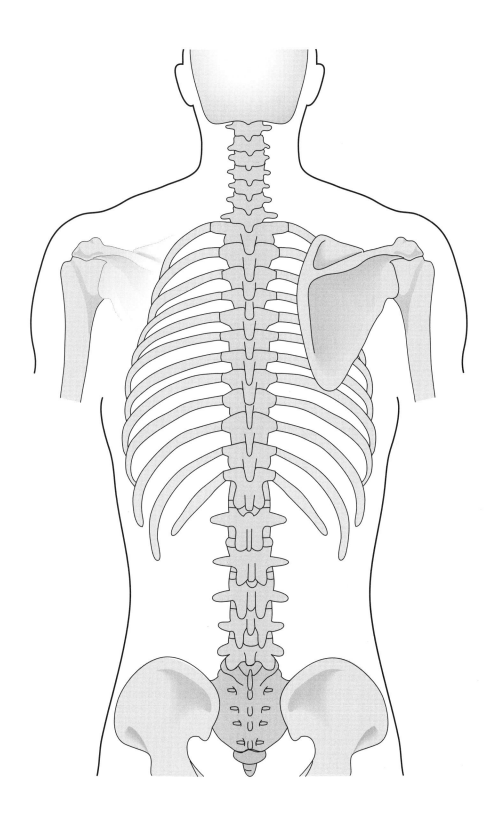

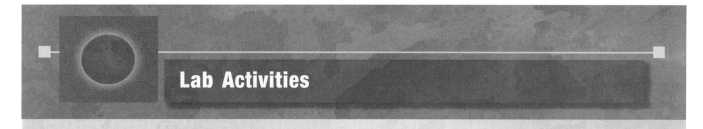

Lab Activities

Lab 9-1: Body Mechanics

Objective: To identify movements associated with improper body mechanics and functional tasks.

Equipment Needed: A lab partner, common ADL equipment, video recorder

Step 1.   With a partner, critique your movements as you engage in a variety of simple common movements or tasks. Videotape the movements for use in activity analysis. Employ proper body mechanics with these movements. Identify joint motions and muscle groups used.

Step 2.   Choose one task (or simple movement) and write an activity analysis, focused on the ROM and strength mechanisms of the lower back. Replay the videotape to assist with assessing the movements.

Step 3.   Choose one activity and "evaluate" it using the *Occupational Therapy Practice Framework's* motor skills, body functions, and body structures to explain the activity.

Lab 9-2: Building Back Models

Objective: To appreciate the flexibility of the lower back.

Equipment Needed: A lab partner, a table top, a variety of objects—clothespins, rubber bands, various sizes of building blocks, Theraband, flexible wire, duct tape, 1/4-inch dowels

Step 1.   Using the objects provided, attempt to build a model of the back, replicating the mobility of the back and noting the flexibility/strength relationship.

Lab 9-3: Palpation of the Landmarks of the Lower Back

Objective: To demonstrate palpation of the landmarks of the lower back

Equipment Needed: A lab partner

Step 1.   Using a skeleton to assist you, palpate the following landmarks on your partner. Make sure your partner is undressed appropriately to be able to palpate the skin directly:

a. Spinous processes of L5–L1

b. Transverse processes of L5–L1

c. Quadratus lumborum

d. Erector spinae

e. Iliac crest

f. ASIS

Step 2.   Switch roles with your partner and repeat step 1.

Lab 9-4: Range of Motion in the Lower Back

Objective: To properly assess range of motion in the lower back.

Equipment Needed: A lab partner, pen/pencil, paper

Step 1.   Using your partner, who should be appropriately undressed, assess the ROM of the lumbar spine in all directions. For each direction, name one structure that will limit the ROM.

Step 2.   Switch roles with your partner and repeat step 1

Chapter 10

THE ABDOMINAL REGION

Objectives

Upon completion of this chapter, the reader should be able to:

- Describe the movements of the abdominal region.

- Locate the major ligaments associated with the abdominal region.

- Describe the functions of the ligaments of the abdominal region.

- Name the major muscles involved in the abdominal region.

- Locate the origin, insertion, and innervation of each major muscle of the abdominal region.

- Explain the action of each major muscle of the abdominal region.

- Describe the palpation of each major muscle of the abdominal region.

Key Words

abdominal aponeurosis	intercostal nerve	transverse abdominal
external oblique	internal oblique	aponeurosis
iliohypogastric nerve	rectus abdominis	transversus abdominis
ilioinguinal nerve	subcostal nerve	
inguinal ligament	thoracolumbar fascia	

INTRODUCTION

During a visit to a health club or spa, observe the number of individuals performing exercises that strengthen the abdominal region. Observe the region as the muscles contract to move the torso in different directions. While making your observations, imagine the numerous joints in the abdominal region that are made up from the spinal region. Also think about the structures and supporting tissues as they provide a strong base of support for the appendicular skeleton.

The abdominal cavity is the region located inferior to the diaphragm and superior to the pelvic region. The muscles of the region are responsible for strong contractions that aid in many activities such as trunk flexion, defecation, and laughing. These movements are made possible by the strong structures that provide stability, including the strong muscles, ligaments, and the bands of aponeurosis that provide support for the muscles of this region.

 NERVOUS INNERVATION

The nerves that innervate the muscles of the abdominal region originate from the ventral ramus of the T9–T12 spinal nerves and the ventral ramus of the L1 spinal nerve. These nerves extend from the ramus and branch into the intercostal, subcostal, iliohypogastric, and ilioinguinal nerves.

Intercostal and Subcostal Nerves

The **intercostal nerves** that branch from the ventral ramis of the T9–T11 spinal nerves and the **subcostal nerve** stemming from the spinal nerve T12 innervate the rectus abdominis muscle of the anterior abdominal cavity (Figure 10-1). Each of these nerves originates on the posterior surface of the abdominal region and extends laterally, bisecting the transversus abdominis and internal oblique muscles. As the nerves track in the anterior direction, they track toward the more superficial layer of the abdominal muscles. By doing so, the intercostal and subcostal nerves provide appropriate innervation of all of the rectus abdominal region muscles.

Iliohypogastric and Ilioinguinal Nerves

The **iliohypogastric** and **ilioinguinal nerves** originate from the ventral ramis of the spinal nerves T12 and L1 (see Figure 10-1). Both nerves are located more distally to the intercostal and subcostal nerves and, therefore, extend inferiorly, innervating the lower reaches of the abdominal cavity. Immediately after the ventral ramus, the two nerves branch, with the iliohypogastric branching superiorly to the ilioinguinal nerve. From the branch, each nerve bisects the transversus abdominis and internal oblique muscles. As the nerves track in the anterior direction, they extend in this direction and innervate all of the muscles of the abdominal cavity. Table 10-1 summarizes innervation of the abdomen.

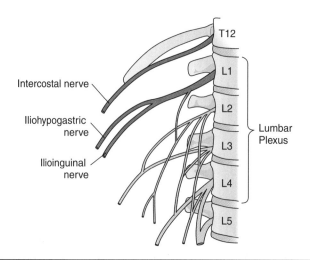

Figure 10-1   *Intercostal and Subcostal Nerves*

Table 10-1 *Innervation of the Abdominal Region*

Nerve	Affected Anterior Muscles	Affected Lateral Muscles
Intercostal	Rectus abdominis	External oblique, internal oblique, transversus abdominis
Iliohypogastric	None	External oblique, internal oblique, transversus abdominis
Ilioinguinal	None	External oblique, internal oblique, transversus abdominis

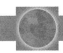 MOVEMENT OF THE ABDOMINAL REGION

The movements of the abdominal region create actions that cause gross movements of the trunk. Unlike the muscles of respiration, the abdominal muscles cause movements that occur in all three planes. Flexion, extension, and hyperextension movements all occur in the sagittal plane around a frontal axis. During these movements, the superior region moves toward the inferior region; for example, when an individual performs an abdominal crunch or a sit-up. Lateral bending movements occur in the frontal plane around a sagittal axis; for example, when you bend sideways to scratch the lateral surface of the thigh. The final movements of the abdominal region occur as the muscles cause its rotation. These movements occur in the transverse plane around a vertical axis. As you learn the different movements referenced in Table 10-2, perform these movements to help you better understand their actions.

Table 10-2 *Movement of the Abdominal Region*

Movement	Description
Trunk Flexion	Forward bending of the trunk
Trunk Rotation	Twisting of the trunk to either side of the body
Lateral Flexion	Bending the trunk to either side of the body
Abdominal Compression	Decreasing the size of the abdominal cavity

 STABILITY OF THE ABDOMINAL REGION

The stability of the abdominal region is created by many bands of fascia and strong ligaments. This connective tissue covers large portions of the abdominal region and, in conjunction with the abdominal muscles, account for the contractions of the muscles of the abdominal region. Furthermore, the structures provide a sound base of support for which the rest of the muscles of the superior and inferior appendicular skeletons pulls on while performing activities of daily living.

Linea Alba

The linea alba is a thick band of connective tissue that runs from the xiphoid process of the sternum to the pubic symphysis (Figure 10-2). It is the central anterior line of the body that serves as an attachment point for the external oblique, internal oblique, and transversus abdominis muscles. This anatomical reference line also signifies the midline of the body that separates the body into right and left halves along the sagittal line. Locate the linea alba as it runs along the center of the rectus abdominis from the xiphoid process to the symphysis pubis.

Inguinal Ligament

Located in the region where the hip joint bends is the **inguinal ligament**, spanning from the anterior superior iliac spine to the pubic tubercle (see Figure 10-2). This broad band of tissue serves as an attachment point for the internal oblique and transversus abdominis muscles.

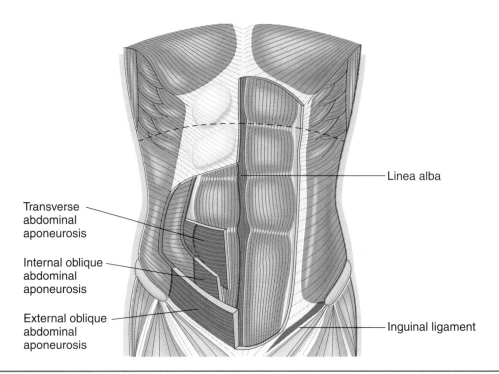

Transverse abdominal aponeurosis

Internal oblique abdominal aponeurosis

External oblique abdominal aponeurosis

Linea alba

Inguinal ligament

Figure 10-2   *Linea Alba*

Abdominal Aponeurosis

The **abdominal aponeurosis** is a flat band of connective tissue that provides support to the abdominal region. The abdominal aponeurosis has two layers. The most superficial layer (see Figure 10-2) is the external oblique abdominal aponeurosis, which attaches the external oblique abdominal muscles to the linea alba. The underlying layer (see Figure 10-2) is the internal oblique abdominal aponeurosis which attaches the internal oblique abdominal muscles to the linea alba.

Transverse Abdominal Aponeurosis

The **transverse abdominal aponeurosis** spans from the lateral border of the transversus abdominis muscle to the abdominal aponeurosis (see Figure 10-2). This band of connective tissue also secures the transversus abdominis muscle to the abdominal wall.

OTA Perspective

Strong abdominal musculature is necessary to "balance" out the strength of the (lower) back. Weak abdominal muscles (e.g., due to obesity or pregnancy) may contribute to LBP (review Chapter 9 as necessary). Decreased muscle tone, hypotonicity, or increased muscle tone, hypertonicity, in the abdominal musculature will affect trunk movements and, therefore, postural control. At times binders or braces are worn to support either the back or the abdomen, or both, which may compensate for the weak musculature, provide support during healing, maintain safety during necessary movements, prevent unwanted movement, or alleviate pain. Abnormal muscle tone might be a result of which diagnoses? CVA, TBI, CP, or SCI? (Look up the abbreviations you are not already familiar with.)

Thoracolumbar Fascia

The **thoracolumbar fascia** is a fibrous membrane that supports the abdominal region. The fascia spans from the lumbar vertebrae to the iliac crest and lower ribs. The fascia attaches laterally to the transversus abdominal muscles and mimics the support of the transverse abdominal aponeurosis on the medial side of the transversus abdominal muscles.

Xiphoid Process

The xiphoid process is located at the inferior end of the sternum. Its main function is to provide an attachment point for the linea alba and rectus abdominis muscle.

 ## MUSCLES OF THE ABDOMINAL REGION

The abdominal region has four muscles that provide movements for the trunk and create compression of the abdominal cavity. These muscles are located on the anterior and lateral surfaces of the abdominal region and are the external oblique, internal oblique, rectus abdominis, and transversus abdominis muscles.

External Oblique

The **external oblique** muscle is a rhomboid-shaped muscle with fibers extending inferiorly from the last nine ribs toward the iliac crest and connect to the abdominal aponeurosis and then to the linea alba (Figure 10-3). When both sides of the muscle contract, they cause trunk flexion. However, when only one side contracts at a given time, the result is lateral trunk flexion. When the external oblique contracts with the spinal rotators, it causes trunk rotation to the opposite side. The external oblique can be palpated on the anterior lateral abdomen.

Name:	External Oblique
O:	Ribs 4–12
I:	Iliac crest and abdominal aponeurosis to the linea alba
N:	8–12 intercostal nerves
A:	Lateral flexion, trunk rotation, and abdominal compression
P:	Anterior lateral abdomen

Internal Oblique

The **internal oblique** muscle is a rhomboid-shaped muscle with fibers extending diagonally in the superior direction from the inguinal ligament and iliac crest toward the ribs and abdominal aponeurosis and then to the linea alba (Figure 10-4). When both sides contract at the same time, they cause trunk flexion. Much like the external oblique muscle, when only one side contracts at a time it causes lateral trunk flexion. When the internal oblique contracts with the spinal rotators, they cause rotation of the trunk to the same side. The internal oblique can be palpated on the lateral abdomen.

Name:	Internal Oblique
O:	Inguinal ligament, iliac crest, and thoracolumbar fascia
I:	Ribs 9–12 and abdominal aponeurosis to the linea alba
N:	8–12 intercostal nerves
A:	Lateral flexion, trunk rotation, and abdominal compression
P:	Anterior lateral abdomen

Rectus Abdominis

The **rectus abdominis** muscle is a rhomboid-shaped muscle (Figure 10-5) with tendinous intersections. It is located superficial to the oblique muscles on the anterior portion of the abdominal region on either side of the linea alba. The rectus

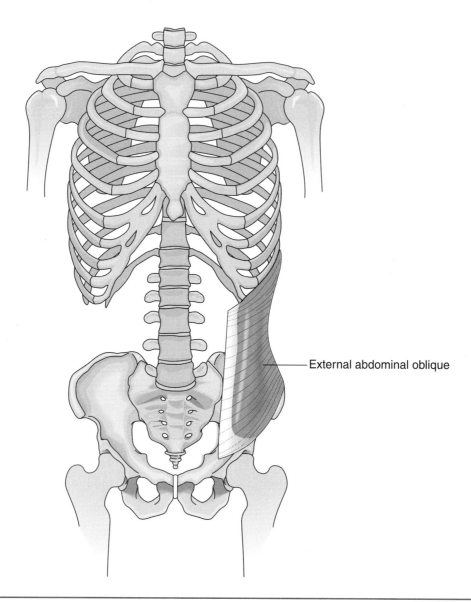

Figure 10-3 *External Oblique*

abdominis originates on the pubis and runs toward the xiphoid process. When it contracts it causes trunk flexion and abdominal compression. It can be palpated at the midline of the abdomen.

Name:	Rectus Abdominis
O:	Pubis
I:	Cartilage of 5–7 ribs, xiphoid process
N:	7–12 intercostal nerves
A:	Trunk flexion and abdominal compression
P:	Midline of the abdomen

Transversus Abdominis

The **transversus abdominis** muscle is a fan-shaped muscle (Figure 10-6) located on the lateral sides of the rectus abdominis. The fibers run horizontally from the inguinal ligament, thoracolumbar fascia, and the lower six ribs and attach to the abdominal aponeurosis and then to the linea alba. When the transversus abdominis contracts, it causes abdominal compression and trunk stability. This muscle is deep to the rectus abdominis muscle and is not easily palpated.

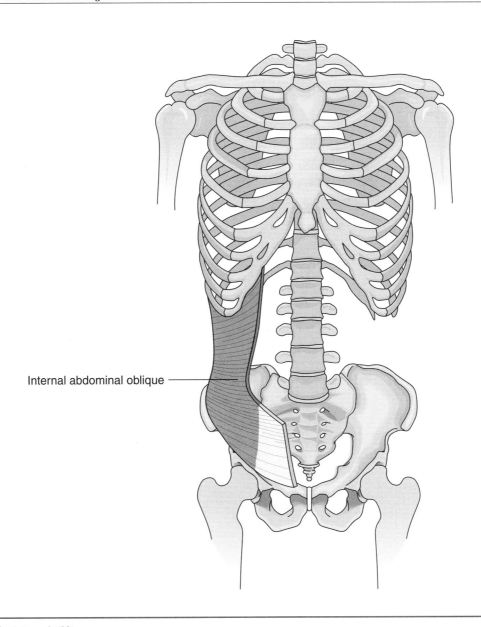

Internal abdominal oblique

Figure 10-4 *Internal Oblique*

Name: Transversus Abdominis
O: Inguinal ligament, iliac crest, thoracolumbar fascia, and lower six ribs
 I: Abdominal aponeurosis to the linea alba
N: 7–12 intercostal nerves
A: Abdominal compression
P: None

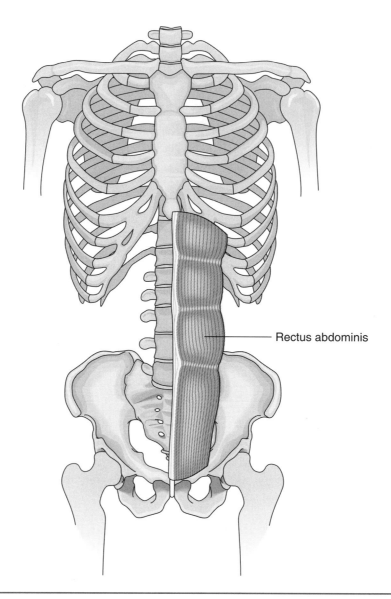

Rectus abdominis

Figure 10-5 *Rectus Abdominis*

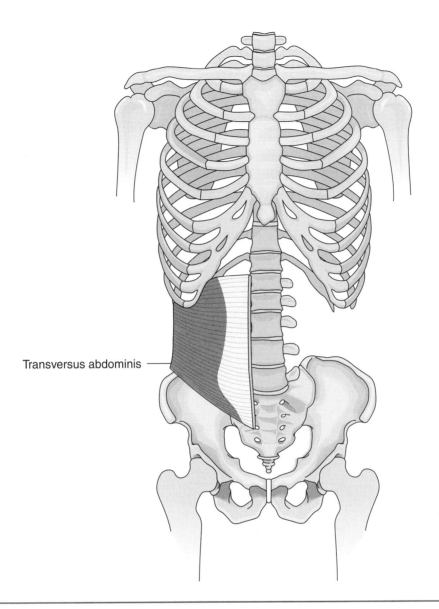

Transversus abdominis

Figure 10-6 *Transversus Abdominis*

OTA Perspective

Sensorimotor approaches are utilized for the OT evaluation and treatment of persons with neurological impairments. Rood, Brunnstrom, and Bobath (also the names of the theorists) are common models of practice and subsequent treatment methods used when working with and caring for clients with CNS dysfunction. Although these are complex theoretical works, with accompanying treatment methods and goals, very basically, the theory and intervention supporting motor retraining serves to facilitate normal movement and use of the affected side, develop more normal postural mechanisms, and inhibit abnormal reflexes and movement patterns. One aspect is postural control, incorporating effective use of the abdominal musculature. For the OTA student who is interested in learning more about these models of practice, and the relationship to the study of kinesiology, research into sensorimotor approaches is recommended. Interviewing an occupational therapist who specializes in this area of clinical practice and observing client treatment sessions will also provide a richer appreciation and understanding.

KEY CONCEPTS

- The movement of the abdominal region creates gross movements of the trunk. Abdominal muscles cause movements in all three planes.
- There are many ligaments in the abdominal region: the linea alba, inguinal ligament, and the abdominal aponeuroses.
- The ligaments of the abdominal region provide a base of support for the muscles of the abdominal region to attach to.
- The abdominal region has four major muscles: the external oblique, the internal oblique, the rectus abdominis, and the transversus abdominis.

BIBLIOGRAPHY

Luttgens, K. (2000). *Kinesiology: Scientific basis of human motion* (9th ed.). Madison, WI: McGraw-Hill.

Marieb, E. (2003). *Human anatomy & physiology* (6th ed.). Menlo Park, CA: Addison Wesley Longman.

Minor, M. (1998). *Kinesiology laboratory manual for physical therapist assistants*. Philadelphia: F. A. Davis.

Stone, R. (1990). *Atlas of the skeletal muscles*. Dubuque, IA: Wm. C. Brown.

WEB RESOURCES

- The site www.nismat.org/ptcor/abdominal shows safe abdominal exercises developed by physical therapists.
- Go to www.marylandsportsmedicine.com/imagepages for pictures of the abdominal region.
- For features of injuries that occur to the abdominal region, go to www.nlm.nih.gov/medlineplus/ency/article/003136.htm. This Web site includes the etiology, signs and symptoms, treatment, and diagnosis of those injuries.

(These Web addresses were current as of February 2004.)

REVIEW QUESTIONS

Fill in the Blank

Provide the word(s) or phrase(s) that best completes the sentence.

1. The _____ muscle runs horizontally.

2. The rectus abdominis originates at the _____ and inserts on the _____.

3. There are _____ muscles in the abdominal region.

4. The linea alba runs from _____ to the _____.

5. The action of _____ _____ aids in sneezing, coughing, and defecation.

Multiple Choice

Select the best answer to complete the following statements.

1. The contraction of the _____ muscle(s) cause lateral trunk flexion.
   a. rectus abdominis
   b. transversus abdominis
   c. internal oblique
   d. external oblique

2. The muscles that cause trunk rotation are the _____ .
   a. external oblique
   b. internal oblique
   c. transversus abdominis
   d. external oblique and internal oblique

3. When sneezing or coughing, the most active muscle(s) is/are the _____ .
   a. external oblique
   b. internal oblique
   c. transversus abdominis
   d. rectus abdominis
   e. transversus abdominis and rectus abdominis

4. The muscle that is easiest to palpate is the _____ .
   a. external oblique
   b. internal oblique
   c. transversus abdominis
   d. rectus abdominis

5. The muscle in the abdominal region that originates only on the lower ribs is the _____ .
 a. external oblique
 b. internal oblique
 c. transversus abdominis
 d. rectus abdominis

Matching

Match each of the following descriptions with the appropriate term.

_____ **1.** Runs from the ASIS to the pubic crest	A.	External oblique
_____ **2.** Posterior/lateral connective tissue	B.	Lateral trunk flexion
_____ **3.** Distal sternum	C.	Inguinal ligament
_____ **4.** Movement to one side	D.	Abdominal aponeurosis
_____ **5.** Superior to rectus abdominis	E.	Abdominal compression
_____ **6.** Occurs when coughing	F.	Thoracolumbar fascia
_____ **7.** Anterior connective tissue	G.	Internal oblique
_____ **8.** Horizontal connective tissue	H.	Xiphoid process
_____ **9.** Most superficial muscle	I.	Linea alba
_____ **10.** Runs from the xiphoid to the pubis aponeurosis	J.	Transversus abdominis

Critical Thinking

1. For years sit-ups were the preferred method of strengthening the abdominal region. Recent evidence suggests that full sit-ups may be contraindicated and detrimental to the lower back region. Why do you think this is? What are alternative ways to strengthen the abdominals?

2. Imagine a person swinging a golf club. Do the abdominals play a part in this motion? Name some exercises to prescribe to a patient or client who wants to improve his or her golf swing and core body strength.

3. Research the attachments of the thoracolumbar fascia. Discuss the role of the fascia and discuss the treatment of restricted fascia.

4. Review Table 10-2 regarding the movements of the trunk. If you have not already done so, stand up and mimic those movements. Does it seem fairly "easy" to replicate the movement and to grossly identify the muscle involved? Do you think you could instruct someone to perform those same movements? If you have done any research on sensorimotor treatment approaches (used with adults, children, and infants), you probably feel a little overwhelmed with their complexity. It may seem like it is a large leap to get from one (e.g., instructing someone to perform trunk flexion) to the other (e.g., positioning for maintained stretch in an elongated position, which is part of Rood's theory). So how will you get there? Are you even interested in learning more about this specialty treatment area of OT? Speculate on what you might do, or be expected to know, compared to the supervising occupational therapist.

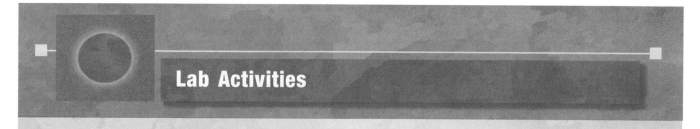

Lab Activities

Lab 10-1: Brace and Binders

Objective: To utilize the Internet as a resource for researching equipment and instructions for their use.

Equipment Needed: Internet access, pen and paper if findings are to be recorded

Step 1. Use your "Internet skills" to find sites that supply abdominal binders. Which ones appear to be best for providing stability for weak abdominal muscles?

Step 2. Find out what TLSO means, and what they are. Also find the instructions for donning (putting on; *doffing* means taking off) this particular brace.

Step 3. For the student who is interested in learning more, change the donning instructions so that they are applicable to someone with a cognitive impairment, someone with decreased U/E strength, or someone with poor postural control (all scenarios are common in OT clinical practice).

Lab 10-2: Stand/Sit Transfer

Objective: To relate abdominal muscle movements with standing movements.

Equipment Needed: Various surfaces from which to rise (e.g., hardback chair, sofa, tub bench, soft arm chair, etc.), pillows or extra padding

Step 1. From a sitting position, stand up and return to sitting. Do this several times. Pay close attention to what your back (skeletal system and muscles), your abdominal muscles, your legs, your arms, and your head and neck all do individually to contribute to this complex movement.

Step 2. Can you "take away" any one component? How does this change the movement? Is it a "safe" movement?

Step 3. Place a pillow over your abdomen, as if you were pregnant or obese, or attempt to mimic hypotonicity of your abdominal muscles. How does this "impairment" affect the "stand up from sitting" movement? Over time, how might continuing to replicate this movement with this impairment affect safety? What are the muscles that are compensating for the impaired ones? General posture? Pain? Occupational performance? Discuss your findings and speculations with the instructor and your classmates.

Lab 10-3: Bony Landmarks and Muscles of the Abdominal Region

Objective: To identify and properly palpate the bony landmarks and muscles of the abdominal region.

Equipment Needed: A lab partner, pen/pencil, paper

Step 1. With your partner in the supine position, palpate the following landmarks:

■ ASIS
■ Xiphoid process
■ Ribs 8–10 laterally, in line with the axilla
■ Pubic symphisis

Step 2. Using the same partner, palpate the following muscles, instructing your partner how to facilitate a contraction in these muscles as you palpate:

■ Rectus abdominis
■ External oblique
■ Internal oblique

■ Tranversus abdominis—palpate at the medial aspect of the ASIS deeply, and have your partner gently take his or her bellybutton to the floor, performing a pelvic floor contraction at the same time. If the palpating finger is pushed anteriorly, your partner is using too much oblique activity. A gentle tightening should be felt under the palpating finger.

Step 3. Using a Swiss ball, teach your partner an exercise program to strengthen the trunk muscles. Include exercises for the abdominals and the back extensors.

Step 4. Switch roles with your partner and repeat steps 1 through 3.

Chapter 11

POSTURE ASSESSMENT AND INTERVENTION

Key Words

anterior pelvic tilt	genu valgus	plumb line
flat-back posture	genu varus	posterior pelvic tilt
forward head posture	kyphosis-lordosis posture	swayback posture
genu recurvatum	military-type posture	

INTRODUCTION

Proper posture assessment is a critical component of the evaluation and treatment prescription for every patient. It is also part of the ongoing reassessment for progression for the patient as rehabilitation proceeds. Posture evaluation helps the therapist determine the stress and strain placed on soft tissue, joints, and bones through habitual faulty alignment. Posture evaluation also provides initial information on potential problems with muscular length and weakness balances influencing or created by faulty habitual postures. Further evaluation of joint mobility, muscle flexibility, and strength is required for a comprehensive determination of the patient's status, but it is beyond the scope of this chapter. Before addressing proper postural assessment and the four basic postures, a quick review of anatomical planes is required.

Review of Anatomical Planes

Three anatomical planes are used in all discussions of anatomy: posture, kinesiology, and basic movement. All three planes can be assessed at multiple points along the body. For posture, the coronal point of each plane is considered, determining the center point of each plane such that their intersection would be at the center of body mass. The frontal plane divides the body into anterior and posterior structures. The sagittal plane divides the body into right and left structures, whereas the transverse or horizontal plane divides the body into top and bottom, or superior and inferior, structures. In standard postural assessment performed in a standing position, the frontal plane is used in assessment from the anterior and posterior views of the patient. The sagittal plane is assessed in side views of the patient. Because of possible differences between right and left positioning, both sides must be assessed. The horizontal plane is assessed indirectly in the standing position when the alignment of the scapulae or pelvic girdle is assessed for protraction or retraction, or limbs are assessed for internal or external rotation. The transverse plane can also be assessed in the supine or prone position, along with the frontal plane. All planes may be assessed in the sitting position for patients who have balance challenges or if the upper quadrants of the body are being assessed for faulty sitting posture problems (such as in workspace ergonomic evaluations or fitting for wheelchair alignment).

PRINCIPLES OF POSTURE EVALUATION

It is highly recommended that all novices of postural evaluation utilize a **plumb line** to assist in visualizing the coronal plane for the frontal and sagittal views. A plumb line is a piece of string with a weight on the bottom that is suspended from the ceiling of a clinic. The patient is asked to stand beside the plumb line facing either the string (for the anterior view) or the adjacent wall (sagittal view). For all views, the plumb line is aligned in orientation to the feet. This is the most stable point of reference. The orientation of all other structures is influenced by the position of the feet in relation to the plumb line. In the sagittal view, the proper alignment of the plumb line begins just slightly anterior to the lateral malleolus. In the ideal posture, the remaining plumb line orients slightly anterior to the knee joint axis, slightly posterior to the axis of the hip, along the bodies of the cervical and lumbar vertebrae, through the shoulder joint, and through the external auditory meatus. In the frontal view, the plumb line reference point is midway between the patient's heels. The easiest way to find this midpoint is by using diagrams of feet properly positioned on the floor or by positioning the patient's feet equally on either side of the clinician's foot that is aligned with the plumb line. The plumb line will then fall midway between the lower extremities, through the midline of the pelvis, sternum, and skull.

The clinician can decide whether assessment of a patient's posture will proceed from the feet superiorly or from the head inferiorly. Often this decision is guided by the needs of a patient and from the complaints and mechanism of injury gleaned from the patient interview. Generally, clinicians choose to begin their evaluation from the frontal view, with the patient facing the clinician. This facilitates any initial instructions that the clinician must give and allows a continuation of the process of forming a trusting relationship with the patient. While the patient remains in place, the clinician then proceeds to the assessment from the posterior view. In this manner, the patient's position does not change, and comparisons of segmental positioning from anterior to posterior are valid. After the posterior view is assessed, the patient can be repositioned for assessment in the frontal plane. It is highly recommended that if the complaint is unilateral, the nonaffected side is evaluated first followed by the affected side. This allows for comparison of the affected side to a standardized normal and to the patient's habitual posturing.

OTA Perspective

Ankylosing spondylitis is a chronic spinal inflammatory disease that usually begins between the ages of 17 and 35. The disease is more common and more serious in males; it is present in women but usually in a milder form.

The pathology of the disease begins with inflammation of the ligaments and joint capsules of the joints of the spine and usually starts in the sacroiliac joint. The inflammation slowly progresses up the spine and is followed by calcification and ankylosis of the joints.

As the calcification occurs, the spine becomes gradually stiffer and adopts a fixed flexed posture. The thoracic kyphosis becomes more pronounced, the lumbar spine curvature is lost, and the forward head posture can become significant. Pain is usually localized within the spine, and morning stiffness is a significant feature. Involvement of peripheral joints can occur in 50% of the cases, and the rheumatoid factor is negative. Diagnosis is usually made by the clinical features, an X-ray, and a blood test. Treatment consists of anti-inflammatory medication and ongoing PT to prevent further loss of range of motion and to maintain strength.

Frontal Plane Evaluation

From the frontal view the clinician evaluates the head position for rotation or side bending, shoulders and scapulae for elevation or depression, and protraction or retraction. Protraction and retraction of the scapulae are more readily evaluated from the posterior view, comparing the medial borders of the scapulae in their relation to the thoracic spine. Protraction (movement away from the vertebrae) of the scapulae will appear as abduction, often with notable differences between the affected side and the unaffected side in the case of unilateral injury or disease. Winged scapulae will appear to have prominent inferior angles.

Spinal curves are assessed for neutral positioning of the spinous processes or a scoliosis (lateral curvature in either a "C" or "S" formation). The pelvis is evaluated through palpation of the anterior superior iliac spine (ASIS) and the posterior superior iliac spine (PSIS). Through palpation of these landmarks the clinician can determine iliac elevation, drop, or lateral tilt. The elevation or drop can be confirmed by palpation of the iliac crest.

The greater trochanters of the femur can be compared to assess a possible leg length difference. Knees are assessed for genu valgus or varus and patellar alignment. **Genu valgus** is commonly referred to as "knock knees," a terminology used in some texts on posture. The knees are positioned toward midline, forming an "L," with the angle of "L" being the knee and the arms being the femur and tibia. **Genu varus** is determined as the knees are positioned laterally. Patellar alignment can be assessed in the frontal view for proper positioning in relation to the knee joint to rule out positional malalignment such as patella alta. Ankles and feet are evaluated in the frontal plane for pronation or supination, assessed by the positioning of the medial malleolus and longitudinal arch. A pronated foot appears to have a flattened longitudinal arch with medial positioning of the medial malleolus. A supinated foot appears to have a high arch and may have lateral positioning of the medial malleolus. Heel position from the posterior view will also validate the assessment from the anterior view.

Sagittal Plane Evaluation

From the sagittal view, the clinician evaluates the head for neutral positioning of the external meatus over the shoulder. When the head appears to be aligned anteriorly to the ideal position, a syndrome of faulty alignment, called "**forward head posture**" (FHP), will be apparent. This is a common fault in many postures, incorporating hyperextension of the atlanto-occipital joint, excessive extension of the upper cervical spine, and flexion of the lower cervical and upper thoracic spine. The patient appears to have a prominent jaw line and flattened cervical spine. The patient's mouth may also drop open, secondary to alignment changes in the temporomandibular joint, or appear to be clenched in an attempt to keep the mouth closed. A less common faulty posture is axial extension, causing flattening of the cervical lordosis and posterior positioning of the head in relation to the shoulder.

Protraction and retraction of the scapular girdle also are evaluated from the sagittal view. This view also allows for assessment of normal, minimal, or excessive spinal kyphosis and lordosis. Pelvic tilt is assessed through determination of the relationship of either the ASIS and PSIS or the ASIS and pubic symphysis. A neutral pelvic tilt has a 10-degree angle between the ASIS and the PSIS. Greater than 10 degrees indicates a **posterior pelvic tilt**, and less than 10 degrees indicates an **anterior pelvic tilt**. Another way to assess pelvic tilt is based on the vertical line created between the ASIS and pubic symphysis when the pelvis is in neutral tilt. If the line tilts posteriorly toward the spine, the pelvis is in posterior tilt. If the line tilts anteriorly away from the body, the pelvis is in anterior tilt. Posterior pelvic tilt occurs concurrently with decreased lumbar lordosis. An anterior tilt is associated with increased lumbar lordosis. Knee position evaluated in the sagittal plane is related to increased flexion or extension of the knee joint. **Genu recurvatum** refers to hyperextension of the knee joint. And, finally, ankles are evaluated for habitual dorsiflexion, plantar flexion, or neutral positioning at 90 degrees.

Transverse Plane Evaluation

From the transverse plane, the clinician evaluates rotation of the upper extremities, lower extremities, and pelvis. The greater trochanter and knees can be palpated for assessment of hip internal or external rotation. This assessment continues down to the knee joints, using patellar position in orientation to the front: a patella facing medially indicates internal rotation, and, a patella facing away from midline indicates external rotation. Internal or external rotation of the upper extremities is assessed in a similar manner with the greater tuberosities and cubital region of the elbow. The anatomical position has the body in full external rotation of the upper extremities; however, most people hold their extremities in a neutral position with palms into the thighs. Internal rotation of the arm is often associated with scapular protraction or forearm pronation, or both. Rotation of the ilia of the pelvis is also assessed from the transverse plane. Internal rotation of the ilia is called an "inflare" and appears as ASIS that are too close to midline. External rotation is called an "outflare" and appears as ASIS that are too far from the midline.

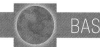 BASIC POSTURES

Ideal Segmental Alignment

An ideal segmental alignment is characterized with the head in a neutral position with no forward or backward posture and the cervical spine with a normal lordosis (Figure 11-1). Scapulae are flat against the thorax and in neutral positioning. The thoracic spine shows normal kyphosis, and the lumbar spine shows normal lordosis. The pelvis is in neutral positioning with the ASIS in a vertical plane with the symphysis pubis. Hips and knees are neither flexed nor extended, and the ankle joints are in a neutral 90-degree angle creating a vertical alignment of the legs.

In the sagittal view all of the anterior and posterior muscles are in balance. The abdominals pull upward and the legs pull downward, positioning the pelvis in neutral. Activation of back extensors and abdominals provide core stability of the trunk.

From the posterior view the head is in a neutral position without side bending or rotation (Figure 11-2). (A slight right side bend is seen in the picture.) The cervical, thoracic, and lumbar spines are all straight, although Figure 11-2 shows the cervical spine slightly side bent to the right. The scapulae are in a neutral position with the medial borders almost parallel and about 3 to 4 inches apart. The pelvis is level with both PSIS in the same plane. Hip joints are level and in neither abduction nor adduction. No genu valgus or varus is apparent, and feet are parallel with a slight toeing out. Achilles tendons are vertical, indicating that neither pronation nor supination is present, although Figure 11-2 shows that a slight pronation may be possible.

In ideal posture, the trunk flexor, hip adductor, opposite abductor, tibialis posterior, foot flexor, and opposite foot everter muscles are all active to hold the trunk, pelvis, and legs in a stable position. Legs and trunk muscles must be balanced contralaterally to hold the pelvis in a neutral position and to maintain standing and sitting balance. Slight variations from neutral alignment are not uncommon and should not be considered to be abnormal. Handedness is seen as a slight depression of the shoulder girdle on the dominant side and a slight elevation of the pelvis on the same side.

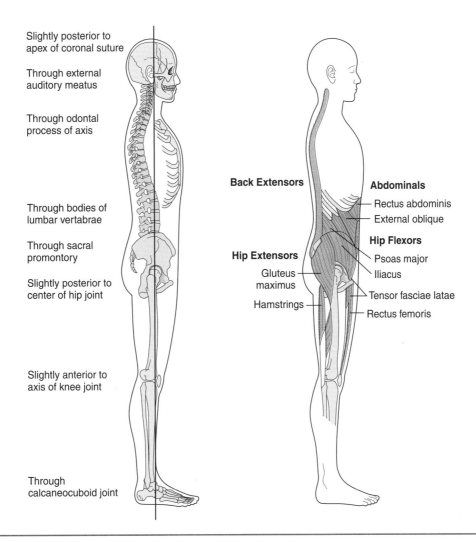

Figure 11-1 *Ideal Segmental Alignment: Side View*

Kyphosis-Lordosis Posture

Kyphosis-lordosis postures are highlighted by a forward head positioning, causing hyperextension of the upper cervical spine, flexion of the lower cervical spine, and flexion of the upper thoracic spine (Figure 11-3). The thoracic spine shows increased kyphosis throughout (increased flexion), and the lumbar spine shows increased lordosis (hyperextension). The scapulae are abducted and protracted. The pelvis is in an anterior tilt, causing hip flexion and slight hyperextension of the knees. The ankle joints are in slight plantar flexion owing to the backward inclination of the legs.

When studying Figure 11-3, note the shortened muscles of the neck extensor muscle group and one-joint hip flexors. The low back muscles are likely to be short, but if they are strong, no length change may happen. In a sitting position, the low back muscles are stretched while the one-joint hip flexors shorten, so low back muscle shortness may be seen less often than one-joint hip flexor shortness. Neck flexors are elongated as well as the erector spinae of the thorax, external obliques, and hamstrings. The rectus abdominis may not be elongated owing to the depression of the chest from increased thoracic kyphosis.

Swayback Posture

Swayback posture is often mistaken as kyphosis-lordosis posture because of the common use of the term *swayback* to describe the sagging back of old horses (Figure 11-4). There are significant differences between the two postures that can be readily seen by the clinician. The term *swayback* refers to the trunk position in relation to the plumb line. The thoracic spine is elongated and has displaced (swayed) posteriorly to the plumb line. The lumbar spine is in decreased lordosis (flexion), which is related to a posterior tilt of the pelvis. This posterior pelvic tilt creates hyperextension of the hip joints with a forward displacement of the pelvis to stabilize body weight against the posterior displacement of the trunk. The knees are hyper-

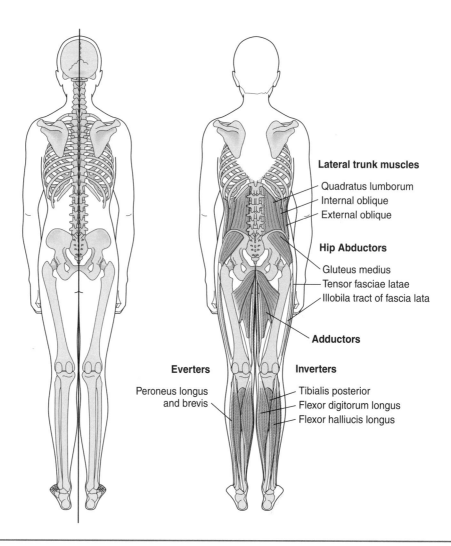

Lateral trunk muscles
Quadratus lumborum
Internal oblique
External oblique

Hip Abductors
Gluteus medius
Tensor fasciae latae
Illobila tract of fascia lata

Adductors

Everters
Peroneus longus
and brevis

Inverters
Tibialis posterior
Flexor digitorum longus
Flexor halliucis longus

Figure 11- 2 *Ideal Alignment: Posterior View*

extended, allowing the ankles to remain in a neutral position. As seen with the kyphosis-lordosis posture, the head is in a forward position with concurrent changes in the cervical spine.

One-joint hip flexors are elongated and weakened, as are the external obliques, upper back extensors, and cervical flexors. The hamstrings and upper fibers of the internal obliques are shortened. The low back extensors are strong but not shortened.

Flat-Back Posture

As with the kyphosis-lordosis and swayback postures, a **flat-back posture** incorporates a forward head position with concurrent changes in the cervical and upper thoracic spine (Figure 11-5). The lower thoracic spine and lumbar spine are straight, having lost their normal curves. The resultant, or concurrent, pelvic position is a posterior pelvic tilt. The hips and knees are extended. Occasionally, the knees are slightly bent instead of extended, as with many elderly patients. The ankles are in slight plantar flexion.

One-joint hip flexors are elongated and weak, and the hamstrings are short and strong. Although the back muscles are elongated, they may or may not be weakened.

Military-Type Posture

At first glance, **military-type postures** appear to be close to an ideal posture (Figure 11-6). However, the lumbar spine shows increased lordosis (hyperextended), the pelvis is in an anterior tilt, and the knees are slightly hyperextended. The head is in neutral or may show axial extension and a reduction of the cervical lordosis.

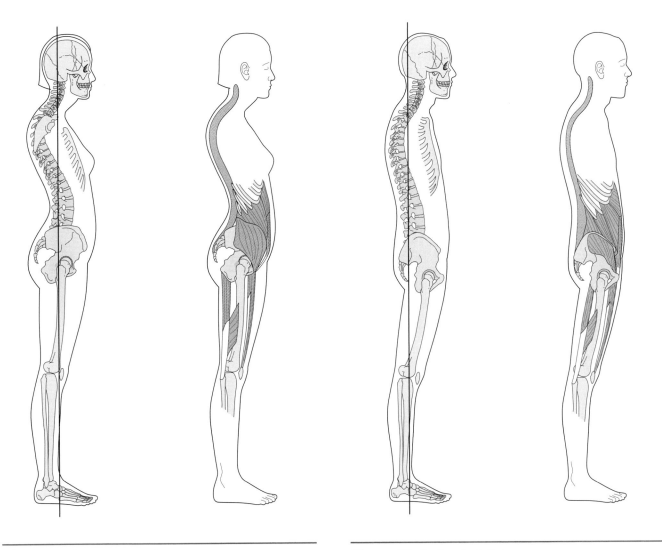

Figure 11-3 *Kyphosis-Lordosis Posture*

Figure 11-4 *Swayback Posture*

OTA Perspective

"Positioning" and "seating assessments" are very common areas of OT clinical practice. The text's description of what is "normal" posture is thorough and ideal. The OTA student should practice mimicking the typical and the abnormal postures. It is imperative to have a good understanding of what is anatomically correct posture—many of the clients treated in OT practice will *not* have this ideal posture and will, therefore, have resulting issues in occupational performance. Numerous diagnoses have accompanying postural concerns—Parkinson's, SCI, CVA, MS, CP, MD, pelvic and hip fractures, OA, JRA, post-polio syndrome, and so on. (Look up the abbreviations with which you are not familiar.) From what you already know about these diagnoses, can you mimic the typically demonstrated abnormal postures?

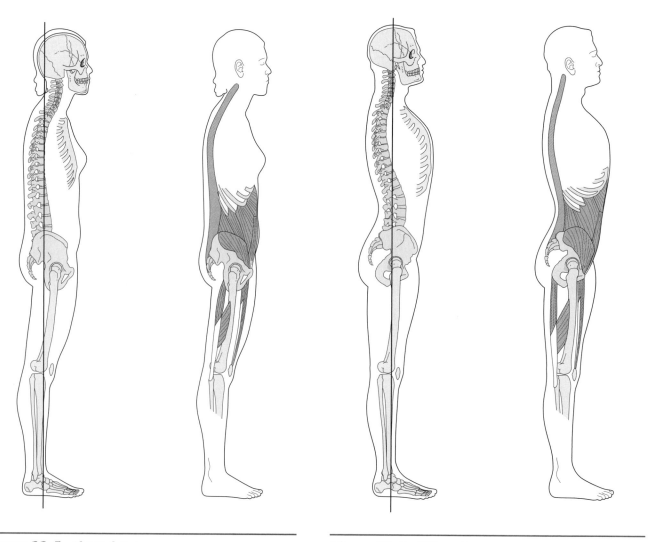

Figure 11-5 *Flat-Back Posture*

Figure 11-6 *Military-Type Posture*

The rectus abdominis muscle is often elongated and weak, whereas the hamstrings are slightly elongated and may or may not be weak. Low back extensors and one- and two-joint hip flexors are shortened and strong.

POSTERIOR VIEW ASSESSMENT

This demonstration of alignment in the posterior view often shows frequently seen postural faults (Figure 11-7). The head tends to be in neutral without side bend or rotation owing to the adjustments made in the spine to allow the head to be centered. However, in Figure 11-7, the model shows a slight side bend and rotation to the right. The cervical spine is straight, but the thoracolumbar curve is convex toward the left. This causes the right shoulder to be low and the pelvis to have a lateral tilt, appearing high on the right. Body weight has shifted toward the right of the plumb line. The right hip joint is in adduction and medial rotation, with compensatory left hip abduction to balance to body shift. The knees appear to be straight. Compensations are seen in the feet with slight left pronation resulting from postural deviation of the body to the right.

Similar to the thoracolumbar convexity toward the left, left lateral trunk muscles will be elongated and weak. Also elongated and weak are the right hip abductors (particularly the gluteus medius), left hip adductors, right peroneus longus and brevis, and left tibialis posterior and foot flexors. The muscles on the opposite side will be short and strong. This is the posture that may be apparent in small amount for handedness.

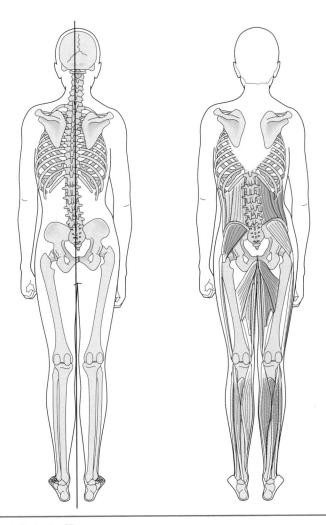

Figure 11-7 *Faulty Alignment: Posterior View*

 POSTURE THROUGH THE LIFE SPAN

Posture begins to develop as early as the third prenatal trimester. Movements of the fetus to change position, rotate, and roll are postural changes that continue until positioning for birth. During the first 3 months of life, an infant is fully flexed in both prone and supine positioning. Trunk and extremities are in full flexion until about 4 to 6 months of age, when the infant begins to lift his or her head up. At this point cervical lordosis begins to develop, as does thoracic extension. Early development of lumbar lordosis also begins at this time. With assistance infants also begin to sit up. Erect sitting with lumbar lordosis is present between 6 and 8 months of age, along with early standing with the upper trunk and shoulder girdle positioned behind the feet so balance assistance is needed. By 7 to 9 months, the child has three spinal curves and can sit and be independent while performing quadriped activities. By 10 to 12 months, standing is also independent, with flat feet, accentuated lumbar lordosis (up to 30–40 degrees), protruding abdomen, and arms in a "high guard" position of abduction, external rotation, and elbow flexion for balance.

Lumbar lordosis begins to reduce by 2 to 3 years of age. The protruding abdomen is normal for children until about 10 to 12 years of age, when the child's waist becomes smaller. The longitudinal arch of the foot develops by 6 to 7 years of age, about the time when genu valgus seen in most children resolves. Posture becomes close to the ideal segmental alignment by adolescence, although this is also when most faulty postural habits begin to emerge.

Over time, an individual's posture remains very flexible and changes consistently secondary to activities, lifestyle and health. As a person enters the senior years of life, posture becomes very dependent on continued mobility, activity level, health, and genetics. Typically, elderly individuals display postures very similar to a young child with a wide base of support, flexed knees and hips, flattened lumbar spine, increased thoracic kyphosis, and an inclination forward of the vertical plane of the plumb line. Elderly adults often have a forward head posture related to health issues such as decreased vision, osteoporosis, and habitual changes in posture that developed through life.

OTA Perspective

"OT for w/c eval" ("occupational therapy for wheelchair evaluation") is a common physician order written for clients who live in a nursing home. One place to start the evaluation is with a posture assessment—ideally in standing, sitting, and lying prone and supine. Unfortunately, in reality, the evaluation will be conducted without gathering information from all four positions and will likely rely on what the OT practitioner observes while the client is in a sitting position. A more complete posture assessment may be hindered by the client's limited physical capacities (e.g., unable to stand), by the progression of the disease (e.g., joint contractures), by complaints of pain or fatigue with position changes or prolonged assessment time, by cognitive impairments affecting direction following abilities, or by the client's developmental status (e.g., a young child who does not comprehend the reason for the assessment and, therefore, is sometimes or often "noncompliant" in attending and following commands). A "w/c eval" can be further complicated by time and money constraints from the funding source, by limited availability of trial equipment, or by vendor accessibility. These are not meant to discourage the OT practitioner from doing his or her best, nor are they excuses for performing a less-than-adequate posture assessment. They are, however, real life challenges that need to be incorporated into providing OT skilled services. Knowledge of "normal" posture and posture and movement changes typical to a specific disease or maturation stage will greatly contribute to a successful posture assessment as part of an "OT for w/c eval."

 INTERVENTION

The primary goal of postural interventions is to reduce the strains and stresses on musculoskeletal structures created by poor postural habits. To achieve this goal the core muscles of the trunk must be strong, properly coordinated, under control, and have the endurance to work throughout the day. The primary muscle groups targeted include the abdominals, particularly the transversus abdominis and abdominal obliques; the trunk extensors, and the scapular stabilizers, particularly the lower trapezius because the upper trapezius is often overworked. In addition to these primary muscles, any muscle groups determined to be elongated and weak from a postural evaluation are added into the program. All postural exercises are performed with minimal resistance and progressive repetitions to build endurance. Just enough resistance should be used to provide assistance in stimulating muscle activity but not enough to overwhelm the client's ability to use proper form, technique, and motor control. Clients should receive exercises to be performed in the supine, prone, sitting, and standing positions because postural control is necessary in all of these positions.

The first core exercise that all clients must receive is isometric control of the transversus abdominis muscle. The client is taught to pull the "belly button" toward the spine as the visual and sensory cue to activate the transversus abdominis. This isometric contraction must then be maintained as the client moves the trunk or the limbs through various exercises. This can be achieved through abdominal curl-ups, straight leg raises, arm exercises, or functional movements such as transitions from sit to stand or lifting.

A second core exercise includes activation of the lower trapezius muscles with proper motor control through movement and positioning of the scapulae. The lower trapezius is an important component in the force couple of scapular stabilizers and is often one of the muscles determined to be weak in postural evaluation. To activate the lower trapezius the scapulae are pulled medially and inferiorly. This is facilitated by verbal cuing and also by concurrent and separate activation of the middle trapezius. Proper timing and activation of the lower trapezius can be achieved during exercises such as arm raises, curl-ups, and trunk extensions.

Trunk extension or isometric activation of the erector spinae and other trunk extensors are critical components of postural exercises and awareness. These exercises can be initiated if the prone leg or arm lifts, providing maximal support for the trunk, and then progressed to quadriped, standing, or mobile surfaces. The trunk extensors can also be activated without facilitation from the extremities.

Multiple tools can be used in postural exercises. The most simple tool is an exercise mat for active movement exercises, focusing on moving the body with maximal motor control. Other tools can include Theraband or theratubing, foam rollers, weighted or unweighted therapeutic balls, cam system or isokinetic exercise machines, and the Pilates system. Some of these tools, such as Pilates, require specialized education to properly incorporate them into a rehabilitation program. However, most tools are standard tools in rehabilitation and the clinician is only limited by his or her own experience or creativity.

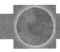

KEY CONCEPTS

- The basic concepts of posture evaluation include observing a patient in all three planes: frontal, sagittal, and transverse. A plumb line and foot lines are used to assess the posture as it relates to abnormalities and muscle imbalance.

- In postural evaluation, there are four major types of posture: kyphosis-lordosis, swayback, flat-back, and military. However, when everything is in its proper place, the term *ideal segmental alignment* is applied.

- Throughout life, the body goes through many types of changes. This is especially true from when we are born through adulthood.

- Once an evaluation of posture has taken place, the OT assistant will write an exercise prescription. These exercises often consist of numerous activities and focus on all of the muscles that affect posture. To incorporate an appropriate exercise routine the OTA may utilize theraband, Pilates, and numerous other exercises to accomplish posture corrections.

BIBLIOGRAPHY

Flynn, T. W. (1996). *The thoracic spine and rib cage: Musculoskeletal evaluation and treatment.* Boston: Butterworth-Heinemann.

Hall, C. M., & Brody, L. T. (1999). *Therapeutic exercise: Moving toward function.* Philadelphia: Lippincott Williams & Wilkins.

Kendall, F. P., McCreary, E. K., & Provance, P. G. (1993). *Muscles: Testing and function* (4th ed.). Philadelphia: Lippincott Williams & Wilkins.

Magee, D. (2002). *Orthopedic physical assessment* (4th ed.). Philadelphia: W. B. Saunders.

Porterfield, J. A., & DeRosa, C. (1995). *Mechanical neck pain: Perspectives in functional anatomy.* Philadelphia: W. B. Saunders.

Sahrmann, S. A. (2002). Does postural assessment contribute to patient care? *Journal of Orthopedic and Sports Physical Therapy, 32,* 376–379.

Twomey, L. T., & Taylor, J. R. (2000). *Physical therapy of the low back* (3rd ed.). Philadelphia: Churchill Livingstone.

REVIEW QUESTIONS

True or False

In the blanks provided, indicate whether each of the following statements is true or false.

_____ **1.** It is common for small children to have a protruding abdomen.

_____ **2.** In frontal plane examination, pronated ankles may make knees appear to be knock-kneed.

_____ **3.** A forward head is a component of the flat-back, kyphosis-lordosis, and swayback postures.

_____ **4.** In ideal posture, the plumb line is posterior to the knee joint.

_____ **5.** Military posture is the ideal alignment of the spine and muscles.

Multiple Choice

Select the best answer to complete the following statements.

1. Right-handed individuals would typically have a _____ .
   a. low right shoulder
   b. low left shoulder
   c. deviation of the head to the right
   d. deviation of the head to the left

2. The lumbar spine has _____ in a swayback posture.
   a. increased lordosis
   b. decreased lordosis
   c. normal lordosis
   d. lateral lordosis

3. A posterior pelvic tilt is associated with a _____ .
   a. long rectus abdominis
   b. short iliopsoas
   c. short rectus abdominis
   d. long semimembranosus

4. Postural assessment in the frontal plane is used to determine _____ .
   a. forward head posture
   b. knock-knees
   c. hyperextended knees
   d. thoracic kyphosis

5. In postural evaluation, a plumb line is used to determine the _____ .
   a. sagittal plane
   b. frontal plane
   c. transverse plane
   d. coronal plane

Critical Thinking

1. In the current climate of health care, OT evaluation and treatment sessions are becoming less frequent and of shorter duration. This necessitates good clinical reasoning, prioritization of client needs, specialization skills for the OT practitioner, and accurate documentation of the need for skilled OT services. In following up with the "OT for w/c eval and treatment as indicated" physician order, numerous factors need to be considered. The first one is obviously the client and his or her goals—the reason for the OT order in the first place. Discuss other potential factors and complexities, including the OT practitioner's expertise, the funding source for purchasing the wheelchair, the likely compliance issues on the client, caregiver(s) and the facility, and the predicted progression of the disease. And then add "ethics" to the discussion.

2. Correct posture is very important for a number of reasons. Imagine that you are discussing this with a 13-year-old adolescent girl with an increased thoracic kyphosis who has been sent to you for postural advice and exercises. The client is unenthusiastic about attending therapy. Describe the advice that you would give her regarding posture and why it is important to correct it at this age.

3. List and describe six exercises that you would give to this 13-year-old client to help correct her kyphosis and any other treatment techniques that you would use to help cue her into improving her posture.

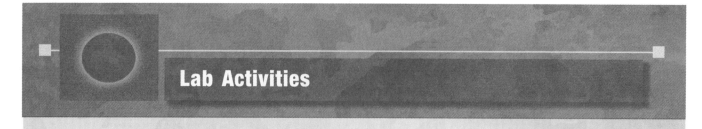

Lab Activities

Lab 11-1: Assessment of Normal Posture

Objective: To properly assess and evaluate proper posture.

Equipment Needed: A lab partner or partners, pen/pencil, paper

Step 1.   Using this chapter, and with your partner suitably undressed, assess his or her posture, starting either at the head or the feet, assessing in all three planes. List all your findings.

Step 2.   Switch to two other partners and repeat step 1.

Step 3.   Teach all of the partners the correct posture for both standing and sitting.

Lab 11-2: Assessment of Ankylosis

Objective: To properly assess and evaluate an abnormality in posture.

Equipment Needed: A lab partner, pen/pencil, paper

Step 1.   Your client is a 23-year-old male who has been recently diagnosed with ankylosing spondylitis. The client has many questions. Explain your knowledge of the disease and then the importance of good posture.

Step 2.   Using your partner, instruct him or her in a program of five exercises that the client should do to strengthen and maintain range.

Step 3.   The client also has questions regarding the athletic activities that he should be doing and those he should be avoiding. Provide an explanation for the activities to participate in and avoid.

Lab 11-3: Postural Assessment

Objective: To compare and contrast normal and abnormal postures.

Equipment Needed: Clinic or classroom setting, disease resource books, pen and paper for writing reaction paper

Step 1.   Research a diagnosis discussed within this chapter with respect to *typically* expected postural involvement.

Step 2.   Respectfully mimic that posture, with only mild impairments. Walk, sit down and stand up again, open the door, don a pullover sweatshirt, climb a flight of stairs, or other similar common ADL. Pay special attention to safety aspects, along with effectiveness and efficiency of completing those tasks, and overall independence.

Step 3.   Now respectfully mimic a greater postural impairment. Can you safely perform the tasks in step 2? Can you do them at all?

Step 4.   Write a reaction paper contrasting normal posture with the postural impairments and actions you experienced.

Lab 11-4: Sitting Position Assessment

Objective: To increase observation skills with regard to identifying postural aspects.

Equipment Needed: A lab partner, chair, pen and paper for writing results and recommendations

Step 1.   With a partner, review the postural aspects of sitting (review this chapter's ideal segmental alignment section), observing the proper posture characteristics in your partner. Observe these aspects from the frontal plane, the sagittal plane, and the transverse plane.

Step 2.   Have your partner assume a sitting posture consistent with one of the diagnoses discussed in this chapter. Observe the aspects of that sitting position from the frontal plane, the sagittal plane, and the transverse plane.

Step 3.   Together with your partner, make recommendations for improving the posture—whatever appears to coincide with what you know about postural aspects and the diagnosis you chose.

Step 4.   If you are interested in learning more, observe your partner in a standing or prone/supine position, both for normal posture and when mimicking a postural impairment, and in all three planes.

Chapter 12

RESPIRATION

Key Words

active expiration	external intercostal	phrenic nerve
active inspiration	forced expiration	pre-expiration
carbon dioxide	homeostasis	pre-inspiration
central tendon	inferior border of the rib	superior border of the rib
costal cartilage	inspiration	thoracic cavity
diaphragm	internal intercostal	
expiration	oxygen	

INTRODUCTION

Take a moment to observe the respiration processes of taking in air (inspiration) and expelling air (expiration) as an individual is relaxing. Now take another step further and think about inspiration and expiration when the body is placed under stressful conditions such as exercise. Are the same muscles that cause respiration movements involved in both situations, or are there additional muscles that contract to help with the processes of respiration during exercise?

Respiration is a process through which the muscles of the thoracic cavity expand and constrict the chest cavity of the body, allowing **oxygen** (O_2) to transport into the bloodstream and **carbon dioxide** (CO_2) to be removed from the bloodstream.

Respiration occurs in the **thoracic cavity** of the body as the muscles of inspiration and expiration contract to change the volume (or space) of the thoracic cavity. The thoracic cavity is made up of a collection of ribs (costae) and costal cartilage that are firmly attached to the sternum in the anterior, the thoracic spine in the posterior, and the diaphragm muscle in the inferior region of the thoracic cavity. Several muscles are involved in the process of respiration while the human body is at rest.

Once physiological parameters are changed involving O_2 uptake and CO_2 removal, additional muscles are required to maintain the physiological functions of the human body and to maintain **homeostasis**.

PHASES OF RESPIRATION

Throughout the day, physiological demands for O_2 and CO_2 change as the body moves from one condition or activity to the next. As a result, there are four phases of passive respiration: pre-inspiration, inspiration, pre-expiration, and expiration. **Pre-inspiration** is a static phase that precedes inspiration. **Inspiration** is the active phase of air intake that is characterized by the expansion of the thorax. **Pre-expiration** is a static phase that precedes expiration and follows inspiration. **Expiration** is the active phase of air outflow that is characterized by the decrease in the thoracic volume.

In addition to the passive processes of respiration, there are two active phases of respiration that occur when the body actively forces air in and out of the thoracic cavity: **active inspiration** and **active expiration**. During both phases additional muscles (synergists) assist in the exchange of O_2 and CO_2.

Inspiration

During inspiration, the action of the diaphragm muscle accounts for about one third of the volume change associated with inspired air, with the external intercostal and scalene muscles also being active. The actions of these muscles, the diaphragm to the inferior, the external intercostals to the anterior, and the scalene muscles superior to the thoracic cavity, pull on the ribs, causing the volume in the thoracic cavity to expand (Figure 12-1). As a result, the actions of these muscles expand the lungs, causing air to be inspired into the lungs. Take, for example, a syringe that is being filled with a fluid for injection. As the fluid is drawn, the volume within the syringe changes, causing the fluid to be taken into the syringe.

During periods of increased physiological O_2 demands on the body, such as exercise, synergist muscles aid in inspiration movements. Mainly, the sternocleidomastoid and levator scapula muscles increase the efficiency and exchange of O_2 uptake. By recruiting these muscles, forced inspiration occurs as the volume of the thoracic cavity further increases, allowing a greater amount of O_2 to be taken up by the lungs.

Expiration

Expiration is a passive process at rest when the muscles of inspiration simply relax (see Figure 12-1). Take the syringe example once again. If the syringe was full of fluid, and a weight was applied to the plunge, the volume within the syringe would change as the fluid was removed. In the lungs, when the muscles of respiration relax, the pressures exerted on the thoracic cavity collapses, causing the expiration of air.

During conditions when there is an increased physiological demand on the body, **forced expiration** occurs as the diaphragm and intercostal muscles are activated along with a variety of other synergist muscles. Mainly, the abdominal muscles contract to increase pressures exerted on the thoracic cavity. The recruited muscles (transverse abdominis and oblique abdominals) are covered in Chapter 10, The Abdominal Region.

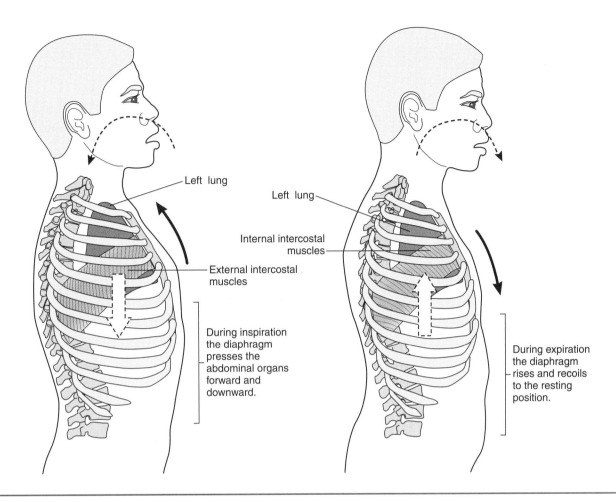

Figure 12-1 *Inspiration and Expiration*

Left lung

External intercostal muscles

During inspiration the diaphragm presses the abdominal organs forward and downward.

Left lung

Internal intercostal muscles

During expiration the diaphragm rises and recoils to the resting position.

 MAJOR THORACIC REGION LANDMARKS ASSOCIATED WITH RESPIRATION

Many different anatomical structures are associated with the thoracic region as it relates to respiration. These structures provide sound attachment points for the muscles that cause respiration movements.

Central Tendon

The **central tendon** is a flat tendon located in the central region of the diaphragm muscle (Figure 12-2). The tendon is broad, making up the middle superior region of the abdominal wall. The central tendon can be found inferior to the middle and inferior lobe of the left lung, the middle lobe of the right lung, and the heart. All of the muscle fibers of the diaphragm run toward this central tendon. As the muscle fibers pull on the central tendon, they cause the **diaphragm** to contract in the inferior direction. As a result, the diaphragm flattens in the inferior direction and the volume at the inferior region of the thoracic cavity increases.

Costal Cartilage

Costal cartilage is located on the anterior surface of the thoracic cavity at the end of each true rib (1–7) and false ribs (8–10) and firmly attaches them to the sternum (Figure 12-3). The costal cartilage is made of elastic hyaline cartilage that expands and contracts as the chest rises and falls during respiration. If this arrangement were not present or made with solid bone, the thoracic cavity would not have the ability to rise and fall, which would greatly inhibit respiration.

OTA Perspective

As a clinical OT practitioner, the OTA will treat clients with respiratory system diseases. Although most of these diseases primarily affect the internal organs (e.g., lungs, trachea), they secondarily affect the musculoskeletal structure of the chest and neck, which, in turn, affects the client's psyche; living, working, and playing environments; and social connections.

Lung diseases may ultimately cause a "barrel-chest" appearance and overdeveloped neck and shoulder muscles. These accessory breathing muscles are compensating for a compromised diaphragm muscle and loss of elasticity in the intercostal muscles. Because of the nature of the disease, people with an advanced respiratory disease use their accessory breathing muscles more than those without a respiratory diagnosis. The respiratory musculoskeletal structure must work hard during inhalation and exhalation when there is poor gas exchange in the alveoli of the bronchial structure. People with a respiratory disease also tend to use other compensatory means of assisting the inhalation/exhalation process such as taking a semireclined position, propping against a table or counter to limit the amount of upper body muscle work needed for breathing, or relying on gravity-assisted positions to compensate for weak musculature.

An understanding of the respiratory and cardiovascular systems—both from kinesiology and anatomy and physiology perspectives—will assist the OTA when working with clients with cardiopulmonary diagnoses.

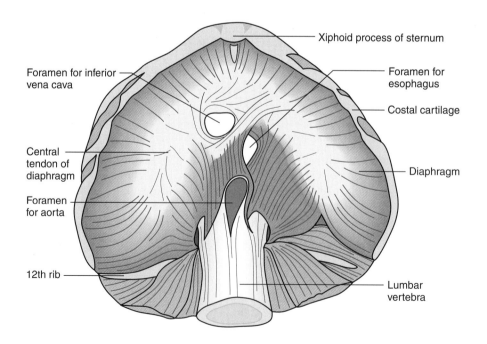

Figure 12-2 *Central Tendon*

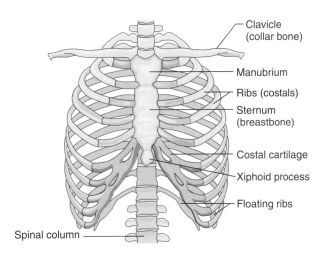

Figure 12-3 *Costal Cartilage*

Transverse Processes

The transverse processes of the vertebrae are bony landmarks that project in the lateral direction from each of the vertebrae. The importance of the transverse processes to the muscles of respiration is linked to the additional surface area that each landmark provides for muscle attachments. Mainly, the scalene muscles have an origin attachment on the transverse processes of C3–C6 and insert on the ribs. From this origin location the muscles are able to pull on the ribs during forced inspiration to increase the volume of the thoracic cavity.

Superior and Inferior Borders of the Rib

The **superior borders of the ribs** and the **inferior borders of the rib** are the insertion points for the intercostal muscles. These broad surfaces run from the anterior region of each costal bone and track laterally to the posterior costal region. These broad attachments provide a large surface area for the muscles of respiration.

Rib fractures can occur in a variety of ways, such as a direct blow to the rib or a fall on the rib. A fit of coughing in a more elderly patient can cause a spontaneous rib fracture, or the fracture can be secondary to metastases.

Signs and symptoms of rib fractures include pain with deep breathing or coughing, localized tenderness to palpation or springing of the rib, and a positive X-ray. Isolated fractures seldom require treatment beyond pain medication and rest. Rib fractures are initially very painful but should be pain-free by 8 weeks.

Complications of rib fractures include a flail chest, in which there is a loss of integrity of the chest wall and a part of the rib cage moves independently from the rest of the ribs. This can be caused by a fracture of a rib in two places. Because this is a much more serious condition, it may involve artificial ventilation of the patient. Rib fractures may also penetrate the chest wall and cause severe respiratory problems.

 NERVOUS INNERVATION

Three major nerve groups innervate the muscles that are responsible for respiration processes. The first of these nerve groups are the intercostal nerves, which originate from the ventral rami of the thoracic nerves T1–T11. A second nerve, the phrenic nerve, originates from the ventral rami of spinal nerves C3–C5. Finally, the lower cervical nerve innervates the scalene muscles.

Intercostal Nerves

Eleven pairs of intercostal nerves innervate the internal and external intercostal muscles. These nerves originate from the ventral rami of thoracic nerves T1–T11. Each of the 11 pairs of intercostal nerves is found just inferior to the associated rib and between the internal and external intercostal muscles. The nerves extend from the rami and extend laterally and medially to their termination points near the sternum. This arrangement allows each of the intercostal nerves to innervate each associated intercostal muscle.

Phrenic Nerve

The **phrenic nerve** originates at the ventral rami of the cervical nerves C3–C5 (Figure 12-4). From this origin, the nerve tracks between the anterior and middle scalene muscles at their midpoint and begins extending in the inferior direction. After the phrenic nerve tracks inferiorly, the nerve runs deep to the first rib and into the thoracic cavity. From here the nerve passes to the lateral sides of the heart and terminates at the diaphragm. This arrangement allows the phrenic nerve to innervate the diaphragm muscle and cause the contractions associated with respiration. Table 12-1 summarizes the innervation related to respiration.

Table 12-1   *Innervation Related to Respiration*

Nerve	Affected Anterior Muscles	Affected Lateral Muscles	Affected Posterior Muscles
Intercostal	External intercostals Interior intercostals	None	None
Phrenic	Diaphragm	Diaphragm	Diaphragm
Lower Cervical	Anterior scalene	Middle scalene	Posterior scalene

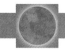

MOVEMENT OF RESPIRATION

The movements of respiration occur at multiple joints as described in the landmark section of this chapter. Although there are numerous joints associated with the thoracic region, the movements are nonlinear and, therefore, do not cause motions that occur in the sagittal, frontal, or transverse plane. Perform the movements referenced in Table 12-2 to help familiarize the movements that occur in the thoracic cavity.

Table 12-2   *Movements Related to Respiration*

Movement	Description
Inspiration	Expansion of the thorax
Expiration	Depression of the thorax
Forced Inspiration	Quick, deep, maximum inspiration
Forced Expiration	Quick, deep, maximum expiration

Asthma is a common condition that frequently affects children and adults. Characteristics of the disease include bronchospasm of the airways of the lungs, causing wheezing and breathlessness. Asthma may be related to allergies such as dust mites, pollens, and certain foods, or it can be induced by exercise. A family history also may be present. Acute attacks are common and can be very serious; the patient will have a wheeze, significant shortness of breath, and use of accessory muscles of respiration. As the attack subsides mucus secretions build up in the airways, resulting in a productive cough. Treatment in the acute phase consists of the use of bronchodilators orally, intravenously, or by inhalation. Prophylactic treatment with an inhaler daily can help prevent acute attacks.

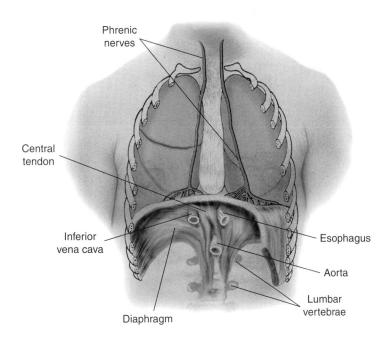

Phrenic
nerves

Central
tendon

Inferior
vena cava

Esophagus

Aorta

Lumbar
vertebrae

Diaphragm

Figure 12-4 *Phrenic Nerve*

 MUSCLES OF RESPIRATION

External Intercostals

The **external intercostal** muscles are rhomboidal in shape and are located between the ribs running from anterior to posterior (Figure 12-5). They possess short parallel fibers that slant inferiorly and medially running from the origin located on the inferior border of a superior rib to the insertion on the superior border of an immediately inferior rib. The action of the external intercostal muscles is to elevate the ribs, making the thoracic cavity larger, which aids in inspiration.

External intercostal muscles can be palpated between the ribs in the intercostal spaces on the anterior aspect of the body. The origin is on the inferior border of the superior rib, and insertion is on the superior border of the inferior rib.

Name:	External Intercostals
O:	Rib above
I:	Rib below
N:	Intercostal nerve
A:	Elevation of the ribs and inspiration
P:	Between the ribs on the anterior aspect of the body

Internal Intercostals

The **internal intercostal** muscles are rhomboidal in shape and are located deep to the external intercostals (Figure 12-6). The internal intercostal muscles have short parallel fibers that slant inferiorly and laterally from the origin on the inferior border of the rib superior to the insertion on the superior border of the immediately inferior rib. The intercostal muscles depress the ribs, making the thoracic cavity smaller, which aids in expiration processes.

Internal intercostal muscles cannot be palpated because they are deep to the external intercostal muscles. The origin is on the superior border of the rib below and insertion is on the inferior border of the rib above.

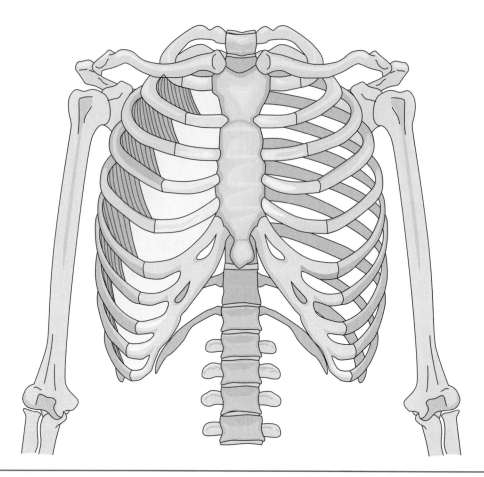

Figure 12-5 *External Intercostals*

Name: Internal Intercostals

O: Rib below

I: Rib above

N: Intercostal nerve

A: Depression of the ribs and expiration

P: Difficult to palpate

Diaphragm

The diaphragm is a dome-shaped muscle located between the thoracic and abdominal cavities (Figure 12-7). On contraction, the diaphragm depresses the central tendon, which flattens the muscle, causing the inferior region of the thoracic cavity to flatten, thus aiding in inspiration movements.

Palpation of the diaphragm is not possible because it is too deep to the muscles and bones of the abdominal and thoracic cavities. The origin of the diaphragm occurs in several places. The xyphoid process is the anteriormost origin, the inner surfaces of the lower six ribs and their respective cartilages are the costal origins, and the first three lumbar vertebrae are the posteriormost origins. The diaphragm inserts on the central tendon.

Name: Diaphragm

O: Ribs, xyphoid process, and vertebrae of the lumbar spine

I: Central tendon

N: Phrenic nerve (C3–C5)

A: Inspiration

P: Impossible to palpate

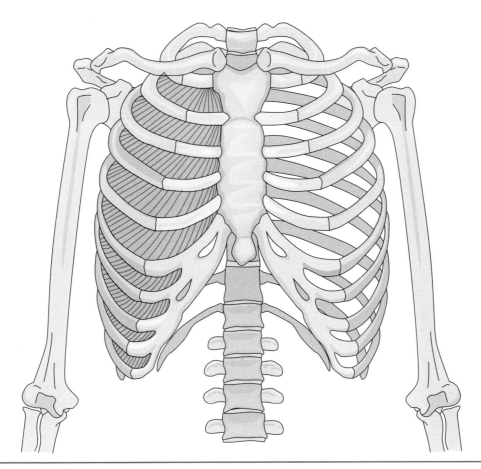

Figure 12-6 *Internal Intercostals*

Scalene

The scalene muscles are a collective group of strap muscles located on the anterolateral aspect of the neck (Figure 12-8). The scalene muscles act as synergists for inspiration. The origin of the anterior scalene is on the transverse processes of cervical vertebrae C3–C6 and inserts on the anterior border of the first rib. The origin of the intermedial scalenes occurs on the transverse processes of cervical vertebrae C2–C7 and inserts on the upper surface of the first rib. The origin of the posterior scalenes is on the transverse processes of cervical vertebrae C4–C6 and inserts on the outer surface of the second rib.

The scalene muscles may be palpated by placing the hand on the lateral aspect of the neck while taking a deep breath. Try to differentiate between the three parts in between the sternocleidomastoid and the trapezius muscles.

Name:	Scalenes
O:	Anterior: C3–C6 transverse processes
	Intermedial: C2–C7 transverse processes
	Posterior: C4–C6 transverse processes
I:	Anterior: first rib
	Intermedial: first rib
	Posterior: second rib
N:	Ventral rami of the cervical nerves
A:	Inspiration
P:	Anteriorly on the lateral neck

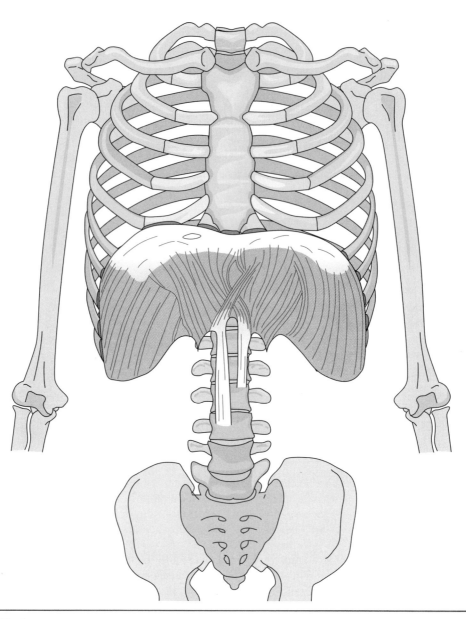

Figure 12-7 *Diaphragm*

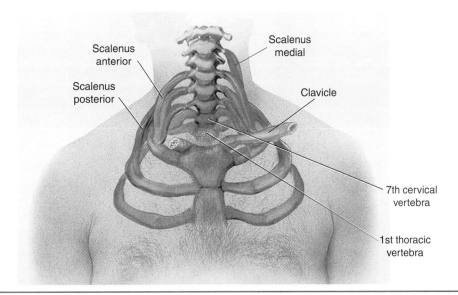

Figure 12-8 *Scalenes*

 KEY CONCEPTS

■ An increase and decrease in the lung volume allows for oxygen and carbon dioxide to exchange. These movements are made possible by the sympathetic innervation of the diaphragm, scalene, and intercostal muscle groups.

■ The nerves that innervate the muscles of respiration are both cranial and spinal nerves that cause the various motions noted with respiration.

■ There are four major muscles that provide the movements associated with the respiration process: scalene, internal intercostal, and external intercostal muscle groups, and the diaphragm. The primary muscle contractions of the diaphragm muscle cause the actions of passive respiration. The diaphragm, however, in association with the synergist muscles, allows for the actions that cause active respiration.

 BIBLIOGRAPHY

Luttgens, K. (2000). *Kinesiology: Scientific basis of human motion* (9th ed.). Madison, WI: McGraw-Hill.

Marieb, E. (2003). *Human anatomy & physiology* (6th ed.). Menlo Park, CA: Addison Wesley Longman.

Minor, M. (1998). *Kinesiology laboratory manual for physical therapist assistants*. Philadelphia: F. A. Davis.

Stone, R. (1990). *Atlas of the skeletal muscles*. Dubuque, IA: Wm. C. Brown.

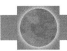 WEB RESOURCES

• The site www.nlm.nig.gov/medlineplus/copdchronicobstructivepulmonarydisease features the etiology of chronic obstructive pulmonary disease, including signs and symptoms, treatment, and diagnosis.

• Go to www.lungusa.org/diseases/lungemphysema.html for an overview, A & P, coping with, and signs and symptoms of emphysema.

(These Web addresses were current as of February 2004.)

REVIEW QUESTIONS

Fill in the Blank

Provide the best word(s) or phrase(s) that completes the sentence.

1. The scalene muscle group provides _____ movements.

2. Inspiration uses the _____ intercostal muscles.

3. The diaphragm is a _____ shaped muscle.

4. There are _____ phases of respiration.

5. The _____ nerve innervates the diaphragm muscles.

Multiple Choice

Select the best answer to complete the following statements.

1. The muscle that attaches to the superior border of the rib below is the _____ .
   a. scalene anterior
   b. diaphragm
   c. internal intercostal
   d. external intercostal

2. The _____ muscle is the most superficial.
   a. scalene intermedial
   b. diaphragm
   c. internal intercostal
   d. external intercostal

3. The diaphragm separates the _____ cavities.
   a. pelvic and abdominal
   b. abdominal and thoracic
   c. thoracic and pelvic
   d. mediastinum and thoracic cavity

4. The phrenic nerve innervates the _____ muscle.
   a. scalene anterior
   b. diaphragm
   c. internal intercostal
   d. external intercostal

5. The _____ muscle inserts on the second rib.
   a. scalene anterior
   b. scalene posterior
   c. scalene intermedial
   d. internal intercostal

Matching

Match each of the following descriptions with the appropriate term.

_____ **1.** Decrease in thoracic cavity size

_____ **2.** Top surface of the rib

_____ **3.** Synergist muscles used for inspiration

_____ **4.** Static phase that precedes inspiration

_____ **5.** Connects the ribs to the sternum

_____ **6.** Part of the diaphragm

_____ **7.** Cavity that is responsible for breathing

_____ **8.** Increase in thoracic cavity size

_____ **9.** Muscle that lies between the ribs

_____ **10.** Lateral projection of vertebrae

A. Costal cartilage

B. Inspiration

C. Central tendon

D. Thorax

E. Expiration

F. Transverse process

G. Scalenes

H. Internal intercostals

I. Pre-expiration

J. Superior border of the rib

Critical Thinking

1. Draw a diagram depicting the movement of the diaphragm muscle during inspiration and expiration.

2. Using your knowledge of the spinal cord and nervous system, explain or speculate why damage to the spinal cord above C3 would be seriously detrimental to respiration.

3. Are respiratory and cardiac diseases preventable? "Stop smoking," "get enough exercise," "avoid air pollutants," and "manage stress" are frequently heard as "words of wisdom" to those wishing to live a healthier life. Do you smoke? Do you exercise regularly? Should you be "practicing what you preach?" Do you think that how you live your life affects the impact you make when you are educating clients on ways to live theirs? Part of good intervention with a client with a cardiopulmonary diagnosis is education. Are you responsible for educating a client with a total hip replacement (THR), arthritis, or Parkinson's disease about the potential risks of continuing to smoke and living a sedentary lifestyle? Would you educate these clients on deep-breathing techniques? Is this type of education a skilled OT service and, therefore, billable?

4. Research and describe bucket handle and pump handle motion of the ribs. Describe which ribs do each motion and describe a pathological condition that would reduce both of these motions.

5. Research chronic obstructive pulmonary disease. Describe the following:

   a. Etiology

   b. Age and sex of the patient

   c. Signs and symptoms

   d. Treatment

   e. Role of OT

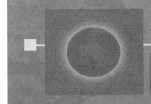

Lab Activities

Lab 12-1: Deep Breathing

Objective: To observe inhalation and exhalation in yourself and in a partner. In simple terms, explain "what is happening" (refer to the inspiration and expiration sections as necessary). Teach your partner deep-breathing techniques—diaphragmatic breathing (or belly breathing) and pursed-lip breathing.

Equipment Needed: Comfortable surfaces such as a mat or a recliner

Step 1.   Take a *deep* breath. *Slowly* exhale. Do it a couple more times. Observe this deep breathing in your partner. What is happening?

Step 2.   Teach your partner "diaphragmatic breathing" or belly breathing—a common technique taught to clients with a respiratory disease.

Step 3.   Follow directions as your partner teaches you "pursed-lip breathing"—another common deep-breathing technique.

Step 4.   Explain "when" one should use these deep-breathing techniques.

Lab 12-2: Assessment of Rib Fractures

Objective: To properly evaluate an injury resulting in a rib fracture.

Equipment Needed: A lab partner, pen/pencil, paper

Step 1.   Your patient sustained a rib fracture 10 weeks previously and still has reduced rib expansion. Assess your partner's upper rib expansion by palpating bilaterally over the anterior chest wall over the upper ribs and having him or her take a deep breath in and out.

Step 2.   Repeat the same process, assessing the middle and lower ribs, palpating laterally in line with the axilla.

Step 3.   The patient has reduced expansion of the left lower ribs with inhalation. Teach your partner how to increase his or her rib expansion in two different positions.

Lab 12-3: Identification of Landmarks Related to Respiration

Objective: To properly identify the landmarks of respiration.

Equipment Needed: A lab partner, pen/pencil, paper, skeleton

Step 1. Using a skeleton to assist you, palpate the following bony landmarks on your partner:

Partner lying supine:

Sternum—superior aspect, angle of Louis, and the xiphoid process

Clavicle

2nd rib anteriorly

sixth rib laterally in line with the axilla

Partner lying prone:

eighth rib posterior angle

T10 spinous process

Part III
Muscles of the Inferior Appendicular Skeleton

Chapters 13-16

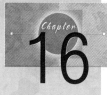

Chapter 13

THE HIP JOINT

Key Words

acetabulum
adductor brevis
adductor longus
adductor magnus
adductor tubercle
anterior inferior iliac spine
anterior superior iliac spine
biceps femoris
femoral neck
femoral nerve
fibular head
gemellus inferior
gemellus superior
gluteus maximus
gluteus medius
gluteus minimus
gracilis
greater trochanter
iliac crest
iliac fossa
iliacus

iliofemoral ligament
iliopsoas muscle
ilium
inferior gluteal nerve
inferior ramus of pubis
ischial tuberosity
ischiofemoral ligament
ischium
lateral condyle
lateral epicondyle
lateral epicondyle of the tibia
lesser trochanter
linea aspera
lumbosacral plexus
medial condyle
medial condyle of the tibia
medial epicondyle
obturator externus
obturator foramen
obturator internus

obturator nerve
pectineus
piriformis
posterior inferior iliac spine
posterior superior iliac spine
pubic symphysis
pubis
pubofemoral ligament
quadratus femoris
ramus of the ischium
rectus femoris
sartorius
sciatic nerve
sciatic notch
semimembranosus
semitendinosus
superior gluteal nerve
tensor fasciae latae
tibial plateau
tibial tuberosity

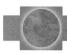

INTRODUCTION

The attachment point for the inferior appendicular skeleton to the axial skeleton occurs at the hip joint, where the head of the femur articulates with the acetabulum of the hip, making up the acetabulofemoral joint. Because of the complex movements that occur in this region and the stress of human movement, the 21 muscles that are located in this region provide strength and support as the extremities move through a full range of motion. Often, the muscles that cause the movements located around the hip joint have an origin on an anatomical landmark of the pelvis and an insertion on the distal end of the femur or proximal end of the tibia or fibula. Therefore, in this region there are both single and multijoint muscles that cause the complex movements of the hip joint.

MAJOR LANDMARKS OF THE HIP JOINT

The bones that are important to the contractions that occur around the hip joint include the pelvis, femur, tibia, and fibula. Each of these bones increases the surface area for the muscle attachment. Additionally, the pelvis provides specific landmarks that form passageways that allow the nerves to pass into the inferior extremities.

The Pelvis

The pelvis is a flat rounded bone that contains many different anatomical landmarks, increasing the surface area for large numbers of muscles to attach to, much like the scapula of the shoulder girdle. In Chapter 5 you learned that the pelvic bone is divided into three distinct regions: the **ilium**, **ischium**, and **pubis** (Figure 13-1). The ilium region is located most superior and runs from an anterior and lateral to posterior position, the ischium region is located inferior and posterior, and the pubic region is located inferior and anterior. Unlike many bones, there is not a distinct boundary line that separates each region from the next.

Landmarks of the Ilium Beginning with the anterior surface of the ilium, there are two distinct bone landmarks that are important to the attachment of the anterior muscles of the hip joint. The most simple landmark to locate is the **anterior superior iliac spine** (ASIS), which is the point of the pelvis located on the anterolateral surface of the ilium. The ASIS is an important landmark for the identification of the abdominal skinfold in body composition and the biomechanical measurement of Q-angle. Located inferior to the ASIS lies the **anterior inferior iliac spine** (AIIS) where the rectus femoris muscle originates.

Moving in the posterior and medial direction from the ASIS, locate the large rounded superior border of the ilium known as the **iliac crest**. The true identification of the iliac crest runs between the ASIS and the **posterior superior iliac spine** (PSIS). This region of the pelvic bone is located where the hands are placed when the hands are "on the hips." The iliac crest is important because of the large amount of surface area that it provides for muscle attachments of the abdominal region, anterior hip, and posterior hip. Inferior to the crest is an area that is depressed into the bone called the **iliac fossa**. The fossa increases the surface area by deepening the anterior surface of the ilium. This structure allows for a large origin attachment site for the anterior hip muscles.

Located inferior and medial to the iliac crest are two additional "spines" that increase the surface area for muscle attachments of the posterior hip. The more superior of these structures is the PSIS. Moving inferiorly to the PSIS lies the **posterior inferior iliac spine** (PIIS). Both the PSIS and PIIS increase the surface area of the posterior hip and provide part of the origin location for the gluteus maximus and gluteus medius muscles. Inferior to the PIIS, note a large indentation into the ilium. This indentation is known as the **sciatic notch**, which allows the sciatic nerve to track toward the inferior regions of the inferior appendicular skeleton.

The articulation surface on the pelvis for the hip joint is the **acetabulum**. The acetabulum is a deep spherical-shaped structure that increases the stability of the articulation between the head of the femur and the hip. Lining the superficial wall of the acetabulum is the labrum of the acetabulum, which increases the stability of the hip joint by increasing the surface area of the joint capsule. In addition, the deep concave shape and articulation with the convex femoral head creates a union that provides strong stability that is difficult to separate.

Landmarks of the Ischium The ischial region of the pelvis begins inferior to the sciatic notch and runs anterior to the body of the pubis. The posterior and inferior regions of the ischium make up the posterior and inferior walls of the **obturator foramen**. These "holes" in the pelvic bones allow the **obturator nerve** to track toward the muscles of the inferior regions of the inferior appendicular skeleton.

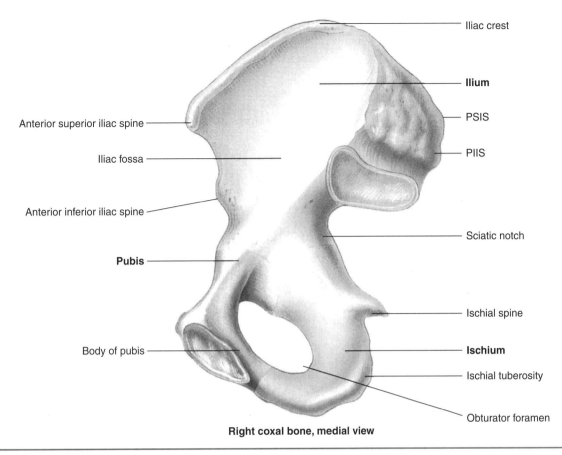

Iliac crest

Ilium

PSIS

PIIS

Anterior superior iliac spine

Iliac fossa

Anterior inferior iliac spine

Sciatic notch

Pubis

Ischial spine

Ischium

Body of pubis

Ischial tuberosity

Obturator foramen

Right coxal bone, medial view

Figure 13-1   *Landmarks of the Pelvis*

Located on the posterior surface of the ischium are several distinct landmarks that increase the surface area for muscle attachment. The first of the ischial landmarks is the **ischial tuberosity** projecting off the body of the ischium. This landmark is important because it provides a strong attachment for the hamstring muscles. Located on the inferior surface of the ischium is the **ramus of the ischium**. This structure also provides additional surface area for the hamstrings muscle group.

Landmarks of the Pubis   The pubic region of the pelvis attaches the two pelvic bones together at the **pubic symphysis** at the medial surface of the pelvic region. These amphiarthroses joints increase the stability that is provided for the inferior appendicular skeleton. Although this is a well known fact, the pubic region also contains several landmarks that increase the surface area of the pelvis for muscle attachment.

Starting where the ischium ends at the posterior region of the pubis and moving anteriorly lies the first of the structures that increases the surface area of the inferior pubis. This region makes up the anterior portion of the obturator foramen. This part of the pubis also provides the attachment site for the gracilis, adductor magnus, and adductor brevis muscles. Moving medially from the **inferior ramus of the pubis** is the symphysis pubis. The superior ramus of the pubis runs from the superior region of the pubic symphysis in the lateral direction to the ischium. This section of the pubis makes up the superior region of the obturator foramen and provides an attachment for the adductor muscle group of the hip.

Landmarks of the Femur

The landmarks of the femur are important to the origin and insertion for the single-joint muscles of the hip and knee joints. The location of several landmarks also aids in the production of forces that occur in the given areas.

Starting at the proximal end of the femur, locate the head of the femur (Figure 13-2). This extremely convex structure articulates with the acetabulum of the pelvis, making up the acetabulofemoral joint. In normal circumstances, the femoral head is held in place by numerous ligaments that increase the stability of the joint. Located lateral to the femoral head is the **femoral neck**. This portion of the femur projects the head outward and increases the surface area of the region for muscle attachment.

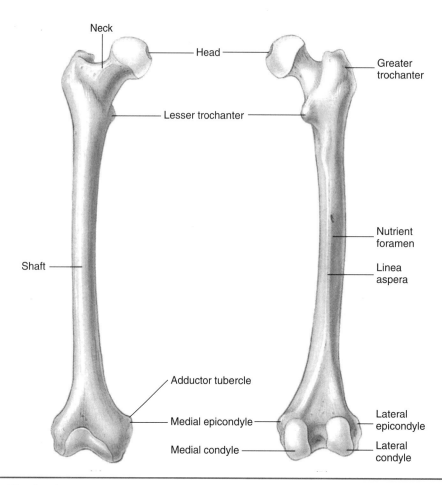

Figure 13-2   Femoral Landmarks

Located lateral to the femoral neck is the **greater trochanter** of the femur. This rectangle-shaped projection increases the surface area for the insertion of the gluteal muscle group. If you track the bone in the medial and inferior directions, you will locate the smaller **lesser trochanter** of the femur. The lesser trochanter also increases the surface area of the femur and is the insertion for the iliopsoas muscle.

If you now follow the diaphysis of the femur along the posterior surface, locate the ridge formation that projects outward in the posterior direction. This line is called the **linea aspera** of the femur. Palpate this structure and realize that many muscles that cause actions around the knee and hip joints attach to this structure. For example, the adductor magnus of the medial hip and the vastus medialis and vastus lateralis of the knee joint originate from this projection.

The distal region of the femur has five specific landmarks that are important to human movement. Locate the first of these structures by palpating the medial distal surface of the femur. In this location, the **adductor tubercle** projects in the medial direction and provides a projection for the adductor magnus muscle of the medial thigh. Moving distally from this location, you will find the rough surface of the **medial epicondyle** of the femur. The two surfaces of the femur that articulate with it include the **medial** and **lateral condyles**. These articular surfaces function with the medial and lateral meniscus of the knee joint, and the anterior and posterior surfaces provide additional surface area for the muscles of the knee joint. The last component of the femur is the **lateral epicondyle**. Much like the medial epicondyle, the lateral epicondyle is a rough surface that provides additional surface area for origins and insertions.

Landmarks of the Tibia and Fibula

The proximal region of the tibia and fibula provides important landmarks to the muscles that articulate around the hip joint (Figure 13-3). Recall that the tibia is the large medial bone that provides a large amount of support, and the fibula is the smaller bone located on the lateral surface of the leg.

The proximal surface of the tibia provides several landmarks and a large surface area for the insertion of muscles that cause motions of the hip and knee joints. Located on the anterior surface of the tibia is the **tibial tuberosity**. This bone pro-

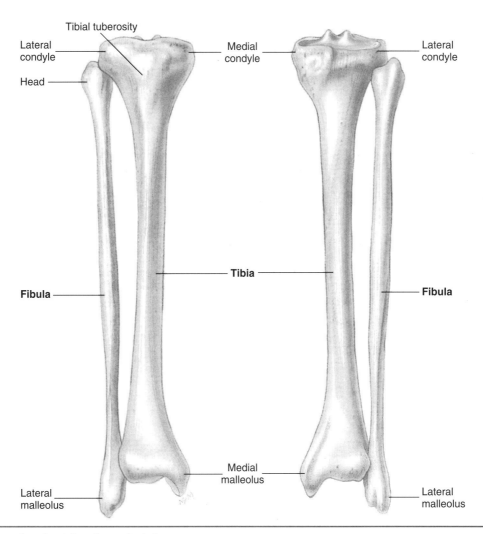

Figure 13-3 *Landmarks of the Tibia and Fibula*

jection secures the patellar tendon and provides a sound attachment for the quadriceps muscle. Moving in the medial direction, you will find the **medial condyle of the tibia**. This broad surface makes up a large area for the insertion attachment of the semimembranosus, sartorius, and gracilis muscles of the anterior hip joint. In addition, the superior surface of the medial condyle provides the inferior support for the joint capsule of the knee joint. Separating the medial and lateral condyles of the femur on the anterior surface of the tibia is the **tibial plateau**. Lateral to this structure lies the **lateral epicondyle of the tibia**, which is the lateral surface for the inferior support for the joint capsule of the knee joint.

The proximal region of the fibula contains the **fibular head**, which is an important attachment point for the muscles of the hip. In fact, this location is the point where the biceps femoris inserts into the fibula.

 NERVOUS INNERVATION

When studying the gross anatomy of the nerves in the human body, understand that there are 31 pairs of spinal nerves containing many nerve fibers (Figure 13-4). Naming the spinal nerves differs in the various regions of the human body. It follows one simple rule: "except for the cervical region, spinal nerves are named from their origin inferior to a given vertebra." For example, the spinal nerve named T7 originates and extends from the spinal cord inferior to the seventh thoracic vertebra. The cervical nerves, on the other hand, follow a different set of rules. Cervical nerves are named from their origin superior to given cervical vertebrae. For example, the second cervical nerve originates superior to the second cervical vertebra. This association holds true until the eighth cervical nerve, the origin of which extends from the inferior to the seventh cervical vertebra.

OTA Perspective

A common scenario requiring OT intervention occurs after a surgical procedure to repair a hip fracture. Knowledge of hip anatomy and joint movement, comprehension of surgical interventions and rehabilitation protocols, and an understanding of the indicated medical management is necessary for providing assessment, treatment, and education of the client with a hip fracture diagnosis. Contributing factors include "who" the client is—what his or her goals are following recovery, attitude toward rehabilitation, pain tolerance, and even the necessary anticipated (and unexpected) psychological adjustments. A comprehensive view provides the best framework for successful intervention to restoring, maintaining, or compensating for safe, efficient, effective, and independent occupational performance.

Lumbosacral Ramus

The nerves that innervate the inferior appendicular skeleton originate at the rami (singular=ramus) of the spinal nerves L2–S3. Each ramus is the branch of the spinal nerve found inferior to the given lumbar and sacral vertebrae. These nerves track inferiorly and form a junction, or plexus, forming the three major nerves of the inferior appendicular skeleton, including the femoral, obturator, and sciatic nerves.

Lumbosacral Plexus

The nerves that innervate the muscles of the hip and thigh originate at the **lumbosacral plexus** and stem from the ventral rami of the spinal nerves L2–S3 (Figure 13-5). The direction of the nerves tracking from superior to inferior dictate the specific muscles they innervate. Four individual nerves and their branches are responsible for innervating the muscles that cause motions around the hip joint: the femoral, obturator, sciatic, and gluteal nerves.

Femoral Nerve The **femoral nerve** originates from the ventral rami of the spinal nerves L2–L4. From the origin of the femoral nerve, it tracks in the inferior direction to innervate the muscles located on the anterior surface of the thigh. As the

OTA Perspective

Osteoarthritis of the hip is a common condition that affects millions of people. Patients complain of pain in the groin, anterior thigh and knee, and over the greater trochanter. Morning stiffness, painful weight bearing, and a limp are the common features. The common deformity is a flexed, adducted, and externally rotated leg. This results in an apparent shortening of the affected side. Real shortening also may be present if there is collapse of the femoral head. Patients describe their inability to do normal ADL and a reduction in their walking distance. Treatment includes PT to relieve pain, strengthening the muscles, and regaining ROM. A total hip replacement surgery is often warranted and frequently has a good outcome.

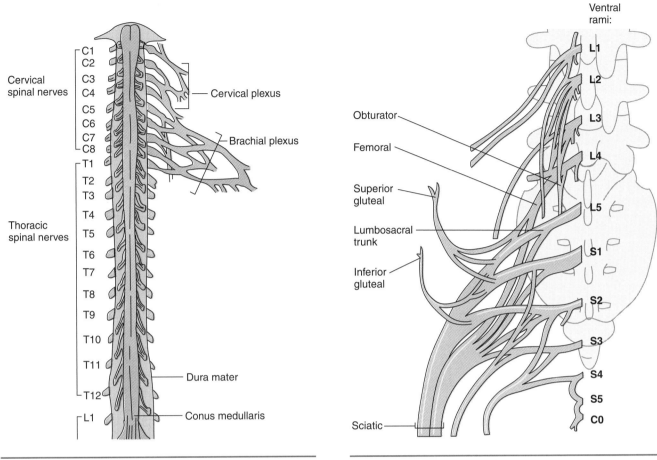

Figure 13-4 *Spinal Nerves*

Figure 13-5 *Lumbosacral Plexus*

nerve tracks to the distal regions of the anterior thigh, it passes between the iliacus and psoas muscles and runs deep to the inguinal ligament. Just distal to the inguinal ligament the nerve further branches into the nerves that innervate the anterior muscle of the thigh region. The individual muscles that the femoral nerve innervates include the pectineus, sartorius, rectus femoris, vastus lateralis, vastus intermedius, and vastus medialis. Further identification of the femoral nerve branches reveals several functional branches, including the saphenous and cutaneous nerves, which are not involved in motor functions of the anterior thigh muscles.

Obturator Nerve A second nerve that originates from the ventral rami of the spinal nerves L2–L4 is the obturator nerve. As the name "obturator" indicates, the nerve tracks through the obturator foramen to the distal region of the thigh. After the obturator nerve passes through the obturator foramen, it tracks deep to the pectineus and adductor longus muscles and superficial to the adductor brevis and adductor magnus muscles. Branches of the obturator nerve innervate the muscles located on the medial surface of the thigh and include the adductor longus, adductor brevis, adductor magnus, gracilis, and obturator externus muscles.

Sciatic Nerve The **sciatic nerve** is the largest of the nonspinal cord nerves and is formed by the ventral rami of the spinal nerves L4–S3. Arguably the most important nerve in the inferior appendicular skeleton, the sciatic nerve has numerous branches which not only stimulate muscles of the thigh but also innervate the muscles that cause actions at the knee and ankle joints. The sciatic nerve tracks from the lumbosacral plexus along the posterior surface of the pelvis and tracks posteriorly to the sciatic notch. After the sciatic nerve is tracked past the sciatic notch, the nerve tracks in the medial direction along the posterior surface of the thigh and can be found deep to the semimembranosus and semitendinosus muscles and superficial to the posterior surface of the adductor magnus muscle. At about half the length of the femur, the sciatic nerve branches into the common peroneal and tibial nerves that are both important nerves to the function of the muscles that cause movements of the ankle joint (these nerves are discussed in further depth in Chapter 15). Although the sciatic nerve is extremely long, its thick body only innervates four muscles before it branches. The sciatic nerve innervates the semimembranosus, semitendinosus, long head of the biceps femoris, and ischiocondylar region of the adductor magnus muscles.

Gluteal Nerves The nerves that innervate the muscles of the hip joint are the **superior** and **inferior gluteal nerves**. Although the nerves track toward the gluteal muscle group, the superior gluteal nerve originates from the ventral rami of the spinal nerves L4–S1, and the inferior gluteal nerve originates from the ventral rami of the spinal nerves L5–S2. From this location, these short nerves run through the sciatic notch and innervate the gluteal muscle group and tensor fasciae latae. The superior gluteal nerve innervates the gluteus medius, gluteus minimus, and tensor fasciae latae, respectively, whereas the inferior gluteal nerve innervates the gluteus maximus. Table 13-1 summarizes the innervation of the hip joint.

Table 13-1 *Innervation of the Hip Joint*

Name of Nerve	Region of Hip/Thigh Affected	Muscles Affected
Femoral	Anterior thigh	Pectineus Sartorius Rectus femoris Vastus lateralis Vastus intermedius Vastus medialis
Obturator	Medial thigh	Gracilis Adductor magnus Adductor longus Adductor brevis Obturator externus
Sciatic	Posterior thigh	Semitendinosus Semimembranosus Biceps femoris Ischiocondylar portion of the adductor magnus
Superior Gluteal	Lateral thigh	Gluteus medius Gluteus minimus Tensor fasciae latae
Inferior Gluteal	Lateral thigh	Gluteus maximus

 ## MOVEMENT OF THE HIP JOINT

The acetabulofemoral joint (hip joint) is a triaxial diarthrodial joint found at the union between the head of the femur and the acetabulum of the pelvis (Table 13-2). During movements of the hip joint, the joint moves through a full range of motion in the sagittal, frontal, and transverse planes. As you learn the different movements referenced in Table 13-2, perform them to help provide you better understand their actions.

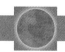 ## STABILITY OF THE HIP JOINT

Because the hip is a large ball-and-socket joint, its ligaments are very strong and provide stability for the motions that occur in this area. Each ligament has a specific function in the movement of the hip and that is to stabilize the joint surfaces from external force. In addition, remember that the hip joint is a synovial joint with a fibrous capsule that spans it. The major reinforcing structures of the hip joint include the iliofemoral, pubofemoral, and ischiofemoral ligaments. All three of these ligaments wrap around the hip joint in a spiral fashion as they attach to the femur (Figure 13-6). In so doing, they create a strong band of fibers that limits hyperextension of the femur.

Iliofemoral Ligament

The **iliofemoral ligament** spans the anterior surface of the hip joint and attaches to the AIIS and proximal medial region of the femur, medial to the greater trochanter. The middle region of the ligament branches and forms an inverted Y shape.

Table 13-2   *Movement of the Hip*

Movement	Axis	Plane	Description
Flexion	Frontal	Sagittal	Decreases angle at the hip; movement of the leg anteriorly
Extension	Frontal	Sagittal	Increases angle at the hip; return of the leg to neutral
Hyperextension	Frontal	Sagittal	Movement of the leg to the posterior side of the body
Abduction	Sagittal	Frontal	Movement of the leg away from neutral in the lateral direction
Adduction	Sagittal	Frontal	Return of the leg to neutral in the medial direction
Diagonal Abduction	Frontal/Sagittal	Frontal/Sagittal	Combination of hyperextension and abduction
Diagonal Adduction	Frontal/Sagittal	Frontal/Sagittal	Combination of flexion and adduction
Horizontal Adduction	Vertical	Transverse	Hip flexed to 90 degrees then adducted
Horizontal Abduction	Vertical	Transverse	Hip flexed to 90 degrees then abducted
Lateral Rotation or External Rotation	Vertical	Transverse	Movement of the entire leg where the foot turns outward
Medial Rotation or Internal Rotation	Vertical	Transverse	Movement of the entire leg that brings the foot back to neutral

Therefore, this ligament is often referred to as the "Y ligament" because of its shape. Because of its position, the Y ligament limits extension, lateral rotation, and medial rotation movements.

Pubofemoral Ligament

The **pubofemoral ligament** spans from the superior ramus of the pubis to the inferior region of the femoral neck. Located inferior to the iliofemoral ligament, the pubofemoral ligament provides anterior and inferior support for the hip joint. The location of the pubofemoral ligament prevents extreme abduction and hyperextension movements of the femur.

Ischiofemoral Ligament

The **ischiofemoral ligament** is the final ligament of the hip joint that spans its posterior surface. The attachment point for the ischiofemoral joint includes the posterior rim of the acetabulum connecting to the posterior region of the femoral neck. In this position, the ischiofemoral ligament limits hyperflexion movements and internal rotation.

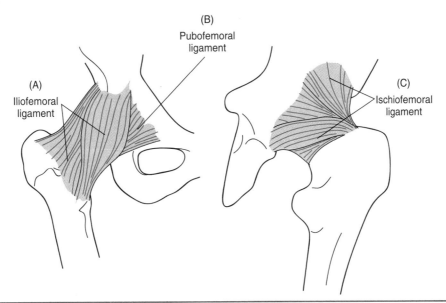

Figure 13-6   *Ligaments of the Hip Joint*

MUSCLES OF THE HIP JOINT

Anterior Muscles of the Hip

The muscles of the anterior hip work together as agonists and synergists to provide the powerful contractions associated with flexion movements that occur in this region. Five individual muscles cross the anterior surface of the hip joint: the iliacus, psoas (iliopsoas), sartorius, rectus femoris, and tensor fasciae latae.

Iliacus and Psoas Muscles Located on the anterior surface of the hip lie the **iliacus** (Figure 13-7) and psoas muscles (Figure 13-8), which, when combined, are referred to as the **iliopsoas muscle**. Because of the anterior position of these muscles, they provide powerful hip flexion movements with each contraction and are commonly referred to as the hip flexors. Both muscles are classified as triangular muscles, with each having a broad origin that inserts into a narrow tendon. When identifying these muscles, notice that they are both extremely deep to the visceral organs. This makes the palpation of these muscles extremely difficult. In fact, the psoas major and minor originate from the anterior vertebral body of T12–L5 and the iliacus muscle originates from the iliac fossa on the anterior surface of the pelvis. The insertion of both muscles narrows into two tendons that insert on the anterior surface of the lesser trochanter.

Name: Iliacus
O: Iliac fossa
I: Lesser trochanter
N: Femoral nerve
A: Hip flexion
P: Too deep to palpate

Name: Psoas Major
O: Anterior and lateral portions of T12–L5 vertebrae
I: Lesser trochanter
N: Ventral rami of L1–L3
A: Hip flexion
P: Difficult to palpate

Sartorius The **sartorius** muscle is the longest muscle in the human body, with an average length of between 2 and 3 feet, depending on the size of the individual. The length of this muscle, however, sacrifices the amount of force that it can

OTA Perspective

Participate in research.

1. Find an illustration of a typical hip anatomy, and draw levels of femoral fractures.

2. Read surgical reports of varying procedures (e.g., ORIF, THR with an Austin-Moore prosthetic device).

3. Examine various "surgical hardware"—pins, rods, plates, and the like.

4. View an X-ray of a noninjured hip, a fractured hip, a hip that was successfully repaired, an abnormally healing hip, and a dislocated hip.

Interview a client following successful (hip fracture) surgery.

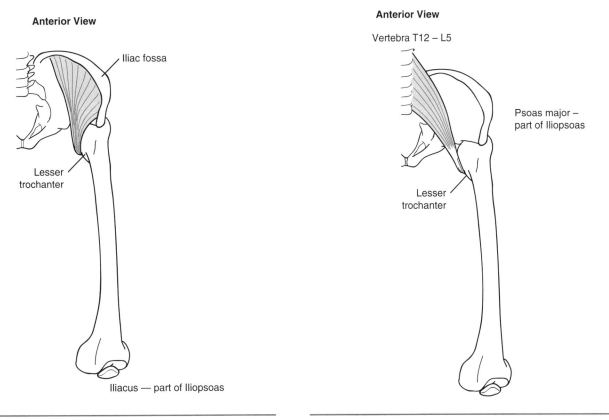

Anterior View

Iliac fossa

Lesser trochanter

Iliacus — part of Iliopsoas

Figure 13-7   *Iliacus*

Anterior View

Vertebra T12 – L5

Psoas major – part of Iliopsoas

Lesser trochanter

Figure 13-8   *Psoas Major*

produce for human movement. It is classified as a strap muscle (Figure 13-9). The origin of the sartorius muscle is located laterally on the ASIS of the ilium. The muscle crosses the middle of the femur and inserts into the proximal medial aspect of the tibia. The direct line of the muscle fibers in the sartorius increases its ability to be flexed and abducted at the same time. This action of the sartorius provides the movement for crossing the legs.

The anterior and superficial location of the sartorius muscle makes it easy to visualize. However, because of its strap nature, the body of the sartorius muscle can be difficult to palpate. The most common place to palpate the sartorius muscle occurs at its distal end, where it inserts into the medial aspect of the tibia. Three muscles have their insertion in this location: the semitendinosus, gracilis, and sartorius. Palpate these muscles posterior to the anteromedial surface of the tibia on the femur when the knee joint is flexed. Here the three muscles can be easily palpated, with the semitendinosus muscle in the most inferior location and the gracilis in the more medial and anterior location. The sartorius muscle is difficult to palpate and can only be found lying between the semitendinosus and gracilis if sufficient pressure is applied to the palpation technique.

Name: Sartorius

O: Anterior superior iliac spine

I: Proximal medial aspect of the tibia

N: Femoral nerve

A: Hip flexion, abduction, and lateral rotation

P: Difficult to palpate

Rectus Femoris   The quadriceps muscle group is located on the anterior surface of the femur and is comprised of the **rectus femoris**, vastus lateralis, vastus intermedialis, and vastus medialis. The only quadriceps muscle that causes actions that occur around both the hip and knee joints, however, is the rectus femoris (Figure 13-10). The rectus femoris is a bipennate-shaped muscle with its origin located on the AIIS. Tracking of the muscle reveals that its long belly runs into the common quadriceps tendon that inserts into the tibial tuberosity via the patellar tendon. Embedded within the insertion lies the patella, which acts as an anatomical pulley that enhances the actions of the quadriceps muscle. The anatomical pulley function of the patella is discussed further in Chapter 14.

The central location of the rectus femoris on the anterior surface of the femur makes this muscle simple to palpate. To palpate the rectus femoris muscle, extend the leg at the knee joint against resistance. Starting superior to the patella, run

Anterior View

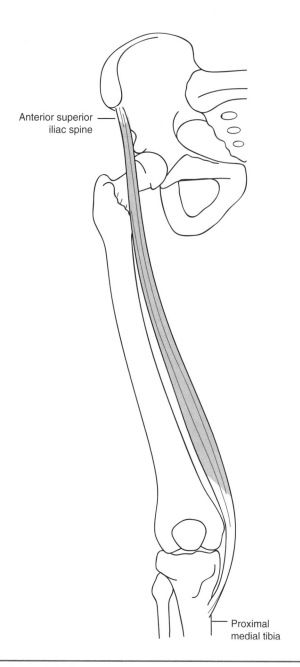

Figure 13-9 *Sartorius*

Anterior View

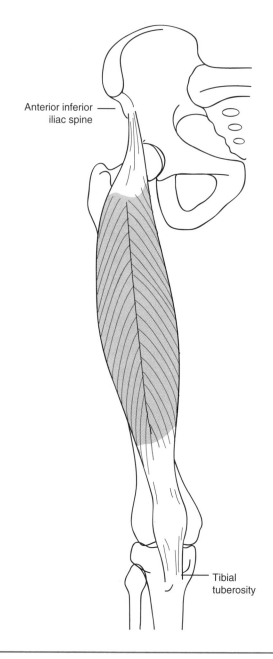

Figure 13-10 *Rectus Femoris*

your fingers in the superior direction towards the middle of the thigh. Located in this spot is the large bulk of the rectus femoris belly in its contracted state.

Name:	Rectus Femoris
O:	Anterior inferior iliac spine
I:	Tibial tuberosity
N:	Femoral nerve
A:	Hip flexion and knee extension
P:	Anterior surface of the thigh

Tensor Fasciae Latae The **tensor fasciae latae** muscle is a fusiform muscle located on the anterior and lateral surface of the hip joint (Figure 13-11). The origin of this muscle crosses anteriorly and laterally to the hip joint and causes a combination of both flexion and abduction motions. An unusual characteristic of the tensor fasciae latae is that the muscle inserts into an extremely long tendonous sheath called the iliotibial tract. In fact, the length of the muscle averages 5 to 10 inches, yet the insertion spans the entire length of the femur inserting into the lateral condyle of the tibia. Although the tensor fasciae latae inserts into the iliotibial tract, it is mainly a strong fascia that covers the lateral surface of the femur.

The tensor fasciae latae muscle can be palpated when the knee is flexed and the leg is abducted from the hip with tension placed on the muscle. Place your fingers on the muscle and note the small surface area that the muscle spans.

After palpating the tensor fasciae latae, palpate the iliotibial tract. To do this, the knee must be relaxed in a flexed position and the toes should point up. Move one hand to the lateral surface of the knee joint located just superior to the fibular head. From this position, move your hand toward the hip along the femoral line and notice the large bulky surface of the vastus lateralis. Just inferior to this muscle is the bulk of the iliotibial tract.

Name:	Tensor Fasciae Latae
O:	Anterior superior iliac spine
I:	Lateral condyle of the tibia via the iliotibial tract
N:	Gluteal nerve
A:	Hip flexion, abduction, and slight medial rotation
P:	Lateral hip anterior to the hip joint

Medial Muscles of the Hip

The muscles that cross the hip joint on the medial surface provide powerful adduction contractions and stabilize the joint through a wide variety of motions, including walking, running, biking, and swimming. Much like the anterior hip muscles, five individual muscles cross the medial surface of the hip joint: the adductor magnus, adductor longus, adductor brevis, pectineus, and gracilis muscles.

The Adductor Group Each of the muscles in the adductor group is triangular in shape with a narrow origin attached to the ischium and pubic regions of the pelvis and a broad insertion located on the femur (Figure 13-12 A–C). When the

Anterior View

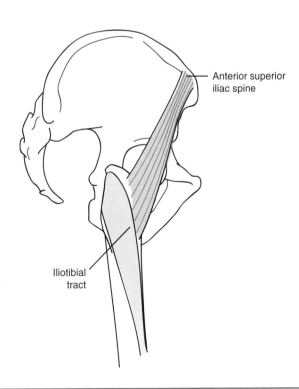

Anterior superior iliac spine

Iliotibial tract

Figure 13-11 *Tensor Fasciae Latae*

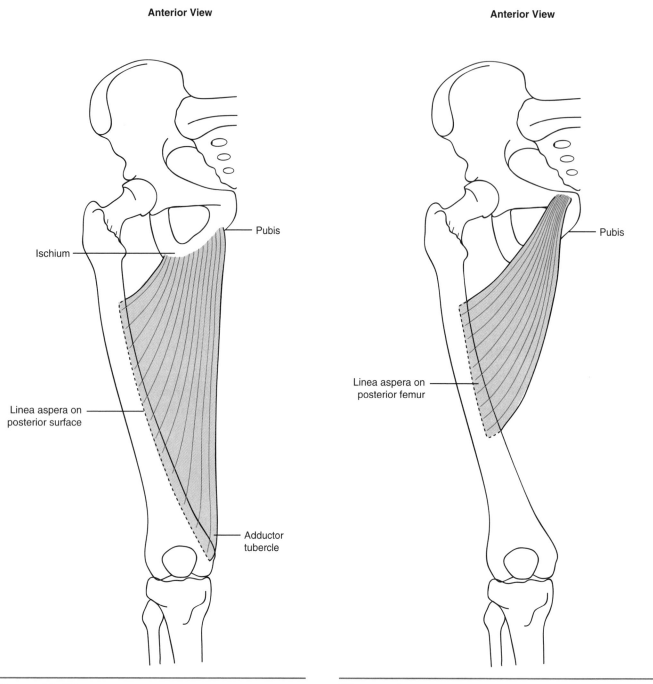

Anterior View

Anterior View

Figure 13-12 *(A) Adductor Magnus*

Figure 13-12 *(B) Adductor Longus*

muscle group is identified, the **adductor brevis** is the most superior muscle and the **adductor magnus** covers the largest surface area. Both the adductor magnus and adductor brevis, however, lie deep to the adductor longus muscle. Because the adductor group muscles are single joint, they are not prone to active insufficiency and provide strong contraction through a full range of motion.

Of the muscles in the adductor group, the **adductor longus** is the only muscle that can be palpated. To palpate the adductor longus, have an individual lie on his or her back with the hip abducted and knee bent. From here you can observe the proximal origin on the ischium of the pelvis. Palpate the belly of the adductor longus by tracing the muscle down the femur in a distal and lateral manner.

Name: Adductor Magnus

O: Ischium and pubis

I: Adductor tubercle and linea aspera

N: Obturator nerve and sciatic nerve

A: Hip adduction

P: Too deep to palpate

Name: Adductor Longus

O: Pubis

I: Middle third of the linea aspera

N: Obturator nerve

A: Hip adduction

P: Medial aspect of the middle half of the thigh

Name: Adductor Brevis

O: Pubis

I: Pectineal line and proximal linea aspera

N: Obturator nerve

A: Hip adduction

P: Too deep to palapte

Pectineus The **pectineus** muscle is a small strap-shaped muscle located superior to the adductor magnus and adductor brevis muscles (Figure 13-13). This muscle has its origin on the superior ramus of the pubis, with the belly of the muscle tracking laterally from here and inserting into the pectineal line on the proximal femur. The pectineus muscle is found deep to the sartorius and femoral artery and vein. Because of the deep location of the pectineus, palpation of this muscle is extremely difficult.

Name: Pectineus

O: Superior ramus of the pubis

I: Pectineal line of the femur

N: Femoral nerve

A: Hip flexion and adduction

P: Difficult to palpate

Gracilis The **gracilis** muscle is a strap-shaped, multijoint muscle (Figure 13-14). With the origin located on the body of the pubis and the insertion on the proximal medial surface of the tibia, the gracilis is one of the longest muscles in the human body. The position of the gracilis is superficial to the adductor longus and adductor brevis and lateral to the semimembranosus muscle of the posterior thigh. Tracking of the muscle to the insertion on the proximal medial tibia reveals that its insertion is anterior to the insertion of the semitendinosus muscle.

To palpate the gracilis, have an individual sit in a chair with the knee joint relaxed and the foot in dorsal flexion. Locate the insertion of the gracilis by palpating the tendon of the semitendinosus muscle, which is the most inferior and distinct tendon on the posteromedial surface. Once the tendon of the semitendinosus muscle has been located, move your fingers in the superior direction 1 cm and feel the insertion of the gracilis, which is deep in this location. Follow the insertion tendon in the direction of the hip and then palpate the muscle of the gracilis in the medial thigh.

Name: Gracilis

O: Body of the pubis

I: Anterior medial surface of the proximal end of tibia

N: Obturator nerve

A: Hip adduction

P: Medial thigh in the posterior and medial directions

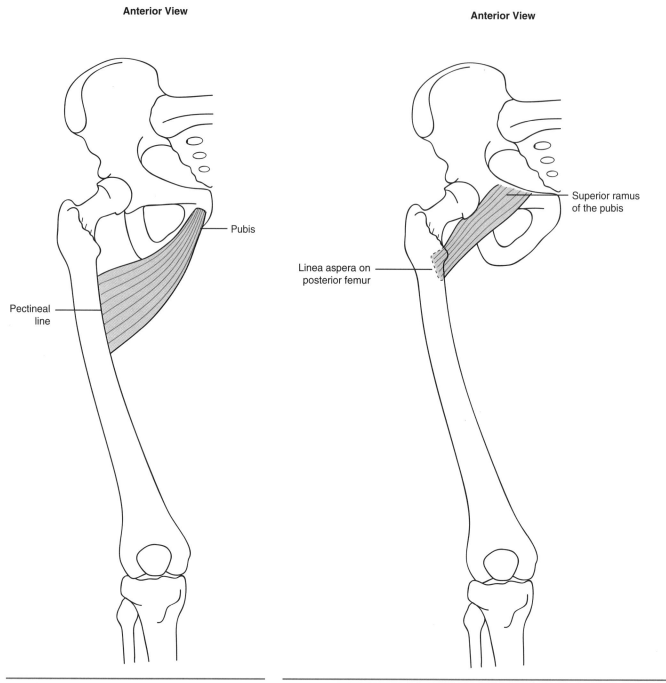

Figure 13-12 *(C) Adductor Brevis*

Figure 13-13 *Pectineus*

Posterior Muscles of the Hip

The posterior hip muscles are a combination of single- and multijoint muscles. The fusiform and triangular shape of these muscles ensures a combination of strong muscle contractions and their ability to move the hip and knee through a full range of motion. The multijoint muscles that make up the hamstrings muscle group include the biceps femoris, semimembranosus, and semitendinosus. The single-joint muscles, on the other hand, consist of the gluteus maximus, gluteus medius, and gluteus minimus. The multijoint muscles of the posterior hip are the semimembranosus and semitendinosus.

Semimembranosus and Semitendinosus The **semimembranosus** (Figure 13-15) and **semitendinosus** (Figure 13-16) are both fusiform muscles that originate on the ischial tuberosity of the ischium and insert on the medial sur-

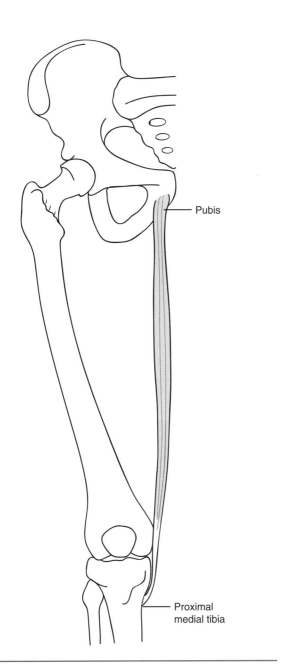

Anterior View

Pubis

Proximal
medial tibia

Posterior View

Ischial
tuberosity

Medial
condyle

Figure 13-14 *Gracilis*

Figure 13-15 *Semimembranosus*

face of the tibia. On identification of these muscles, the semimembranosus lies deep to the semitendinosus. Additionally, a tendon sheath exists in the middle of the belly of the semitendinosus. Contractions of the semimembranosus and semitendinosus cause knee flexion and hip extension. The long length of both of these muscles causes situations in which the muscles can become actively insufficient when flexion occurs at the knee joint and extension occurs at the hip joint at the same time.

When attempting to palpate the semimembranosus and semitendinosus, realize that the semimembranosus is difficult to palpate because of its deep location to the semitendinosus. The semitendinosus, on the other hand, can be palpated from the belly on the posteromedial surface of the femur to the insertion on the medial surface of the proximal tibia. To locate the insertion, remember that three muscles, the semitendinosus, gracilis, and sartorius, can be easily palpated on the posteromedial surface of the knee joint with the tendons of these three muscles located together. The semitendinosus muscle tendon's location is the most inferior of the three muscle's tendons when the knee is flexed. To palpate the belly of the semitendinosus muscle, follow the tendon in the direction of the hip and palpate the belly of the muscle.

Name: Semimembranosus

O: Ischial tuberosity

I: Medial condyle and posterior surface of the tibia

N: Sciatic nerve

A: Hip extension and knee flexion

P: Difficult to plapate

Name: Semitendinosus

O: Ischial tuberosity

I: Anterior and medial surface of the proximal tibia

N: Sciatic nerve

A: Hip extension and knee flexion

P: Posteromedial surface of the femur

Biceps Femoris On the lateral side of the semimembranosus and semitendinosus lies the **biceps femoris** muscle (Figure 13-17). This muscle contains two individual fusiform muscles that share one common tendon that inserts into the head of the fibula. Although the muscles share one common tendon, the origins for the two heads of the biceps femoris are located in two totally separate areas. The long head of the biceps is a two-joint muscle. The origin of the long head lies lateral to the semitendinosus and superficial to the semimembranosus. This makes the long head more susceptible to active insufficiency during muscle contractions occuring around the hip and knee joints. The short head, however, is a single-joint muscle that only crosses the knee joint on the posterior surface. The origin of the short head spans the distance of the distal half of the linea aspera on the posterior surface of the femur. The location of the short head is deep to the long head, which makes its palpation difficult.

To palpate the biceps femoris muscle, locate both the common insertion and muscle belly of the long head. To do so, find the tendonous insertion located on the fibular head while the biceps femoris is in a flexed position. From here slide your hand toward the hip following the tendon of the muscle and locate the belly of the biceps femoris muscle, which is on the posterolateral surface of the femur.

Name: Biceps Femoris

O: Long head: ischial tuberosity

        Short head: linea aspera

I: Head of the fibula

N: Long head: sciatic nerve

        Short head: common peroneal nerve

A: Long head: hip extension and knee flexion

        Short head: knee flexion

P: Lateral aspect of the posterior surface of the knee

Gluteal Group The gluteal group consists of three powerful triangular-shaped muscles that cause extension of the hip joint. Although the **gluteus maximus** (Figure 13-18) provides strong extension movements, the **gluteus medius** (Figure 13-19) and **gluteus minimus** (Figure 13-20) cause strong abduction movements. Of these muscles, the gluteus maximus covers a huge surface area and produces the strongest contractions in the human body. The origin of all three muscles is located on the posterior surface of the ilium, with the belly of the muscle covering the posterior to posterolateral surface of the hip joint, and insert on the femur and iliotibial tract.

Palpation of the gluteus maximus is simple because the major portion of the posterior pelvis contains this muscle. Palpate the large bulk of the muscle that inserts into the superior surface of the iliotibial tract. Because of the superficial location of the gluteus maximus, the gluteus medius and gluteus minimus are difficult to palpate. However, one can palpate the superior region of the gluteus medius by palpating just inferior to the iliac crest on the posterior surface of the ilium. In this location, follow the muscle fibers in the inferior direction toward the gluteus maximus.

Name: Gluteus Maximus

O: Posterior sacrum and ilium

I: Posterior femur just distal to the greater trochanter and iliotibial tract

Posterior View

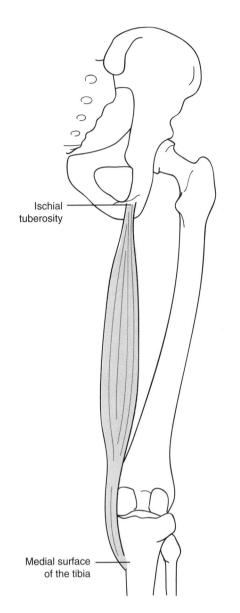

Ischial
tuberosity

Medial surface
of the tibia

Figure 13-16 *Semitendinosus*

Posterior View

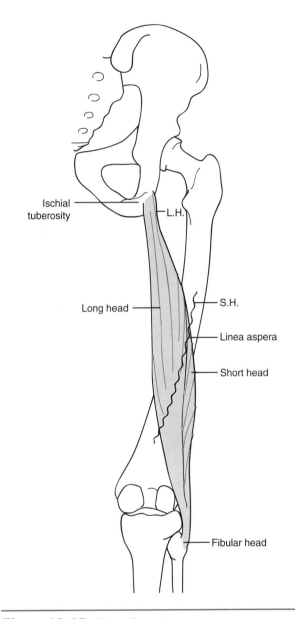

Ischial
tuberosity

L.H.

Long head

S.H.

Linea aspera

Short head

Fibular head

Figure 13-17 *Biceps Femoris*

N:	Inferior gluteal nerve
A:	Hip extension, hyperextension, and lateral rotation
P:	Posterior surface of the buttocks

Name:	Gluteus Medius
O:	Lateral ilium
I:	Greater trochanter
N:	Superior gluteal nerve
A:	Hip abduction
P:	Difficult to palpate

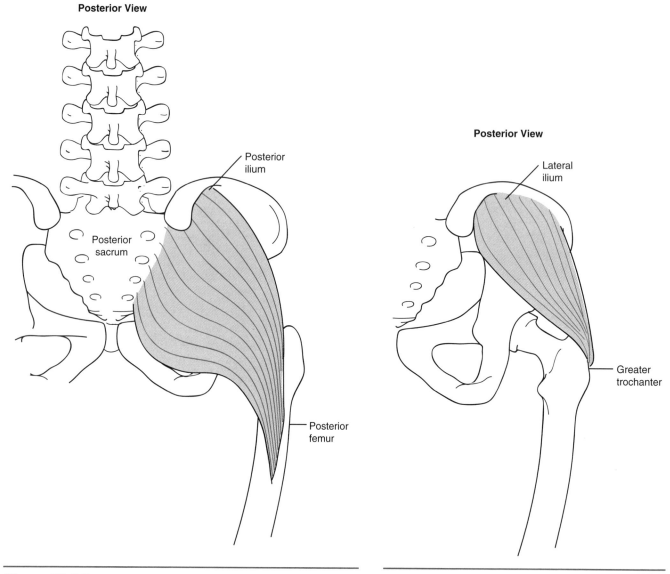

Posterior View

Posterior
ilium

Posterior
sacrum

Posterior
femur

Figure 13-18 Gluteus Maximus

Posterior View

Lateral
ilium

Greater
trochanter

Figure 13-19 Gluteus Medius

Name:	Gluteus Minimus
O:	Lateral ilium
I:	Anterior greater trochanter
N:	Superior gluteal nerve
A:	Hip abduction and medial rotation
P:	Difficult to palpate

Posterior View

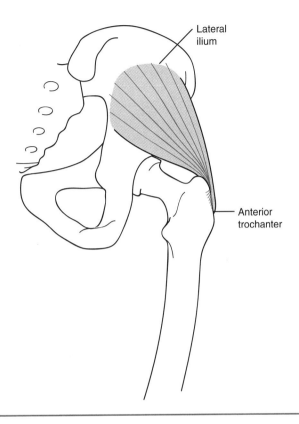

Figure 13-20 *Gluteus Minimus*

Lateral Hip Rotator Muscles

The lateral hip rotator muscles consist of six small strap muscles that lie deep to the muscles of the anterior and posterior muscles of the hip (Figure 13-21 A–F). During human movement, the lateral rotator muscles act together, causing external rotation motions at the hip. The movements of the rotator muscles work in direct opposition to the adductor groups of the hip joint. The most important muscle of the rotator muscles to the allied health field is the piriformis, which is the strongest and largest of the internal rotators. The six lateral rotator muscles include the **piriformis**, **quadratus femoris**, **obturator internus**, **obturator externus**, **gemellus superior**, and **gemellus inferior**. Because of the location of the six deep rotatores, palpation of these muscles is extremely difficult.

Name:	Piriformis
O:	Sacrum
I:	Greater trochanter
N:	Anterior ramus nerve
A:	Lateral rotation of the hip
P:	Difficult to palpate

Name:	Quadratus Femoris
O:	Ischial tuberosity
I:	Intertrochanteric crest
N:	Quadratus femoris nerve
A:	Lateral rotation of the hip
P:	Difficult to palpate

Posterior View

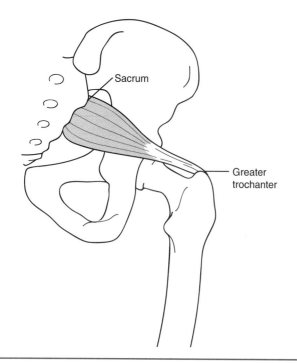

Figure 13-21 *Six Lateral Rotatores: (A) Piriformis*

Posterior View

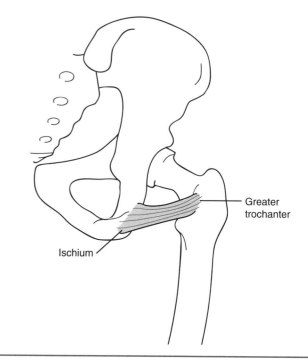

Figure 13-21 *Six Lateral Rotatores: (B) Quadratus Femoris*

Posterior View

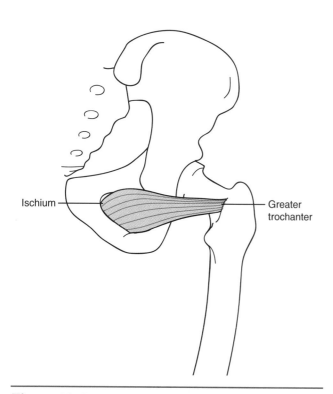

Figure 13-21 *Six Lateral Rotatores: (C) Obturator Internus*

Posterior View

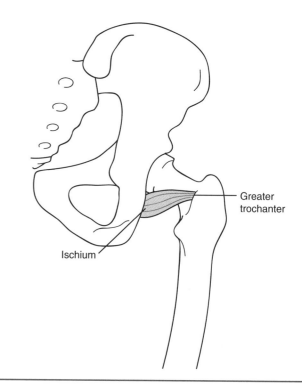

Figure 13-21 *Six Lateral Rotatores: (D) Obturatur Externus*

Posterior View

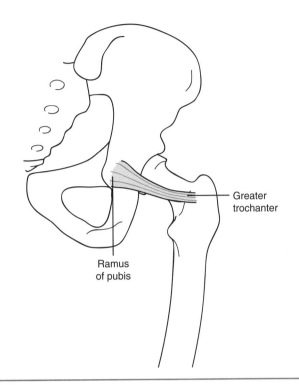

Figure 13-21   *Six Lateral Rotatores: (E) Gemellus Superior*

Posterior View

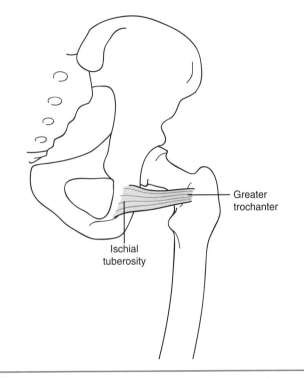

Figure 13-21   *Six Lateral Rotatores: (F) Gemellus Inferior*

Name:	Obturator Internus
O:	Ramus of the pubis and ischium
I:	Trochanteric fossa
N:	Obturator nerve
A:	Lateral rotation of the hip
P:	Difficult to palpate

Name:	Obturator Externus
O:	Ramus of the pubis and ischium
I:	Greater trochanter
N:	Obturator internus nerve
A:	Lateral rotation of the hip
P:	Difficult to palpate

Name:	Gemellus Superior
O:	Ischium
I:	Greater trochanter
N:	Obturator internus nerve and quadratus femoris nerve
A:	Lateral rotation of the hip
P:	Difficult to palpate

Name: Gemellus Inferior

O: Ischium

 I: Greater trochanter

N: Obturator internus nerve and quadratus femoris nerve

A: Lateral rotation of the hip

P: None

KEY CONCEPTS

∎ The hip joint is a triaxial joint that allows motion in three planes. These motions include flexion/extension, adduction/abduction, internal/external rotation, horizontal adduction/horizontal abduction, and circumduction.

∎ The major landmarks of the pelvis, femur, and tibia are all important for the origins and insertions of the muscles that cause movements around the hip joint. Remember that the pelvis is divided into three areas: the iliac, ischium, and pubic regions.

∎ The ligaments of the hip provide stability for the anterior, lateral, and posterior regions of the hip.

∎ When learning the major muscles of the hip, group them together by anatomical location. Remember that the quadriceps muscle group is located in the anterior surface of the hip, the adductor group is located in the medial surface, the hamstrings group is located in the posterior surface, and the gluteal group is located in the lateral surface. Additionally, study the six lateral rotator muscles and become familiar with their function in human movement.

BIBLIOGRAPHY

Hoppenfeld, S. (1976). *Physical examination of the spine and extremities.* London: Prentice Hall International.

Luttgens, K. (2000). *Kinesiology: Scientific basis of human motion* (9th ed.). Madison, WI: McGraw-Hill.

Minor, M. (1998). *Kinesiology laboratory manual for physical therapist assistants.* Philadelphia: F. A. Davis.

Smith, L. K., Weiss, E. L., & Lehmkuhl, L. D. (1996). *Brunnstrom's clinical kinesiology* (5th ed.). Philadelphia: F. A. Davis.

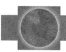

WEB RESOURCES

• Orthopedics.about.com/cs/hipreplacement is a Web site that features pictures and discussions regarding hip replacement surgery.

• The site www.ortho-u.net/oo4/51.htm features many different injuries that occur to the hip joint. It also includes a discussion about treatment modalities and diagnostic procedures.

(These Web addresses were current as of February 2004.)

REVIEW QUESTIONS

Fill in the Blank

Provide the word(s) or phrase(s) that best completes the sentence.

1. The _____ nerve passes through the _____ foramen to innervate the most inferior muscles of the inferior appendicular skeleton.

2. The most superficial muscle of the anterior thigh is the _____ muscle and is classified as a _____ muscle.

3. The adductor magnus muscle mainly provides _____ movements.

4. The main action of the _____ _____ is extension of the hip joint only.

5. The gracilis muscle is located _____ to the surface of the hip joint and provides mainly _____ movements.

6. The short head of the biceps is a _____ joint muscle and provides only _____ at the _____ joint.

7. The gemellus superior and piriformis muscles are both members of the _____ muscle group and provide _____ _____ movements.

8. The _____ _____ _____ muscle attaches to the iliotibial tract, which provides a long insertion for this muscle.

9. Both the _____ _____ and _____ _____ provide abduction of the hip when they contract.

10. The _____ muscle of the posterior hip muscles has a tendonous structure in its muscle belly.

Multiple Choice

Select the best answer to complete the following statements.

1. A muscle that originates on the ASIS and inserts into the medial proximal tibia is the _____ muscle.
   a. sartorius
   b. rectus femoris
   c. gluteus maximus
   d. semitendinosus

2. A muscle that has a common tendon that inserts into the tibial tuberosity via the patellar tendon is the _____ muscle.
   a. sartorius
   b. rectus femoris
   c. gluteus maximus
   d. semitendinosus

3. A muscle that provides the action of crossing the legs is the _____ muscle.
   a. sartorius
   b. rectus femoris
   c. gluteus maximus
   d. semitendinosus

4. The most important muscle to understand of the six deep rotator muscles is the _____ muscle
   a. gemellus inferior
   b. gemellus superior
   c. quadratus femoris
   d. piriformis

5. Of the following muscles, the _____ muscle *cannot* be palpated.
   a. rectus femoris
   b. semimembranosus
   c. semitendinosus
   d. biceps femoris

6. A muscle that provides hip extension and knee flexion is the _____ muscle.
   a. rectus femoris
   b. adductor magnus
   c. gracilis
   d. semimembranosus

7. The smallest adductor muscle of the hip joint is the _____ muscle.
   a. adductor magnus
   b. adductor brevis
   c. adductor longus
   d. pectineus

8. The only single-joint muscle of the hamstrings is the _____ muscle.
   a. long head of the biceps femoris
   b. short head of the biceps femoris
   c. semimembranosus
   d. semitendinosus

9. Of the following muscles, the _____ muscle is the only one listed that *can be* palpated.
   a. short head of the biceps femoris
   b. gluteus minimus
   c. pectineus
   d. adductor longus

10. The longest muscle in the human body is the _____ muscle.
   a. gracilis
   b. rectus femoris
   c. gluteus maximus
   d. sartorius

Matching

Match each of the following descriptions with the appropraite term.

_____ **1.** Rounded part of the ilium on the superior surface

_____ **2.** Formation located inferior to the AIIS

_____ **3.** Large hole located in the inferior pelvis

_____ **4.** Articulating surface of the pelvis

_____ **5.** Long ridge on the posterior surface of the femur

_____ **6.** A structure that separates the medial and lateral condyles of the femur

_____ **7.** Insertion of the adductor magnus

_____ **8.** Superior region of the fibula

_____ **9.** Large depression on the anterior surface of the ilium

_____ **10.** Convex articulating surface of the hip joint

A. Obturator foramen

B. Adductor tubercle

C. Tibial plateau

D. Iliac fossa

E. Femoral head

F. Iliac crest

G. Fibular head

H. Linea aspera

I. Acetabulum

J. Sciatic notch

Critical Thinking

1. On a chart organize the muscles of the hip into anterior, medial, posterior, and lateral muscle groups. Label those muscles that are two joint and single joint. Apply the concept of active and passive insufficiency in these two-joint muscles by performing leg extension and leg curl activities. Isolate those muscles that cross two joints and describe the active and passive insufficiency concept as they apply to these muscles.

2. Imagine the activities of daily living, the actions we perform, and the muscles involved at the hip joint while performing these actions. Now imagine a person performing a general strength training routine. Again think of the movements performed and the muscles involved in these movements. Which part of the hip joint may be stronger or used more frequently? What should you as a health care professional address or target to prevent muscle imbalances?

3. On the diagram provided on the following page, label the structures of the hip and proximal femur. On the drawing and a skeleton, locate and label the following landmarks:

   ■ AIIS

   ■ ASIS

   ■ Iliac crest

   ■ PSIS

   ■ PIIS

   ■ Iliac fossa

   ■ Acetabulum

   ■ Ischial tuberosity

   ■ Obturator foramen

   ■ Ramus of the pubis

   ■ Head of the femur

   ■ Greater trochanter

   ■ Lesser trochanter

(continues)

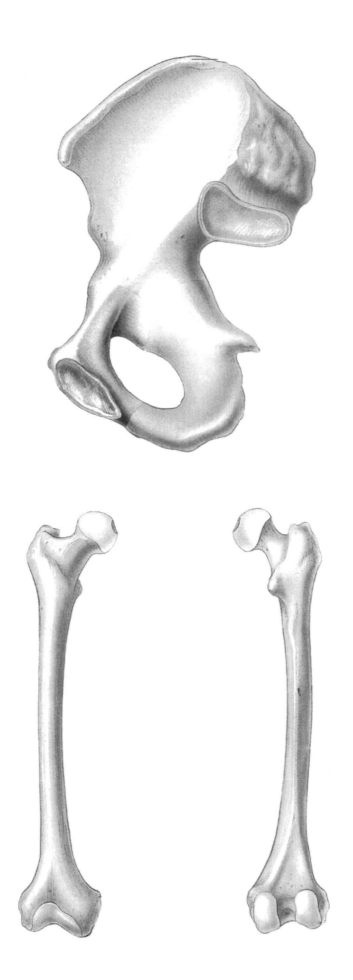

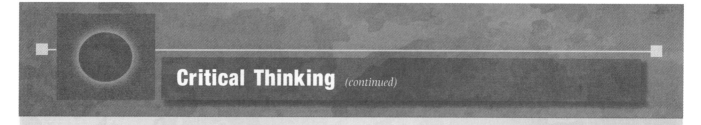

Critical Thinking *(continued)*

4. On the figures provided on the following pages, draw the following major muscles of the hip joint:

- ■ Pectineus
- ■ Adductor brevis
- ■ Adductor longus
- ■ Adductor magnus
- ■ Gracilis
- ■ Semimembranosus
- ■ Semitendinosus
- ■ Biceps femoris
- ■ Tensor fasciae latae
- ■ Gluteus minimus
- ■ Gluteus medius
- ■ Gluteus maximus
- ■ Iliopsoas
- ■ Rectus femoris
- ■ Sartorius
- ■ Sketch the location of the rotator group

5. On the drawings provided in number 4, label the origin, insertion, action, and innervation for each of the muscles.

6. Many factors impact a surgeon's decision regarding the surgical technique used for fracture repair, including the location and severity of the fracture; the patient's physical status, occupation, and age; and the patient's ability to participate in the rehabilitation process. From what you know about cognition, how does a patient's cognitive status impact the rehabilitation process? Can you imagine a situation in which the patient's cognition is so impaired that he or she cannot (safely) maintain the recommended weight-bearing status of the movement precautions? Would the surgeon know this? How? How might this impact the surgeon's decision making (closed reduction vs. open reduction)? What ethical dilemmas might result? How might this impact the patient's living situation?

7. Define the following terms and give an example of a relevant body part and a pathology that responds to it.

Arthroplasty

Arthroscopy

Arthrodesis

Arthrogram

MRI

CT scan

8. Design a handout that includes the home instructions for a patient who has undergone a THA.

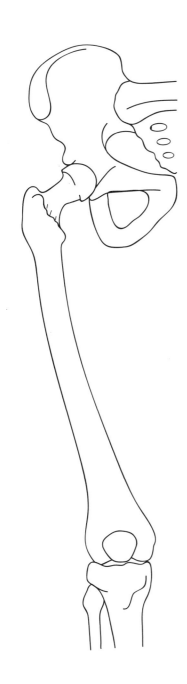

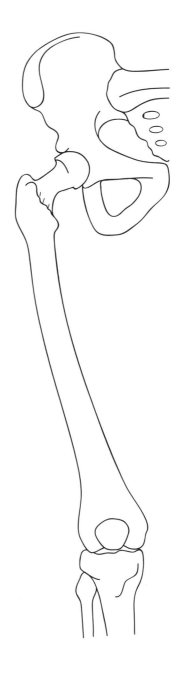

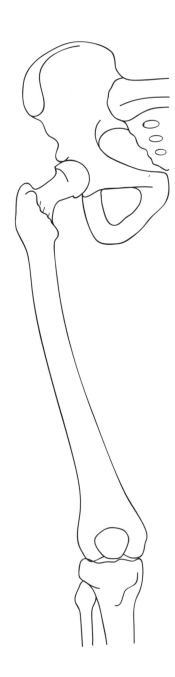
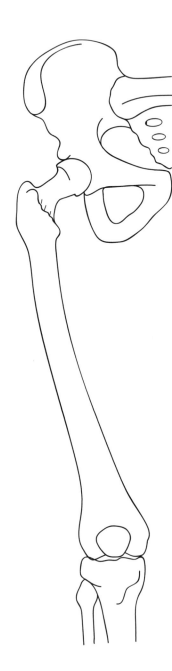

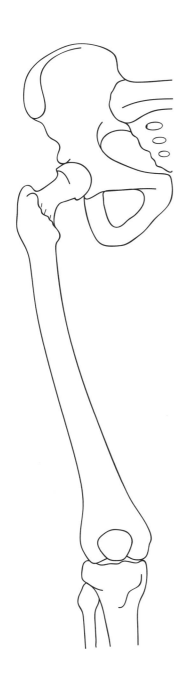

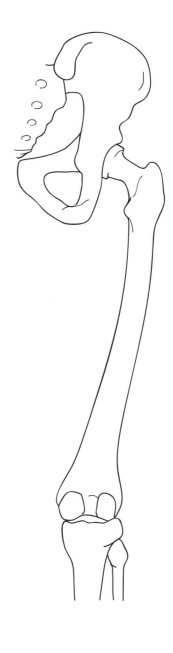

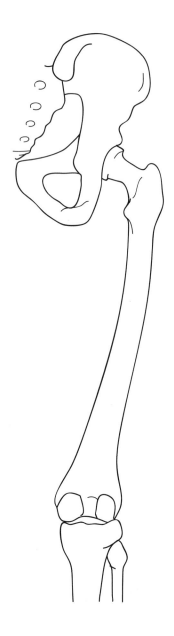
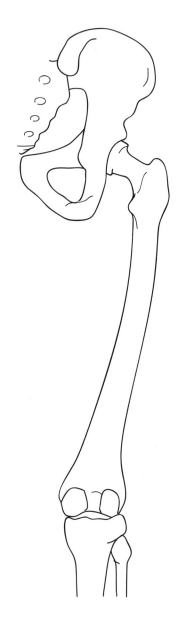

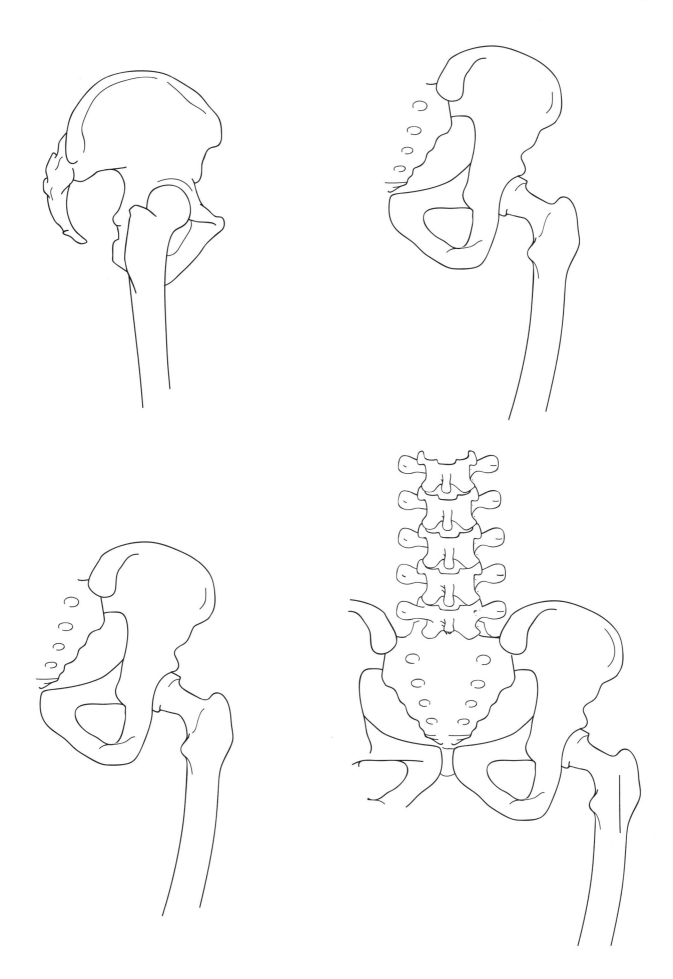

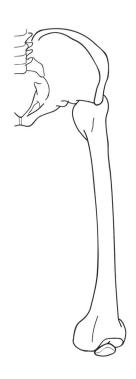

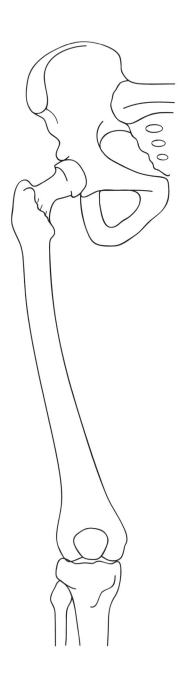

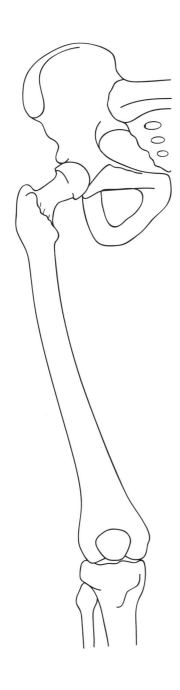

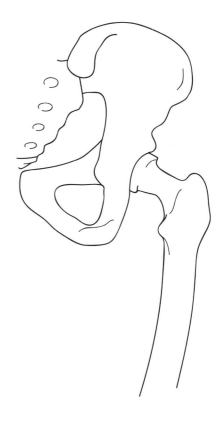

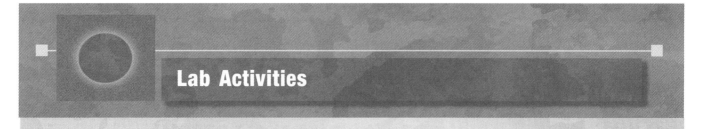

Lab Activities

Lab 13-1: Hip Fractures, Reductions

Objective: To define one method for remediation of hip fractures.

Equipment Needed: Classroom setting for verbal discussion; paper and pencil if answers are to be written out.

Step 1. Define *reduction, closed procedure*, and *open procedure.*

Step 2. Explain weight-bearing restrictions: NWB, TDWB (or TTWB), PWB, WBAT, and FWB.

Step 3. Explain ORIF. (1) What restrictions are imposed by an ORIF procedure? (2) How are they maintained and for how long? (3) What type of compensatory methods may be necessary during the healing process? (4) What happens after the union is healed?

Lab 13-2: Hip Fractures, Prostheses

Objective: To define another method for remediation of hip fractures.

Equipment Needed: Classroom setting for verbal discussion; paper and pencil if answers are to be written out.

Step 1. Define *endoprosthesis* and *bipolar arthroplasty.*

Step 2. Explain "movement precautions."

Step 3. List several personal activities of daily living (PADL) that adhering to movement precautions impacts. Then list several ideas on how to compensate for the lack of the ability to move.

Lab 13-3: Osteoarthritis

Objective: To properly assess for osteoarthritis.

Equipment Needed: A lab partner, pen/pencil, paper, resources

Step 1. Many patients with osteoarthritis of the hip present with a positive Trendelenburg sign. Research the test performed to assess for this disorder.

Step 2. Demonstrate the test on your partner and explain the rationale behind it.

Step 3. Switch and allow your partner to demonstrate the test on you.

Lab 13-4: Total Hip Arthroplasty

Objective: To plan care for the patient recovering from total hip arthroplasty.

Equipment Needed: A lab partner, pen/pencil, paper, walking aids

Step 1. Choose roles as a therapist and a 74-year-old patient who is in the hospital recovering from a total hip arthroplasty (THA).

Step 2. The surgeon has requested WBAT. Decide on what walking aid the patient will be given to assist with ambulation. Describe your criteria for the choice.

Step 3. Teach your partner how to ambulate with the walking aid that you have chosen and how to progress.

Step 4. Switch roles and repeat steps 2 and 3.

Chapter 14

THE KNEE JOINT

Objectives

Upon completion of this chapter, the reader should be able to:

- Describe the movements of the knee.

- Locate the major ligaments of the knee.

- Describe the functions of the ligaments of the knee.

- Name the major muscles of the knee.

- Locate the origin, insertion, and innervation of each major muscle of the knee.

- Explain the action of each major muscle of the knee.

- Describe the palpation of each major muscle of the knee.

Key Words

Achilles tendon
anterior cruciate ligament (ACL)
gastrocnemius
intercondylar eminence
intercondylar fossa
lateral collateral ligament (LCL)

lateral meniscus
medial collateral ligament (MCL)
medial meniscus
menisci
patellar ligament
popliteal ligament
popliteus

posterior cruciate ligament (PCL)
vastus intermedius
vastus lateralis
vastus medialis

INTRODUCTION

Imagine a joint that is under constant stress during every movement of the inferior appendicular skeleton. Visualize the joint structures as they are continually stretched and the support that they provide for the joint time and time again. The joint that best fits this description is the knee joint.

The knee is the largest joint in the human body and is supported on all sides by strong ligaments, muscles, and tendons. During situations when these structures become stretched past a normal limit, they become damaged and lead to the injuries commonly associated with the knee joint.

MAJOR LANDMARKS OF THE KNEE JOINT

The major anatomical structures that are important to the support and strength of the knee joint are found at the distal end of the femur and proximal tibia. A sound knowledge of these landmarks will help you understand the complexity of the largest joint in the human body.

Femur

The distal region of the femur has five specific landmarks that are important to movements of the knee joint (Figure 14-1). Locate the first of these structures by palpating the medial distal surface of the femur. In this location, the adductor tubercle projects in the medial direction and provides a surface for the insertion of the adductor magnus muscle of the medial thigh. Moving distally from this location, locate the rough surface of the medial epicondyle of the femur. The medial epicondyle increases the surface area for the attachment of the muscles and support structures of the knee joint. The two surfaces of the femur that articulate with the tibia are the medial and lateral condyles of the femur. These articular surfaces function with the medial and lateral meniscus of the knee joint, whereas the anterior and posterior surfaces provide additional surface area for attachments of the support structures of the knee joint. On the posterior surface of the femur, notice a large indentation between the two landmarks. This indentation is the intercondylar fossa of the femur, which tracks with the intercondylar eminence of the tibia. The last component of the femur is the lateral epicondyle. Much like the medial epicondyle, the lateral epicondyle is a rough surface that provides additional surface area for origins and insertions of the hip and knee joints and support structures of the knee.

Patella

Positioned on the anterior surface of the knee joint is the patella bone, which is the largest sesamoid bone in the human body (Figure 14-2). Several interesting structural and mechanical facets revolve around the importance of the relationship between the patella and femur to the contractions of the muscles of the inferior appendicular skeleton. When observing the patella, realize that the bone is found within the quadriceps muscle tendon. Palpate your patella and trace the rectus femoris muscle and other quadriceps muscles on the superior surface and the patellar tendon found inferior and inserting into the tibial tuberosity.

For many years, biomechanists have studied the importance of the patella to the strong contractions of the knee joint. These in-depth studies have identified that the position of the patella increases the distance of the contraction of the quadriceps muscles. As a result, biomechanists have identified the patella as a strong anatomical pulley that increases the amount of force produced when these muscles contract. In addition, the third-class lever provided by the patella's position increases the mechanical advantage, which also aids in the strength of the contraction.

Tibia

The bony processes of the tibia are important to both muscle attachments of the hip and knee joints and the support structures of the knee joint (Figure 14-3). To begin observing the anatomical structures of the tibia, locate on a skeleton or drawing the superior surface of the tibia, which is where the femur and tibia articulate with one another. The first thing that should be noticed is that the superior surface of the tibia is similar in shape to the capital letter *B*, with the rounded components making up the posterior surface. This large surface area provides much room for the medial and lateral menisci to sit between the femur and tibia.

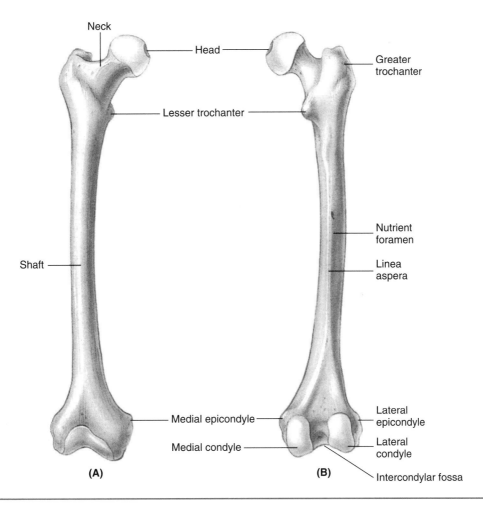

Figure 14-1 *Femur*

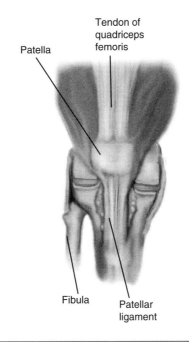

Figure 14-2 *Patella*

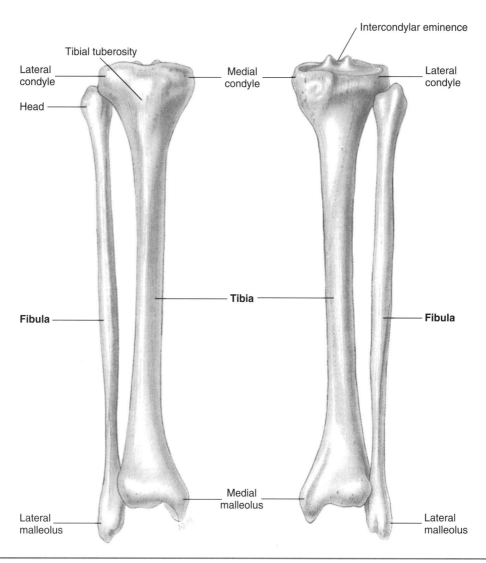

Figure 14-3 *Tibia*

Located on the medial surface of the tibia is the medial condyle, which makes up the medial region of the B shape. This rough structure provides a larger surface for the attachment of the muscles and support structures of the knee joint. Trace the superior surface of the tibia in the lateral direction and locate the intercondylar eminence in the middle of the tibia projecting outward and running from the anterior surface to the posterior surface. The position of the convex **intercondylar eminence** of the tibia enables it to articulate with the concave intercondylar eminence of the femur. During movements of the knee joint, these two structures articulate with one another, increasing the stability of the knee joint as the knee assumes the closed-packed position. Moving laterally from the intercondylar eminence, locate the lateral half of the letter B, which makes up the lateral epicondyle. Much like the medial epicondyle, the lateral epicondyle increases the surface area for origins and insertions of the knee and hip joints and support structures of the knee joint. The final important landmark of the tibia is the large indentation located on its posterior surface where the intercondylar eminence ends. This structure is the **intercondylar fossa** of the tibia.

Fibula

The fibula is the bone located on the lateral surface of the leg. The fibula has one important structure that provides stability of the knee. This important structure is the head of the fibula, which provides a strong attachment point for the lateral collateral ligament.

NERVOUS INNERVATION

Two major nerves innervate the muscles that cause movements at the knee joint. One of these nerves, the femoral nerve, discussed in Chapter 13, continues to track inferiorly to innervate the muscles that cause knee extension. The other nerve is the tibial nerve, which is a branch of the sciatic nerve that innervates the muscles that cause flexion of the knee joint.

Femoral Nerve

In the same location where the femoral nerve branches into the saphenous and cutaneous nerves, just medial to the proximal section of the rectus femoris muscles, the nerve further branches to innervate the muscles that cause knee extension (Figure 14-4). The lateralmost nerves branch to innervate both the vastus intermedius and vastus lateralis muscles. A medial branch tracks deep to the sartorius muscle and innervates the vastus medialis muscle.

Tibial Nerve

Tracking of the sciatic nerve in the distal direction reveals several distinct branches to the posterior inferior appendicular skeleton. This branch occurs approximately one-half the distance of the femur as the sciatic nerve branches into the tibial nerve and the common peroneal (fibular) nerve (Figure 14-5). The common peroneal nerve is important to the muscles of the leg and is discussed in greater depth in Chapter 15.

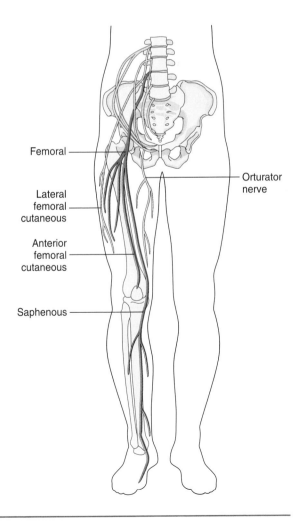

Femoral

Lateral femoral cutaneous

Anterior femoral cutaneous

Saphenous

Orturator nerve

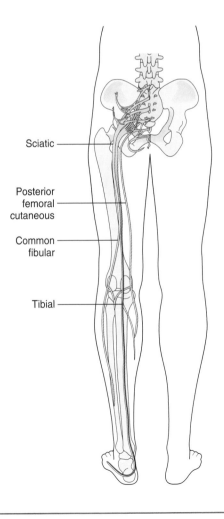

Sciatic

Posterior femoral cutaneous

Common fibular

Tibial

Figure 14-4 *Femoral Nerve*

Figure 14-5 *Tibial and Common Peroneal Nerves*

From the branch at the femur, the tibial nerve can be found deep to the semimembranosus and tracking through the intercondylar eminence of the femur. From here, the nerve runs deep to the gastrocnemius, soleus, and plantaris muscles and superficial to the popliteus muscle as it runs toward the inferior regions of the leg. Because of its posterior location, the tibial nerve innervates the muscles that cause knee flexion such as the gastrocnemius and popliteus muscles. Table 14-1 summarizes the nerves in the knee and the muscles they innervate.

Table 14-1   *Nerves Associated with the Knee Joint Muscles*

Nerve	Affected Anterior Muscles	Affected Posterior Muscles
Femoral	Rectus femoris, vastus lateralis, vastus medialis, vastus intermedius	None
Sciatic	None	Semimembranosus, semitendinosus, biceps femoris
Tibial	None	Gastrocnemius, popliteus

 ## MOVEMENT OF THE KNEE

Often the knee joint is classified as a uniaxial hinge joint that allows motion in only one plane. However, this classification can be misleading. The reason for this is the fact that the knee joint does provide limited biaxial movements by allowing limited motions that occur in the transverse planes in addition to those that occur in the sagittal plane (Table 14-2). Therefore, the actions of the knee joint include flexion and extension movements that occur in the sagittal plane with extremely limited, but vitally important, medial and lateral rotation occurring in the transverse plane.

Table 14-2   *Movement of the Knee*

Movement	Axis	Plane	Description
Flexion	Frontal	Sagittal	Movement of the foot in the posterior direction
Extension	Frontal	Sagittal	Return of the foot to the anatomical position from the posterior direction

 ## STABILITY OF THE KNEE

The joint where the most injuries occur in the human body is at the knee joint because of the support structures of the area and the large forces that are applied to the knee joint on a continual basis (Figure 14-6). The support structures of the knee joint include six ligaments that connect the femur, tibia, and fibula together and two individual cartilaginous structures (**menisci**) that increase the amount of stability for the joint during its continual movements.

Ligaments of the Knee Joint

Many times, the names of the knee joint ligaments are known even before studying the knee joint in a kinesiology class. Therefore, students often have a "leg up" when they learn the names of the ligamentous structures of the knee joint. See if you recognize the name of the first four of the six knee joint ligaments listed, which include the medial collateral, lateral col-

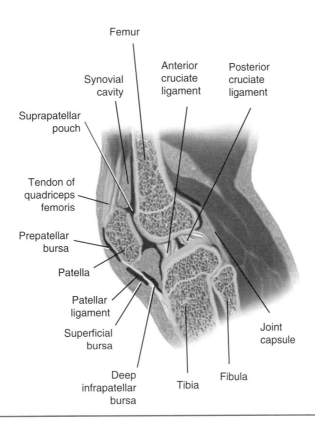

Femur

Anterior cruciate ligament

Posterior cruciate ligament

Synovial cavity

Suprapatellar pouch

Tendon of quadriceps femoris

Prepatellar bursa

Patella

Patellar ligament

Superficial bursa

Deep infrapatellar bursa

Tibia

Fibula

Joint capsule

Figure 14-6 *The Knee Joint*

lateral, anterior cruciate, posterior cruciate, popliteal, and patellar ligaments. As the individual ligaments are discussed, think about the support that each provides for the stability of the knee joint. Of the four ligaments that are often recognized, the collateral ligaments are those that support the medial and lateral surfaces of the knee joint and the cruciate ligaments are those that form a "cross-like" pattern and provide anterior and posterior support.

Medial Collateral Ligament

The **medial** (tibial) **collateral ligament (MCL)** is a flat and broad band ligament that spans the medial surface of the knee joint, spanning from the medial epicondyle of the femur to the medial condyle of the tibia. During human movements such as running and walking, the MCL stabilizes the medial movement of the knee joint when excessive lateral force is applied to it. Therefore, this action limits motions that occur in the frontal and transverse planes.

Because of its position, the MCL is often damaged when excessive force is applied to the lateral surface of the knee joint. For example, imagine a football running back racing down the field with a linebacker in chase. When the running back stops and plants the foot, the linebacker hits the knee on the lateral surface. This increases the force applied to the medial surface of the knee joint. As the MCL is stretched, it attempts to limit the forces that are applied to the joint while providing stability. As a result of excess stress, the MCL is torn and a season-ending injury occurs.

Lateral Collateral Ligament

Located on the lateral surface of the knee joint is the **lateral** (fibular) **collateral ligament (LCL)**. This strong, broad, and cord-like ligament spans from the lateral epicondyle of the femur to the lateral surface of the head of the fibula. Because of its position, the LCL is rarely damaged when compared to the incidence of MCL injuries and provides lateral support for the knee joint. Much like the MCL, the position of the LCL limits movements in the frontal and transverse planes and promotes movements in the sagittal plane.

The reason behind the decreased injury potential of the LCL is because of the lateral position of this ligament. During sport and recreational activities, an excessive force applied to the medial surface of the knee joint is rare when compared to the MCL. However, at times the LCL can be damaged when the knee is planted and as the body weight shifts along the medial surface of the knee. If a great enough force is applied to the medial surface of the knee joint, and the joint moves in the lateral direction, sufficient forces could cause damage to the LCL ligament.

Anterior Cruciate Ligament

The **anterior cruciate ligament (ACL)** is a short band ligament that spans through the deep layers of the knee joint. Positioned to provide anterior support for the knee joint, the ACL spans from an inferior attachment on the intercondyloid eminence of the tibia to a superior attachment on the medial surface of the lateral condyle of the femur. When observing the position of the ACL, realize that the position of the ligament limits excessive sagittal posterior movements of the knee joint while also limiting movements of the knee joint in the frontal and transverse planes.

The ACL is often damaged as many times as the MCL when excessive forces are applied to the joint. In the previous football example imagine instead that the knee joint is being stressed head on along the anterior surface. In this scenario, the running back plants the foot into the ground as the linebacker flies and hits the anterior surface of the knee joint. As this motion occurs, the ACL attempts to limit the posterior movement of the knee joint, which stretches the ACL past its normal length.

Posterior Cruciate Ligament The **posterior cruciate ligament (PCL)** runs from an inferior attachment on the posterior intercondyloid fossa of the tibia to its superior location on the anterolateral attachment of the medial condyle of the femur. The PCL lies posterior to the ACL and is shorter and stronger than the ACL. During movements of the knee joint, the PCL provides posterior support for the knee joint, preventing excessive anterior movements of the knee joint in the sagittal, frontal, and transverse planes. Much like the LCL, the PCL is rarely damaged. In fact, the anterior support provided by the patella enhances the support provided by the PCL ligament and limits anterior movement of the knee joint.

Popliteal Ligament The **popliteal ligament** spans the posterior surface of the knee joint, attaching the posterior surface of the femur and the intercondyloid fossa to the posterior head of the tibia. The popliteal ligament is a broad, flat ligament that protects the knee from hyperextension. For example, when the foot is planted and hit from the anterior direction, the popliteal ligament stretches, preventing posterior movement of the knee joint.

Patellar Ligament Located on the anterior surface of the knee joint is the **patellar ligament**, which spans the anterior portion of the patella, with its superficial fibers running continuous with the central tendon of the patellar tendon. The patellar tendon is a flat and strong ligament that enhances the stability of the anterior surface of the knee joint. Figure 14-7 illustrates the ligaments of the knee.

Cartilage Structures of the Knee Joint

The articular cartilage of the knee joint is composed of fibrous connective tissue that acts as a shock absorber lying between the femur and tibia. These special structures include the lateral and medial menisci.

Medial Meniscus The **medial meniscus** is shaped like the letter *C* and sits on the medial condyle of the tibia (Figure 14-8). On observation of the medial meniscus, notice that its posterior side is thicker than the anterior surface and that the superficial walls of the cartilage span in the superior direction. The concave shape of the medial meniscus enhances the stabil-

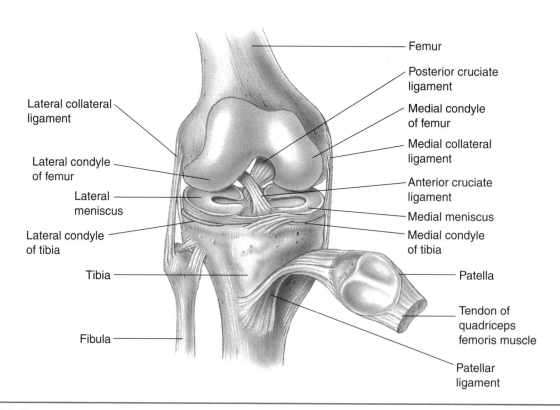

Figure 14-7 *Ligaments of the Knee*

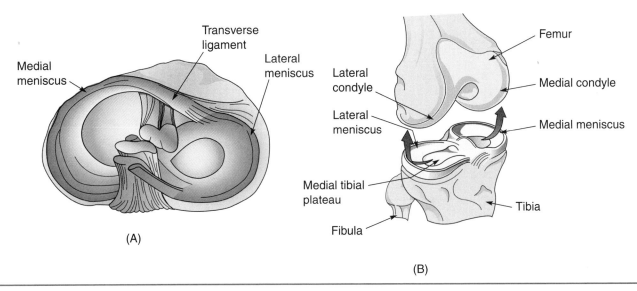

Figure 14-8 *Medial and Lateral Menisci*

ity of the knee joint by articulating with the medial condyle of the femur. This relationship allows the tibia to roll over the distal end of the femur. Because of its position and attachments to the MCL and semimembranosus muscle, the medial meniscus is often damaged as increased rotation forces act on the joint.

Lateral Meniscus The **lateral meniscus** is an incomplete circle-shaped structure that fits into the articular facet of the tibia. Much like the medial meniscus, the lateral meniscus forms a concave shape, with the superficial walls projecting in the superior direction. The convex-shaped lateral condyle of the femur articulates with the lateral meniscus and increases the stability provided by this joint.

Terrible Triad

The term *terrible triad* does not refer to the three amigos or three musketeers but to the most commonly injured structures of the knee joint when excessive forces are applied to it. The structures that make up the terrible triad include the medial meniscus, anterior cruciate ligament, and medial collateral ligament. The term *terrible triad* refers to the common damage to one of these structures and the ensuing damage that occurs to either one or both of the other two structures. For example, when damage occurs to the medial meniscus, often this will cause damage to the ACL and MCL ligaments as well.

 MUSCLES OF THE KNEE JOINT

Although many of the two-joint muscles of the thigh are discussed in Chapter 13, the actions of these muscles are important to the actions that occur around the knee joint. Therefore, several of the muscles that were previously discussed will be mentioned again in table format, only specifying their actions around the knee joint.

Anterior Thigh Muscles

The four anterior muscles that cause actions around the knee joint are grouped together as the quadriceps muscle group and include the rectus femoris, vastus lateralis, vastus medialis, and vastus intermedius. Of these muscles, the rectus femoris is the only two-joint muscle that provides actions around the hip and knee joints. The other three, on the other hand, originate on the femur and cross the knee joint on the anterior surface. Because of the common insertion of these muscles, and the anterior placement of the common tendon, all of the quadriceps muscles work in conjunction with one another and cause extension movements of the knee joint.

OTA Perspective

OT practitioners typically follow a biomechanical approach to restore function after a surgical procedure, adhering to the surgeon's procedures and facility's rehabilitation guidelines (or "clinical pathways"). An evaluation and treatment may begin within days if mobilization is indicated, or after a period of immobilization and healing. Aspects to consider include ROM (active and passive), edema, strength, sensation, and pain, which all impact occupational performance. Review what you already know with regards to assessments for measuring ROM (e.g., goniometer), strength (e.g., manual muscle testing [MMT]), and sensation (e.g., tests to measure sharp/dull, two-point discrimination, and stereognosis). Although these approaches and assessments are considered with regard to knee joint function, they apply to other orthopedic conditions as well.

Rectus Femoris The rectus femoris muscle is the only two-joint muscle of the quadriceps group. Therefore, its expanded description can be found in Chapter 13. However, the anterior position of this muscle causes knee extension around the knee joint.

Name:	Rectus Femoris
O:	Anterior inferior iliac spine
I:	Tibial tuberosity via the patellar tendon
N:	Femoral nerve
A:	Knee extension and hip flexion
P:	Midline of the quadriceps muscle

Vastus Lateralis The **vastus lateralis** muscle is a unipennate muscle found lateral to the rectus femoris (Figure 14-9). An unusual characteristic of the muscle is the posterior location of its broad origin on the lateral lip of the linea aspera. From this location, the muscle wraps around the lateral surface of the femur to the anterior thigh, where the majority of the muscle belly is located. Tracking of the muscle reveals that the tendon of the muscle runs through the patella and inserts into the tibial tuberosity via the patellar tendon. Because of the unipennate shape and single joint that the vastus lateralis muscle crosses, its contractions are strong and forceful.

To palpate the vastus lateralis muscle, locate the patellar tendon superior to the patella and perform the knee extension movement against tension. From the patellar tendon, trace the belly of the muscle toward the hip. As you track the muscle, note the superficial location of the rectus femoris and where the muscle tracks posteriorly and deep to the middle portion of the iliotibial tract. Note that the origin of the vastus lateralis muscle cannot be palpated because of its deep location to the biceps femoris muscle.

Name:	Vastus Lateralis
O:	Linea aspera
I:	Tibial tuberosity via the patellar tendon and lateral aspect of the patella
N:	Femoral nerve
A:	Knee extension
P:	Lateral part of the anterior femur

Vastus Medialis Much like the vastus lateralis muscle, the **vastus medialis** is a unipennate muscle with an origin on the posterior surface of the femur (Figure 14-10). The origin of the vastus medialis muscle is located on the medial lip of the linea aspera of the posterior femur. The belly of the vastus medialis muscle is located on the anterior surface of the thigh and tracks into the common patellar tendon into the tibial tuberosity insertion. Because of its unipennate shape and single joint that this muscle crosses, the contractions of the vastus medialis are also strong and forceful.

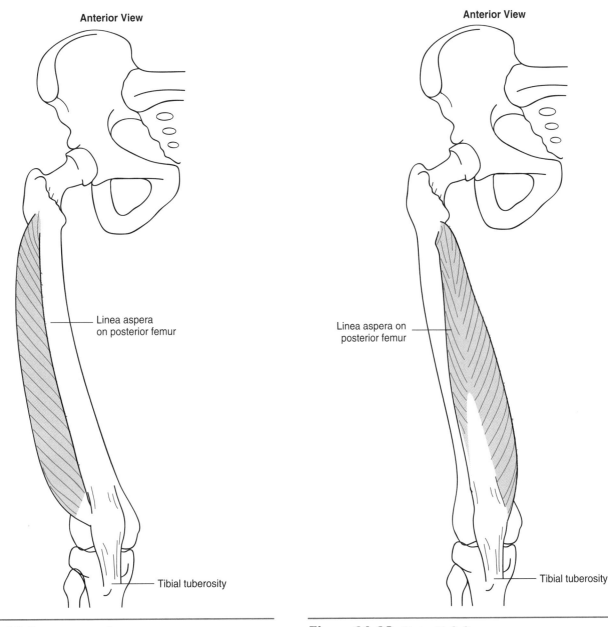

Figure 14-9   *Vastus Lateralis*

Figure 14-10   *Vastus Medialis*

Palpation methods for the vastus medialis muscle are simple and similar to the vastus lateralis. To palpate the vastus medialis, place tension on the leg to cause contractions of the thigh muscles. While the muscle is contracted, locate the medial surface of the patellar tendon superior to the patella. Move your fingers along the tendon to palpate the belly of the muscle in the direction of the hip. After you have located the belly, trace the muscle in the medial direction and notice the track of the muscle as it is positioned deep to the semimembranosus and semitendinosus muscles of the hamstrings group. Remember that the origin of the vastus medialis is impossible to palpate because of its deep position underneath the superficial muscles located in the posterior thigh.

Name: Vastus Medialis

O: Linea aspera

I: Tibial tuberosity via the patellar tendon and the medial aspect of the patella

N: Femoral

A: Knee extension

P: Medial part of the anterior femur

Vastus Intermedius The final muscle of the quadriceps muscle group is the **vastus intermedius**, which has a bipennate shape and is located deep to the rectus femoris muscle (Figure 14-11). The origin of the muscle is located medial to the greater trochanter of the femur and tracks in the distal direction to the common insertion of the tibial tuberosity via the patellar tendon. The belly of the vastus intermedius muscle runs along the major portion of the proximal half of the femur and into a central tendon that tracks toward the patellar tendon. Because of its bipennate shape and single joint that this muscle crosses, the contractions of the vastus intermedius are strong and forceful. Palpation of the vastus intermedius is extremely difficult because of its location deep to the rectus femoris.

Name: Vastus Intermedius

O: Anterior femur medial to the greater trochanter

I: Tibial tuberosity via the patellar tendon

N: Femoral

A: Knee extension

P: Difficult to palpate because it is located deep to the rectus femoris

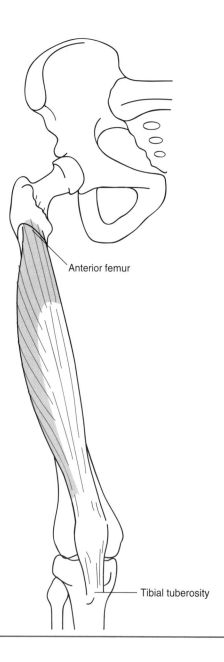

Figure 14-11   *Vastus Intermedius*

Posterior Thigh Muscles

Four muscles of the posterior thigh are discussed in Chapter 13 owing to their two-joint position covering the posterior thigh and hip. These muscles include the semimembranosus, semitendinosus, long head of the biceps femoris, and short head of the biceps femoris. Although a full discussion of the posterior thigh muscles can be found in Chapter 13, the breakdown of each of these muscles follows next.

In addition to the muscles already described, two additional muscles cross the posterior knee joint that causes it to flex. These two muscles are the popliteus and gastrocnemius.

Name:	Semimembranosus
O:	Ischial tuberosity
I:	Posterior surface of the tibia
N:	Sciatic
A:	Knee flexion
P:	Medial aspect of the posterior distal thigh on either side of the semitendinosus

Name:	Semitendinosus
O:	Ischial tuberosity
I:	Anteromedial surface of the proximal tibia
N:	Sciatic
A:	Knee flexion
P:	Medial aspect of the posterior distal thigh slightly above the bend in the knee

Name:	Biceps Femoris
O:	Long head: ischial tuberosity
	Short head: lateral linea aspera
I:	Head of the fibula
N:	Long head: sciatic nerve
	Short head: common peroneal nerve
A:	Long head: hip extension and knee flexion
	Short head: knee flexion
P:	Lateral aspect of the posterior surface of the knee

Popliteus The **popliteus** muscle is a small triangular-shaped muscle located deep to the soleus and gastrocnemius of the posterior leg (Figure 14-12). Unlike many triangular-shaped muscles, the origin of the popliteus muscle on the lateral condyle of the femur is more narrow than the broad insertion located on the posterior surface of the medial condyle of the tibia. This arrangement is unique because the majority of triangular-shaped muscles have broad origins and narrow insertions. For example, the pectoralis major has a broad origin that covers the sternum and middle clavicle and a narrow insertion into the humerus. The origin and insertion arrangement of the popliteus allows the muscle to "unlock" the knee after the knee is in full extension and provides additional support for the flexion movements of the knee.

Because of its small size and its deep location to the gastrocnemius and soleus muscles, the popliteus cannot be palpated.

Name:	Popliteus
O:	Lateral condyle of the femur
I:	Posterior surface of the medial condyle of the tibia
N:	Tibial
A:	Knee flexion
P:	Cannot be palpated because it is deep to the gastrocnemius

Gastrocnemius Located on the posterior surface of the leg in the superior region is the **gastrocnemius** muscle, which is also referred to as the calf muscle (Figure 14-13). This multipennate muscle is extremely strong and crosses two major joints—the knee and ankle joints. The origin of the gastrocnemius lies on the posterior surface of the medial and lateral

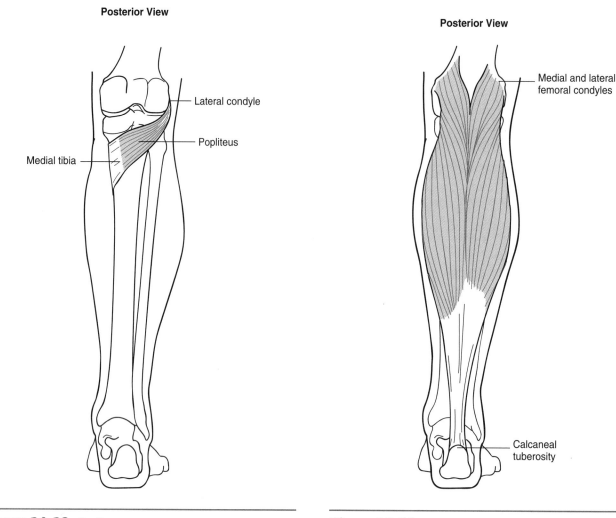

Posterior View

Lateral condyle

Popliteus

Medial tibia

Figure 14-12   *Popliteus*

Posterior View

Medial and lateral
femoral condyles

Calcaneal
tuberosity

Figure 14-13   *Gastrocnemius*

condyles of the femur, with the muscle fibers tracking into a central origin tendon. As the muscle is traced in the inferior direction, two distinct bipennate heads are formed, which run into one common tendon. This tendon is commonly referred to as the **Achilles tendon**, which runs into the calcaneal tuberosity of the calcaneus.

To palpate the gastrocnemius muscle, have an individual sit with the knee joint flexed and the ankle joint in dorsiflexion with the toes pointed toward the ceiling. Locate the "calf" muscle and palpate its belly. When the gastrocnemius muscle is palpated, observe the two distinct heads that are formed. From the belly of the muscle, trace the muscle in the inferior direction to the point where the Achilles tendon inserts into the calcaneal tuberosity.

Name:	Gastrocnemius
O:	Posterior aspect of the medial and lateral condyles of the femur
I:	Calcaneus by way of the Achilles tendon
N:	Tibial
A:	Plantar flexion and knee flexion
P:	Posterior proximal leg

KEY CONCEPTS

■ The knee joint is a uniaxial joint that allows motion in the sagittal plane around a frontal axis; it allows flexion and extension. The knee also allows extremely limited amounts of medial and lateral rotation.

■ Take the time to locate the four major ligaments of the knee. Find the anterior and posterior cruciate ligaments and medial and lateral collateral ligaments.

■ The MCL stabilizes medial movement of the knee. The LCL limits movements in the frontal and transverse planes and promotes movement in the sagittal plane. The ACL provides anterior support for the knee joint, whereas the PCL provides posterior support.

■ Although there are numerous two-joint muscles that cause actions around the knee joint, there are five true knee joint muscles: the vastus medialis, vastus lateralis, vastus intermedius, gastrocnemius, and popliteus.

BIBLIOGRAPHY

Hoppenfeld, S. (1976). *Physical examination of the spine and extremities*. London: Prentice Hall International.

Luttgens, K. (2000). *Kinesiology: Scientific basis of human motion* (9th ed.). Madison, WI: McGraw-Hill.

Minor, M. (1998). *Kinesiology laboratory manual for physical therapist assistants*. Philadelphia: F. A. Davis.

WEB RESOURCES

- To learn more about the anatomy of the knee joint and treatments for knee injuries, visit www.arthroscopy.com.
- Additional information about common knee surgeries and arthritis can be found at www.hipsandknees.com.
- Search for additional Web sites using key terms found in your reading.

(These Web addresses were current as of September 2003.)

REVIEW QUESTIONS

Fill in the Blank

Provide the word(s) or phrase(s) that best completes the sentence.

1. The _____ muscle has an origin on the medial lip of the linea aspera and inserts into the patellar tendon.

2. The _____ muscle has an origin on the lateral lip of the linea aspera and inserts into the patellar tendon.

3. Mechanical observations of the patella reveal that it is a powerful _____ _____ and strong _____ class lever.

4. The calf muscle is also known as the _____ muscle.

5. A muscle that is deep to the rectus femoris is the _____ _____ muscle.

Multiple Choice

Select the best answer to complete the following statements.

1. The ACL provides _____ for the knee joint.
a. posterior support
b. anterior support
c. medial support
d. lateral support

2. The LCL provides _____ for the knee joint.
a. posterior support
b. anterior support
c. medial support
d. lateral support

3. The PCL provides _____ for the knee joint.
a. posterior support
b. anterior support
c. medial support
d. lateral support

4. The MCL provides _____ for the knee joint.
a. posterior support
b. anterior support
c. medial support
d. lateral support

5. The popliteal ligament provides _____ for the knee joint.
a. posterior support
b. anterior support
c. medial support
d. lateral support

Matching

Match the following descriptions with the appropriate term.

_____ **1.** Medial epicondyle of the femur to the medial condyle of the tibia

A. LCL

_____ **2.** Continuous with the patella, and fibers that are continuous with the patellar tendon

B. PCL

_____ **3.** Lateral linea aspera to the patellar tendon

C. MCL

_____ **4.** Posterior surface of the femur and intercondylar fossa to the posterior head of the tibia

D. ACL

_____ **5.** Ischial tuberosity to the head of the fibula

E. Medial Meniscus

_____ **6.** Medial lip of the linea aspera to the patellar tendon

F. Patellar Ligament

_____ **7.** Lateral epicondyle of the femur to the lateral surface of the head of the fibula

G. Biceps Femoris

_____ **8.** Intercondyloid eminence of the tibia to the posterior surface of the medial condyle of the femur

H. Popliteal Ligament

_____ **9.** Intercondyloid fossa to the anterolateral surface on the medial condyle of the femur

I. Vastus Medialis

_____ **10.** Sits on top of the medial condyle of the femur

J. Vastus Laterlis

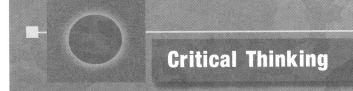

Critical Thinking

1. Imagine all of the different activities that individuals embark on each day. People walk down the street, they run through the park, and some participate in extreme sports. Choose five activities that cause stress to the knee joint. Diagram the support that the different ligaments provide and include a brief description of the forces that would cause damage to the structures of the knee joint during the movements that are described.

2. Observe the arthrokinematics of the knee joint. What occurs at the knee joint when it is in an open and closed-packed position? Describe the motion of the tibia as it tracks around the femur during movement at the knee joint. Is the movement a glide, a spin, or a roll? Explain your answer.

3. Describe the terrible triad in depth. What types of forces are applied to the knee to cause the damage that occurs with the triad structures?

4. On the picture of the knee provided, label the following structures:
   - Medial epicondyle
   - Medial condyle
   - Lateral condyle
   - Lateral epicondyle
   - Median eminence
   - Tibial plateau
   - Medial meniscus
   - Lateral meniscus
   - ACL
   - MCL
   - PCL
   - LCL

5. On the figures provided, draw the following five muscles of the knee joint:
   - Vastus medialis
   - Vastus intermedius
   - Vastus lateralis
   - Popliteus
   - Gastrocnemius

6. On the drawings provided in number 5, label the origin, insertion, action, and innervation for each of the muscles.

7. If fractures occur when the bone's ability to absorb tension, compression, or shearing forces is surpassed, besides trauma, how might a fracture occur (e.g., forceful muscle contractions, bone fatigue, from repeated overloading, bone disease, pathological fractures caused by tumors)? What role can OT practitioners play in prevention and wellness? How does one balance having fun, with natural and logical consequences, with education regarding avoidance or safety with contact sports and with healthy risk-taking? What other factors need to be considered in a wellness and prevention context?

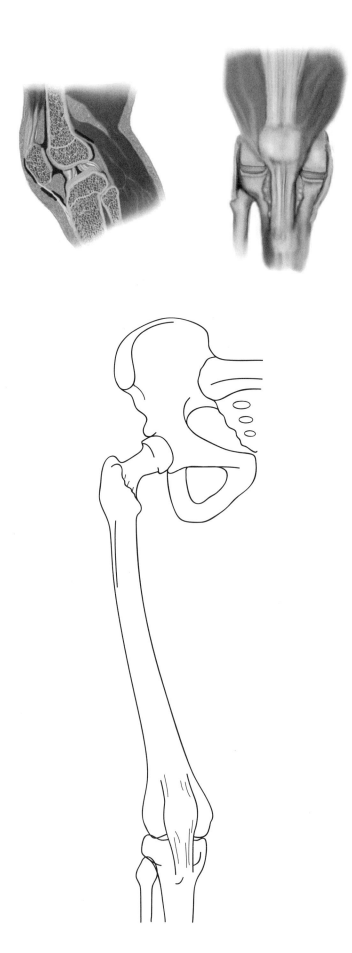

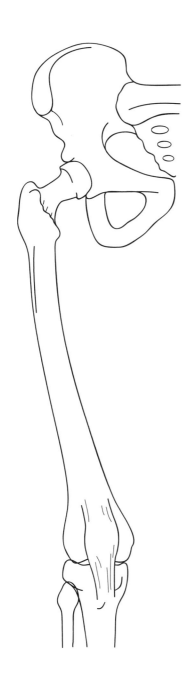

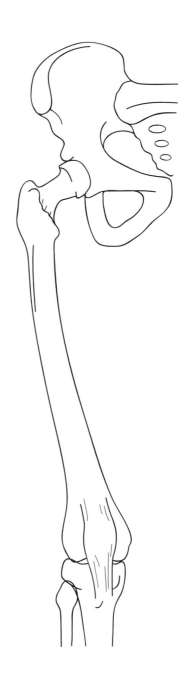

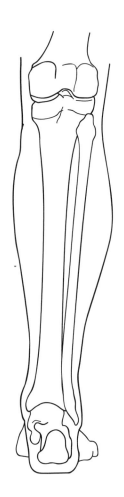

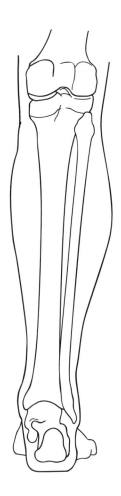

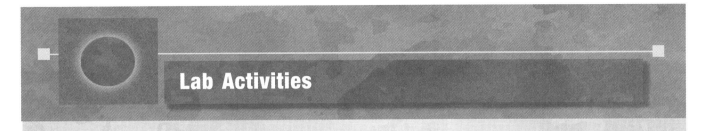

Lab Activities

Lab 14-1: Real or Apparent Shortening

Objective: To assess and evaluate shortening of the leg.

Equipment Needed: A lab partner, tape measure or other measuring devices, pen/pencil, paper, dictionary

Step 1.   Define the terms *real* or *apparent shortening* of the leg.

Step 2.   Measure the leg length of your partner using the following landmarks:

    a. ASIS to medial malleolus

    b. Greater trochanter to medial malleolus

Step 3.   Switch and allow your partner to measure your leg length as in step 2.

Step 4.   Create a situation of apparent shortening of the limb and reassess.

Step 5.   Switch roles and repeat step 4 with your partner.

Step 6.   Discuss the limitations of the measuring techniques. Discuss what would be considered within the norms for a leg length difference. Document your findings.

Lab 14-2: ACL Reconstruction

Objective: To assess and evaluate a patient following ACL reconstructive surgery. This lab involves role-playing a scenario in which a patient 4 weeks post ACL reconstruction is meeting with a therapist.

Equipment Needed: A lab partner, pen/pencil, paper, reference materials

Step 1.   Choose who will role-play the patient and who will role-play the OTA.

Step 2.   Interact and interview the patient regarding his or her experience. Ask questions about the injury and the signs and symptoms the patient is experiencing such as:

    ■ How did you injure your knee?

    ■ What are you feeling in the knee?

    ■ How have you felt since surgery?

    ■ Are you still having pain or weakness?

Step 3.   Examine the patient. Evaluate swelling, ROM, muscle strength, and function of the affected knee.

Step 4.   Design the rehabilitation program for your patient. Outline and explain the short-term and long-term goals of the patient.

Step 5.   Switch roles with your partner and repeat steps 1 through 4.

Chapter 15

THE ANKLE AND FOOT

Key Words

anterior tibiotalar
aponeurosis
calcaneonavicular ligament
calcaneus
cuboid
deltoid ligament
digiti minimi
extensor digitorum longus
extensor hallucis longus
flexor digitorum longus
flexor hallucis longus
flexor retinaculum
hallucis

inferior extensor
   retinaculum
intermediate cuneiform
lateral cuneiform
medial cuneiform
mortise
navicular
peroneus brevis
peroneus longus
peroneus tertius
phalanx
plantar aponeurosis
plantaris

retinaculum
soleus
superior extensor
   retinaculum
superior flexor retinaculum
talus
tenon
tenon-mortise
tibiocalcaneal
tibial nerve
tibialis anterior
tibialis posterior
tibionavicular

INTRODUCTION

The ankle and foot have a collection of several complex anatomical structures, including 26 bones, numerous ligaments, and many tendons, which, when combined together, serve two important functions. The first function is that of support for the entire body and the second function is that of allowing upright movement. Owing to the complexity of the ankle and foot, two important joints allow for the majority of their movements and cause the propulsion of the body forward.

The ankle joint consists of numerous intertarsal joints that allow gliding motions and three distinct diarthrodial joints that allow for range of motion at the ankle. The first of these joints is found at the articulation between the tibia, fibula, and talus. This joint is commonly called the tibiotalar (talocrural) joint and is classified as a **tenon-mortise** joint (peg and socket). Much like in woodworking, where two sections of lumber come together, the medial lateral malleolus forms a socket (**mortise**) that articulates with the peg-shaped talus bone (**tenon**). This arrangement greatly enhances the stability of this region by preventing unwanted lateral and medial movements of the ankle.

The other two joints are found between the articulations of the tarsal bones. Each joint formed by these junctions allows for inversion and eversion movements of the ankle. The first joint is called the subtalar joint, which is at the junction between the talus and calcaneus bones. The second joint is called the midtarsal joint, which is between the junction of the calcaneus and cuboid bones on the lateral side of the foot; on the medial side of the foot is the junction of the talus and navicular bones. The ankle and foot also have many ligaments and tendons, several retinaculums, and 22 muscles. This chapter covers the 12 extrinsic muscles.

 ## MAJOR LANDMARKS OF THE ANKLE AND FOOT

Remember from Chapter 5 that there are seven bones in the hindfoot: the talus, calcaneus, navicular, cuboid, lateral cuneiform, intermediate cuneiform, and medial cuneiform (Figure 15-1). Collectively, these bones are called the tarsals.

Landmarks of the Tarsals

Beginning on the dorsal surface of the foot, the **talus** articulates with the tibia. The **navicular** lies just distal to the talus and articulates with the three cuneiform bones. The three cuneiform bones are labeled 1–3 from medial to lateral (1, **medial cuneiform**; 2, **intermediate cuneiform**; and 3, **lateral cuneiform**) and lie just distal to the navicular, articulating with the first, second, and third metatarsals, respectively. From here, the **cuboid** lies between the **calcaneus** and the fourth and fifth metatarsals.

The view of the plantar surface of the foot shows all seven tarsals and provides the best view of the calcaneus. This bone is also know as the heel bone. The calcaneus provides the insertion point, the calcaneal tuberosity, for both the soleus and the gastrocnemius muscles by way of the Achilles tendon.

Landmarks of the Metatarsals

There are five metatarsal bones located in the midfoot. The first metatarsal bone articulates with the medial cuneiform, the second metatarsal articulates with the intermediate cuneiform, and the third metatarsal articulates with the lateral cuneiform. Both the fourth and fifth metatarsals articulate with the cuboid. The distal metatarsals articulate with their respective phalanges.

Landmarks of the Phalanges

Much like the hand, five individual phalangeal bones make up the forefoot region. By labeling names with the corresponding phalanx, naming the muscles with their insertions into these bones makes identification simple. For example, **hallucis** is the name of the big toe, digitorum refers to any of the toes labeled 2–5 and **digiti minimi** refers to the little toe; therefore, the flexor hallucis longus muscle flexes the big toe and the extensor digitorum longus extends toes 2–5. In addition to individual names of bones, the location of the muscle tendon also reveals the location of the muscle. Notice that all of the phalangeal flexors are located on the plantar surface of the foot and that all extensors are located on the dorsal surface of the foot.

The great toe is the first **phalanx** with two individual phalanx bones. The remaining four phalanges (2–5) have three phalanx bones, each including the proximal, intermediate, and distal phalanx.

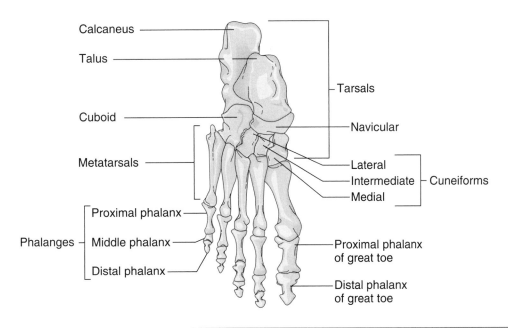

Figure 15-1 *Landmarks of the Tarsals*

NERVOUS INNERVATION

The two major branches of the sciatic nerve, the tibial and common peroneal nerves, innervate the muscles that cause the actions around the ankle joint. The tibial nerve innervates muscles located on the posterior and medial surfaces of the leg, and the common peroneal nerve innervates the muscles located on the anterior and lateral surfaces of the leg.

Tibial Nerve

As the **tibial nerve** tracks in the inferior direction from the intercondylar eminence, it passes deep to the gastrocnemius, soleus, and plantaris muscles and superficial to the popliteus muscle (Figure 15-2). The nerve then runs in the medial direction along the interosseous membrane and wraps around the medial malleolus and tracks into the plantar surface of the foot. After the nerve wraps around the malleolus, it further branches into two distinct nerves: the medial and lateral plantar nerves. Because of the tracking and location of the tibial nerve and its branches, it innervates the soleus, plantaris, flexor digitorum longus, flexor hallucis longus, and tibialis posterior. When studying these nerves, note their location and identify how the nerve tracks to cause muscle innervation.

OTA Perspective

A Syme's amputation is comparable to an ankle disarticulation with the removal of the medial and lateral malleoli and the distal inch of the tibia. This causes the patient to lose what function? A Syme prosthesis is a "plastic syme," which consists of a total-contact plastic socket and solid ankle cushioned heel (SACH) foot; there is no ankle joint.

Does an amputation of the small toes affect function? What function does the great toe provide? What does amputation of the great toe impair? Shoe or toe fillers are used in place of prosthetic devices.

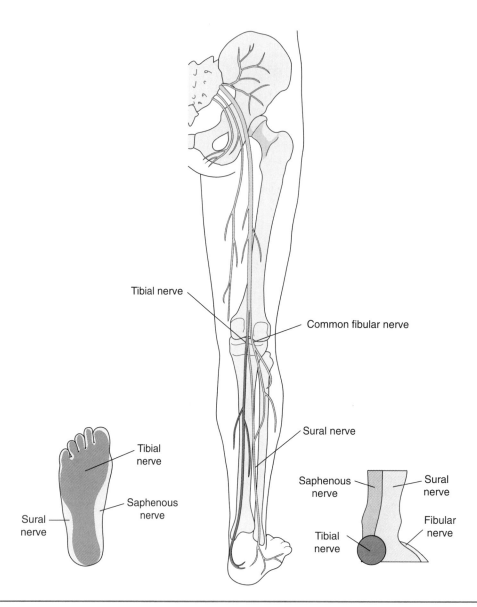

Figure 15-2 *Tibial Nerve*

Common Peroneal (Fibular) Nerve

From the location where the common peroneal nerve branches from the sciatic nerve, it tracks in the inferior and medial directions to the short head of the biceps femoris and deep to the long head of the biceps femoris (Figure 15-3). From this location the common peroneal nerve crosses the knee joint superficially to the lateral epicondyle of the femur. The nerve then continues in the lateral direction and tracks toward the anterior surface as it wraps around the head of the fibula. Finally, the nerve tracks in the inferior direction along the anterior surface of the interosseous membrane and wraps around the anterior surface of the medial malleolus. As the common peroneal nerve continues tracking in the inferior direction, it branches and innervates the tibialis anterior, tertius muscle group, extensor digitorum longus, and extensor hallucis longus muscles. Table 15-1 summarizes the nerves that innervate the foot.

 MOVEMENTS OF THE ANKLE AND FOOT

The movements of the ankle and foot occur at multiple joints and mainly in the sagittal and frontal planes, with little rotation at the talocrural and subtalar joints. Much like the carpals in the hand, the articulations between the tarsal bones pro-

Table 15-1 *Nerves of the Foot*

Nerve	Affected Anterior Muscles	Affected Lateral Muscles	Affected Posterior Muscles
Tibial	None	None	Soleus, plantaris, flexor digitorum longus, flexor hallucis longus, tibialis posterior
Common Peroneal	Tibialis anterior, peroneus tertius, extensor digitorum longus, extensor hallucis longus	peroneus longus, peroneus brevis, peroneus tertius	None

vide gliding motions to increase the ROM of the foot and toes. When learning the different movements referenced in Table 15-2, perform the movements to help you better understand their actions.

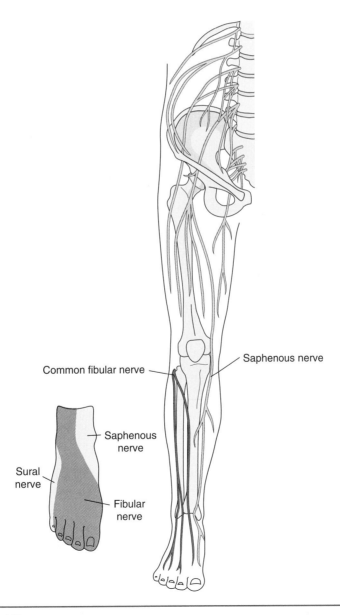

Figure 15-3 *Common Peroneal Nerve*

Table 15-2 *Movements of the Ankle and Foot*

Movement	Axis	Plane	Description
Dorsiflexion or Flexion	Frontal	Sagittal	Dorsal surface of the foot moves toward the anterior surface of the tibia.
Plantar Flexion or Extension	Frontal	Sagittal	Plantar surface of the foot moves away from the anterior surface of the tibia.
Inversion or Adduction or Supination	Sagittal	Frontal	Plantar surface of the foot moves toward the midline of the body.
Eversion or Abduction or Pronation	Sagittal	Frontal	Dorsal surface of the foot moves toward the midline of the body.
Hyperextension (great toe only)	Frontal	Sagittal	Dorsal surface of the foot moves toward the anterior surface of the tibia.

OTA Perspective

A common neurological problem in the lower extremity is "footdrop." This condition presents with a patient who is unable to actively dorsiflex the foot owing to weakness of the ankle dorsiflexors.

The weakness can be caused by a number of factors, among the most common of which are a peroneal neuropathy, direct trauma to the dorsiflexors, compartment syndrome, paralysis following a stroke, sciatic nerve compression from a disk herniation in the lumbar spine, or a diabetic neuropathy.

The condition results in the typical high-stepping gait, with exaggerated hip and knee flexion to enable the foot to clear the ground, and the slap sound of the foot.

 STABILITY OF THE ANKLE AND FOOT

Because the ankle and foot complex consists of a combination of 26 bones, there are many small ligaments that provide stability and support for the articulations between these small bones. There are also bands of flat fibrous connective tissue called **retinaculum** or **aponeurosis**, which aid in the stability of the ankle and foot by bundling muscles together while limiting unwanted movements.

Plantar Aponeurosis

The **plantar aponeurosis** is a flat band of connective tissue located on the plantar surface of the foot connecting the anterior surface of the calcaneus to each of the five phalanges. Because this band covers the width of the foot, it connects to the abductor hallucis muscle on the medial side to the aponeurosis on the lateral side of the foot. Therefore, it provides strength and stability for the bottom of the foot.

Superior Extensor Retinaculum

The **superior extensor retinaculum** is located on the anterior portion of the distal tibia. It attaches the superior region of the lateral malleolus and tracks medially to the tibia just proximal to the medial malleolus (Figure 15-4). This band of connective tissue covers the tendons of the extensor muscles and bundles them together in one central location.

Inferior Extensor Retinaculum

The **inferior extensor retinaculum** is located on the anterior portion of the ankle and foot inferior to the superior extensor retinaculum. This structure has one attachment point on the lateral side of the foot (tuberosity of the fifth metatarsal) and two attachment points on the medial side of the foot. The proximal attachment is on the medial malleolus and the distal attachment is the talus (Figure 15-5). This band of connective tissue covers all of the synovial tendon sheaths of the extensor muscles. It, therefore, allows minimal movement of the tendons laterally or medially and bundles the tendons together at the foot.

Deltoid Ligament

The **deltoid ligament** is located on the medial aspect of the ankle. It is also referred to as the medial ligament and has three parts (Figure 15-6). One end of all three parts of the deltoid ligament attaches to the tibia, whereas the other ends attach to the calcaneus, talus, or navicular individually. Therefore, the deltoid ligaments are individually named the **tibiocalcaneal**, **anterior tibiotalar**, and **tibionavicular**. During human movement, the deltoid ligament provides medial support for the ankle while limiting medial movement of the ankle when a lateral force is applied to the joint.

Plantar Calcaneonavicular Ligament

The plantar **calcaneonavicular ligament** is located on the plantar surface of the foot. This broad, thick ligament attaches the calcaneus to the navicular bone providing support to the talus and the subtalar joint. It is also known as the "spring ligament" owing to its elastic fibers that give this ligament its "bounce."

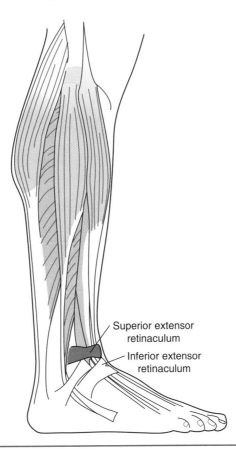

Figure 15-4 *Superior Extensor Retinaculum*

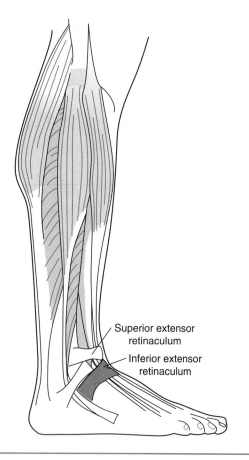

Figure 15-5 *Inferior Extensor Retinaculum*

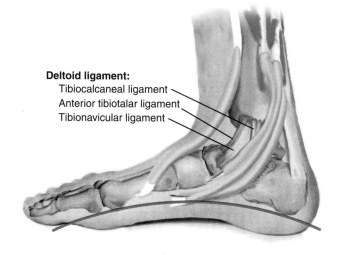

Figure 15-6 *Deltoid Ligament*

OTA Perspective

Traditionally, rehabilitation of the ankle and foot (and the L/E in general) are a PT domain. This makes sense when viewed from the perspective of components—balance, gross motor strength, endurance, coordination, gait, ambulation, and assistive ambulation devices. Also traditionally, splinting is an OT domain, including the ankle and foot. Goals in splinting may include preserving function, preventing deforming contractures, restricting movement or assisting or substituting for movement, and minimizing pain. Diagnoses such as CVA, burns, diabetes, and SCI may result in hypertonicity/hypotonicity, contractures, footdrop, and pain. Review what you know about these diseases and injuries; with those diagnoses in mind, review this chapter for a clinical understanding of the effects of these diseases on ankle and foot function.

Superior Flexor Retinaculum

The **superior flexor retinaculum** attaches the lateral malleolus of the fibula to the calcaneus. It covers the tendons of the peroneus longus and brevis muscles and keeps these tendons from moving out of place.

Flexor Retinaculum

The **flexor retinaculum** attaches the medial malleolus to the calcaneus. It covers the tendons of the tibialis posterior, flexor digitorum longus, and hallucis longus muscles and keeps these tendons from moving out of place.

 MUSCLES OF THE ANKLE AND FOOT

There are 22 muscles in the ankle and foot. This section covers all 12 extrinsic muscles with one exception, the gastrocnemius, which is covered in Chapter 14, The Knee Joint. Extrinsic muscles are those muscles that have a proximal origin on the tibia or fibula and a distal insertion on the tarsals or individual phalanx of the toes.

Anterior Muscles of the Ankle and Foot

The anterior muscles of the ankle and foot work together as agonists and synergists to provide contractions associated with dorsiflexion, eversion, and inversion of the foot. Three individual muscles are located on the anterior aspect of the leg and foot: the tibialis anterior, extensor digitorum longus, and extensor hallucis longus.

Tibialis Anterior   The **tibialis anterior** muscle is a fusiform muscle located on the anterior surface of the tibia (Figure 15-7). The origin of this muscle is on the lateral tibia and interosseous membrane. The tibialis anterior muscle causes dorsiflexion. Because the tibialis anterior inserts on the first cuneiform and first metatarsal, it also causes inversion of the foot.

The tibialis anterior muscle can be palpated easily when the knee is flexed and the ankle joint is in a dorsiflexion position. Place your fingers on the anterolateral aspect of the tibia and perform dorsiflexion at your ankle joint. Note the distal insertion of the tibialis anterior on the dorsal surface of the foot as it inserts into the first cuneiform bone. From this location palpate the muscle in the superior direction and locate the belly of the muscle between the tibia and fibula.

Name:	Tibialis Anterior
O:	Lateral tibia
I:	First cuneiform and metatarsal
N:	Common peroneal nerve
A:	Dorsiflexion and inversion
P:	Lateral aspect of the tibia

Extensor Digitorum Longus   The **extensor digitorum longus** muscle is a unipennate muscle located deep to the tibialis anterior muscle and on the anterolateral surface of the tibia. The origin of this muscle is on the lateral condyle of the tibia, fibula, and interosseous membrane (Figure 15-8) and inserts by the branches of four tendons on the distal phalanges of toes 2–5. As the name "extensor digitorum" implies, the muscle extends the lateral four toes 2–5 and acts as a synergist to provide dorsiflexion and eversion of the foot.

The extensor digitorum longus muscle can be palpated by placing the fingers on the anterior and lateral surfaces of the tibia and then extending the toes. The tendons can be palpated on the dorsal aspect of the foot.

Name:	Extensor Digitorum Longus
O:	Lateral tibial condyle and proximal fibula
I:	Distal phalanges of the lateral four toes
N:	Common peroneal nerve
A:	Extension of the lateral four toes
P:	Tendons can be palpated on the dorsal aspect of the foot

Extensor Hallucis Longus   The **extensor hallucis longus** muscle is a bipennate muscle located deep to the tibialis anterior and extensor digitorum longus muscle (Figure 15-9). The origin of this muscle is on the anterolateral surface of the tibia, and as the tendon tracks past the ankle joint, it slants medially toward the great toe and inserts on the distal phalanx. As the name "extensor hallucis" implies, the muscle extends the great toe. It also acts as a synergist to provide dorsiflexion.

To palpate the extensor hallucis longus muscle, dorsiflex the big toe. Locate the long tendon of the muscle on the dorsal surface of the foot, tracking from the distal phalanx to where it runs deep to the tibialis anterior muscle. Note that the belly of the muscle is deep to the extensor digitorum longus and tibialis anterior and, therefore, cannot be palpated.

Name:	Extensor Hallucis Longus
O:	Anterior fibula
I:	Dorsum of great toe
N:	Common peroneal nerve
A:	Extension of the great toe and ankle dorsiflexion
P:	Tendon can be palpated on dorsum of the great toe

Posterior Muscles of the Ankle and Foot

The posterior muscles of the ankle and foot work as agonists and synergists together to provide contractions associated with plantar flexion, flexion of the toes, and inversion of the foot. Six individual muscles are located on the posterior aspect of the leg: the gastrocnemius, soleus, plantaris, flexor digitorum longus, flexor hallucis longus, and tibialis posterior.

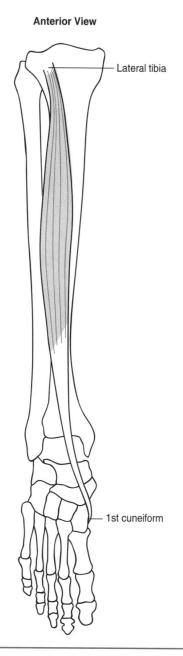

Anterior View

Lateral tibia

1st cuneiform

Figure 15-7 *Tibialis Anterior*

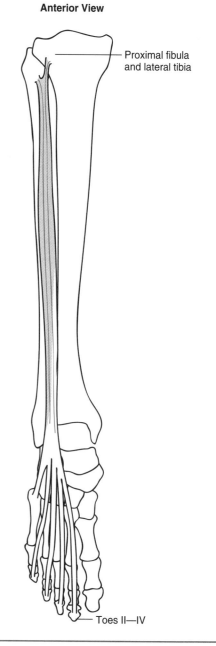

Anterior View

Proximal fibula and lateral tibia

Toes II—IV

Figure 15-8 *Extensor Digitorum Longus*

Gastrocnemius The gastrocnemius is the only two-joint muscle of the posterior leg region. Its expanded description can be found in Chapter 14. The gastrocnemius muscle causes knee flexion and ankle plantar flexion.

Name:	Gastrocnemius
O:	Posterior aspect of the medial and lateral condyles of the femur
I:	Calcaneal tuberosity via the Achilles tendon
N:	Tibial nerve
A:	Plantar flexion and knee flexion
P:	Posterior proximal leg

Soleus The **soleus** muscle is a bipennate muscle located deep to the gastrocnemius, with the belly of the muscle located on the posterior surface of the superior half of the tibia and fibula (Figure 15-10). The soleus originates on the head of the fibula, the lateral and superior half of the surface of the tibia, and the posteromedial surface of the superior half of the fibula. From here the muscle widens to cover the entire posterior surface of the superior half of the leg, tracking into the cal-

Anterior View

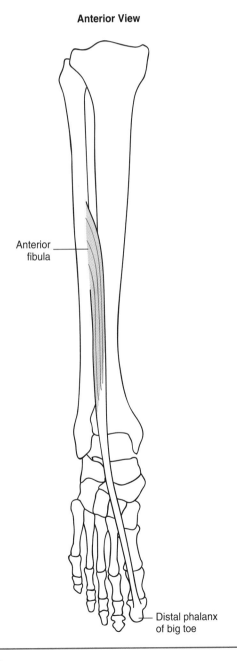

Anterior fibula

Distal phalanx of big toe

Figure 15-9 *Extensor Hallucis Longus*

caneal tuberosity via the Achilles tendon. The soleus muscle plays a large role in the ability of individuals to balance on one foot because it is responsible for plantar flexion and is very active during the reduction of dorsiflexion.

Of the muscles on the posterior aspect of the leg, the soleus and gastrocnemius muscles are the easiest to palpate. The soleus can be palpated on the lateral side of the lower leg deep to the gastrocnemius muscle.

Name:	Soleus
O:	Fibular head and superior half of the posterior tibia and fibula
I:	Calcaneal tuberosity via the Achilles tendon
N:	Tibial nerve
A:	Plantar flexion
P:	Lateral side of the lower leg

Plantaris   The **plantaris** muscle is a small bipennate muscle located deep to the lateral head of the gastrocnemius muscle. It originates on the posterior lateral condyle of the femur and tracks between the condyles of the femur (Figure 15-11). Immediately inferior to the femoral condyles, the muscle narrows into a long tendon, tracking down the medial surface of the soleus where it inserts on the calcaneus via the Achilles tendon. The plantaris muscle assists with plantar flexion and is not always present in human beings. It is too deep and too small to be palpated.

Name:	Plantaris
O:	Posterior lateral condyle of the femur
I:	Calcaneus via the Achilles tendon
N:	Tibial nerve
A:	Plantar flexion
P:	Too deep to palpate

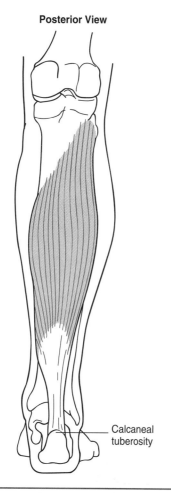

Posterior View

Calcaneal tuberosity

Figure 15-10   *Soleus*

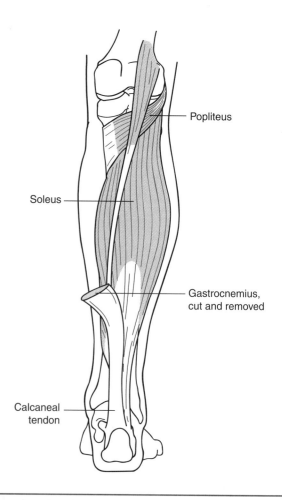

Popliteus

Soleus

Gastrocnemius, cut and removed

Calcaneal tendon

Figure 15-11   *Plantaris*

Flexor Digitorum Longus   The **flexor digitorum longus** muscle is a unipennate muscle located deep to the soleus on the posteromedial aspect of the tibia (Figure 15-12). The origin of the flexor digitorum longus is on the posteromedial surface of the distal half of the tibia, passing posteriorly to the medial malleolus and inserting in the distal phalanges of digits 2–5. As the name "flexor digitorum" indicates, the flexor digitorum longus is responsible for the flexion of digits 2–5. Much like the extensor digitorum longus muscles, the tracking of the flexor digitorum longus on the posterior surface of the medial malleolus increases the forces produced with each muscle contraction.

The flexor digitorum muscle is extremely deep, making it difficult to palpate. However, the insertion tendon can be palpated posterior to the medial malleolus.

Name:	Flexor Digitorum Longus
O:	Posteromedial aspect of the distal half of the tibia
I:	Base of the distal phalanges of the four lateral toes
N:	Tibial nerve
A:	Flexion of the four lateral toes
P:	Tendon can be palpated posterior to the medial malleolus

Flexor Hallucis Longus   The **flexor hallucis longus** muscle is a bipennate muscle located deep to the soleus on the lateral aspect of the leg (Figure 15-13). It originates on the distal half of the posterior fibula and passes behind the medial malleolus, where it inserts into the distal phalanx of the great toe. The flexor hallucis longus muscle is responsible for flexion of the great toe and plays an important role in walking, running, and jumping movements. The strength of this muscle is important for the "push-off" action provided for these activities.

Owing to the deep location of the flexor hallucis longus, this muscle cannot be palpated.

Name:	Flexor Hallucis Longus
O:	Fibula
I:	Great toe
N:	Tibial nerve
A:	Flexion of the great toe
P:	Tendon can be palpated posterior to the medial malleolus

Tibialis Posterior   The **tibialis posterior** muscle is a bipennate muscle located in the deepest position of all posterior leg muscles (Figure 15-14). The tibialis posterior muscle originates from three separate locations: the posterior surface of the fibular head and neck, inferior to the lateral condyle of the tibia and intercondylar eminence of the tibia, and the major portion of the interosseous membrane. The belly then tracks into a central tendon that wraps around the medial malleolus. From this location the tibialis posterior inserts on the plantar aspect of the foot on the navicular and all three cuneiform bones. The tibialis posterior plays a large role in the maintenance of the longitudinal arch. It causes strong inversion and plantar flexion movements of the foot when it contracts.

Owing to the deep location of the tibialis posterior, the muscle cannot be palpated.

Name:	Tibialis Posterior
O:	Interosseous membrane and adjacent surfaces of the tibia and fibula
I:	Navicular and cuneiforms
N:	Tibial nerve
A:	Inversion and plantar flexion
P:	Too deep to palpate

Lateral Muscles of the Ankle and Foot

The lateral muscles of the ankle and foot work as agonists and synergists together to provide contractions associated with eversion of the foot. Three individual muscles are located on the lateral aspect of the leg: the peroneus longus, peroneus brevis, and peroneus tertius. Each of the muscles in the peroneus group provides support on the lateral aspect of the ankle. From a stability prospective, the lateral ankle is the weak side of the ankle joint and is more prone to injury.

Peroneus Longus   The **peroneus longus** muscle is a bipennate muscle covering the lateral aspect of the leg (Figure 15-15). The muscle originates on the head of the fibula, with its central tendon wrapping behind the lateral malleolus to the plantar surface of the foot, where it inserts on the medial cuneiform and first metatarsal. The peroneus longus causes eversion of the foot and assists in plantar flexion. It is most active during the propulsive stage in walking.

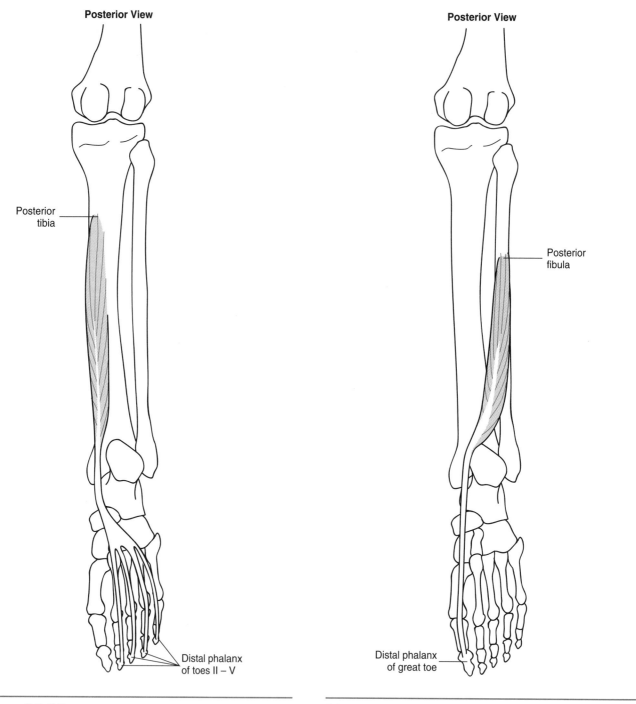

Figure 15-12 *Flexor Digitorum Longus*

Figure 15-13 *Flexor Hallucis Longus*

The belly of the peroneus longus can be palpated just distal to the head of the fibula, and its tendon can be palpated posterior to the lateral malleolus.

Name:	Peroneus Longus
O:	Head of the fibula and lateral condyle of the tibia
I:	Plantar surface of the medial cuneiform and first metatarsal
N:	Common peroneal nerve
A:	Eversion
P:	Distal to the head of the fibula

Peroneus Brevis The **peroneus brevis** muscle is a bipennate muscle located deep to the peroneus longus (Figure 15-16). It originates on the lateral lower half of the fibula, and its tendon passes behind the lateral malleolus and inserts on the base of the fifth metatarsal. The peroneus brevis is a short muscle, as its name implies, and causes eversion of the foot. It also assists with plantar flexion.

The peroneus brevis muscle can be palpated on the lower lateral aspect of the fibula. Its tendon can be palpated just posterior to the lateral malleolus.

Name: Peroneus Brevis
O: Lateral distal fibula
I: Base of the fifth metatarsal
N: Common peroneal nerve
A: Eversion
P: Lower lateral aspect of the fibula

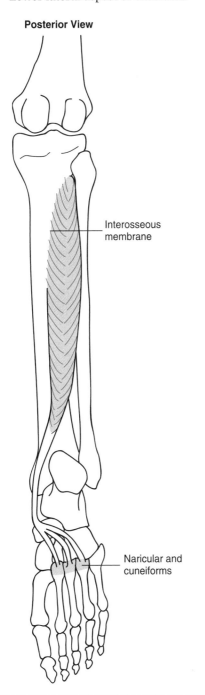

Posterior View

Interosseous membrane

Naricular and cuneiforms

Figure 15-14   *Tibialis Posterior*

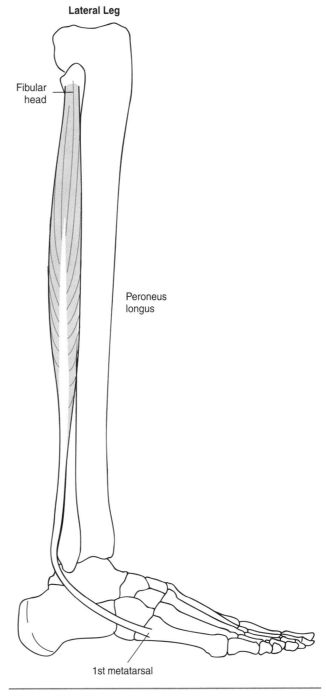

Lateral Leg

Fibular head

Peroneus longus

1st metatarsal

Figure 15-15   *Peroneus Longus*

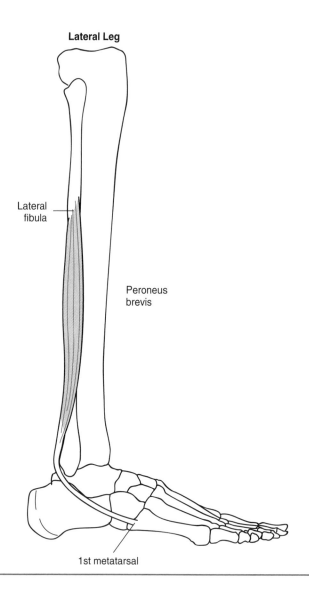

Figure 15-16 *Peroneus Brevis*

Peroneus Tertius The **peroneus tertius** muscle is a bipennate muscle located on the anterior surface of the tibia just lateral and deep to the extensor digitorum longus muscle and lateral to the extensor hallucis longus muscle. Its long central tendon inserts on the base of the fifth metatarsal. Note that the insertion of the peroneus tertius muscle wraps around the anterior surface of the lateral malleolus. This arrangement allows the tendon to act as an anatomical pulley, increasing the amount of force produced with each contraction. Owing to its lateral and dorsal origin insertion position, when the peroneus tertius muscle contracts it provides strong dorsiflexion and eversion movements of the foot.

The small size and deep location of the peroneus tertius makes it extremely difficult to palpate. However, its insertion tendon can be palpated on the dorsal aspect of the foot near the base of the fifth metatarsal.

Name:	Peroneus Tertius
O:	Distal medial fibula
I:	Dorsal surface of the fifth metatarsal
N:	Common peroneal nerve
A:	Dorsiflexion and eversion
P:	Tendon can be palpated at the lateral malleolus

KEY CONCEPTS

■ The ankle/foot complex has several joints and motions. The tibiotalar joint is a uniaxial hinge joint offering only plantar flexion and dorsiflexion in the sagittal plane. Inversion and eversion movements are motions that occur at the subtalar joint.

■ The ankle joint is a complex joint consisting of numerous ligaments and tendons that provide support for the ankle during human movement. Take the time to study the medial and lateral ligaments that provide sound support for the ankle joint during human movement.

■ Remember that there are 22 individual muscles that cause movements at either the ankle or foot. In this chapter, 12 of these muscles have been discussed.

 BIBLIOGRAPHY

Luttgens, K. (2000). *Kinesiology: Scientific basis of human motion.* (9th ed.). Madison, WI: McGraw-Hill.
Minor, M. (1998). *Kinesiology laboratory manual for physical therapist assistants.* Philadelphia: F. A. Davis.

 WEB RESOURCES

• Visit the American Orthopaedic Foot and Ankle Society's Web site at www.aofas.org/ to learn more about injuries and treatment plans for the ankle and foot.

• For information on the field of podiatry and foot problems and additional links in this area, visit www.footandankle.com/ and the American College of Foot and Ankle Surgeons at www.acfas.org/.

• Search for additional Web resources based on key terms used in this chapter.

(These Web addresses were current as of September 2003.)

 REVIEW QUESTIONS

Fill in the Blank

Provide the word(s) or phrase(s) that best completes the sentence.

1. The peroneus muscle group provides _____ movements.

2. The _____ muscle is not present in all humans.

3. When the lateral portion of the foot lifts up, it is called _____.

4. The _____ muscle is the smallest muscle of the ankle and foot.

5. The _____ nerve serves all the muscles on the posterior leg.

6. The main action of the tibialis posterior is _____.

7. The _____ muscle inserts on the dorsal portion of the great toe.

8. The tibialis posterior is located _____ and provides _____ movements.

9. The five tarsal bones are _____, _____, _____, _____, and _____.

10. When the plantar surface of the foot turns toward the midline, it is called _____.

Multiple Choice

Select the best answer to complete the following statements.

1. The muscle that attaches to the base of the fifth metatarsal is the _____ .
   a. peroneus longus
   b. tibialis posterior
   c. soleus
   d. peroneus brevis

2. The most superficial muscle is the _____ .
   a. plantaris
   b. tibialis posterior
   c. soleus
   d. peroneus brevis

3. The synovial tendon sheaths of the extensor muscles are covered distally by the ____.
   a. superior extensor retinaculum
   b. inferior extensor retinaculum
   c. plantar aponeurosis
   d. aponeurosis

4. The structure that supports the longitudinal arch is the _____ .
   a. superior extensor retinaculum
   b. inferior extensor retinaculum
   c. plantar aponeurosis
   d. aponeurosis

5. The largest muscle of the ankle and foot is the _____ .
   a. peroneus longus
   b. tibialis anterior
   c. tibialis posterior
   d. gastrocnemius

6. The most active muscle while balancing on one foot is the _____ .
   a. soleus
   b. gastrocnemius
   c. plantaris
   d. flexor digitorum longus

7. The deepest muscle is the _____ .
   a. peroneus brevis
   b. plantaris
   c. tibialis posterior
   d. extensor digitorum longus

8. The ligamentous structure that provides the greatest support on the medial aspect of the ankle is the _____ .
   a. peroneal retinaculum
   b. inferior extensor retinaculum
   c. flexor retinaculum
   d. deltoid ligament

9. Of the following muscles, the _____ muscle belly *cannot* be palpated.
   a. soleus
   b. flexor digitorum longus
   c. extensor digitorum longus
   d. peroneus longus

10. The phalanx that has less than three bones is _____ .
   a. 4
   b. 3
   c. 2
   d. 1

Matching

Match each of the following descriptions with the appropriate term.

_____ **1.** Heel bone

_____ **2.** Turning the sole of the foot toward the midline

_____ **3.** Great toe

_____ **4.** Name for three bones of the foot

_____ **5.** The top of the foot

_____ **6.** Turning the lateral edge of the foot away from the midline

_____ **7.** Fibrous connective tissue on the bottom of the foot

_____ **8.** Round prominence on the fibula

_____ **9.** The bottom of the foot

_____**10.** Thick band of connective tissue

A. Dorsal

B. Inversion

C. Plantar aponeurosis

D. Retinaculum

E. Plantar

F. Medial malleolus

G. Eversion

H. Calcaneus

I. Hallucis

J. Cuneiform

Critical Thinking

1. One of your clients likes to rollerblade but he or she complains that the lower leg feels fatigued after just a few minutes. What muscles are being utilized during rollerblading, and what are the joint motions involved? Next explain how you would strengthen the muscles involved to aid this person in a more enjoyable exercise session.

2. Analyze the movements, muscles, and joints involved at the ankle for a basketball player performing a jump shot.

3. On the diagram provided below, label the structures of the foot and proximal tibia and fibula. On a skeleton, locate and label the following landmarks:

   ■ Calcaneous

   ■ Talus

   ■ Navicular

   ■ Cuboid

   ■ Cuneiforms

   ■ Metatarsals

   ■ Phalanges

   ■ Medial malleolus

   ■ Lateral malleolus

(continues)

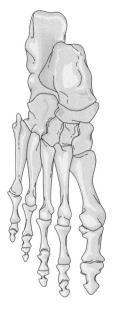

Critical Thinking *(continued)*

4. On the figures provided on the following pages, draw the following major muscles of the foot and ankle joint:

- Gastrocnemius

- Soleus

- Tibialis anterior

- Extensor digitorum longus

- Extensor hallucis longus

- Tibialis posterior

- Flexor hallucis longus

- Flexor digitorum longus

- Peroneus brevis

- Peroneus longus

5. On the drawings from number 4, label the origin, insertion, action, and innervation for each of the above muscles.

6. Define the term *differential diagnosis*. For a patient presenting with footdrop, research five possible causes of the footdrop. For each possible cause, list three other signs and symptoms that would be present to assist in the differential diagnosis. Briefly describe the role of PT in a patient with a permanent foot drop.

7. Describe the advice that you would give to a friend who severely sprained his ankle yesterday. Three weeks later he wants to return to play basketball but is worried about whether he will reinjure his ankle. Describe the advice that you would give regarding avoidance of reinjury.

8. Which works "best" with ankle and foot dysfunction, PT or OT? How does a clinician decide? Is it solely based on facility history and protocol? The diagnoses? The physician or surgeon's treatment order? OT or PT availability? The individual therapist's interest and expertise? The client's ultimate goal? What about billing for equipment used to reach the client's goal(s)? Maybe "best" is a combination of both therapies leading to accomplishing the client's goal(s). How does the treatment team decide? What documentation is written to justify this decision, especially if OT and PT both treat the client's ankle or foot injury and resulting (in)abilities? How is this communicated to the physician or surgeon, the client, and other members of the treatment team? Clinical reasoning drives "how" these questions are answered and "what" type of therapy is provided. Typically, the answers are not "right" or "wrong" but need to be researched and discussed in order to provide quality therapy, physical or occupational, to the client.

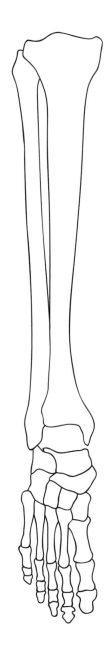
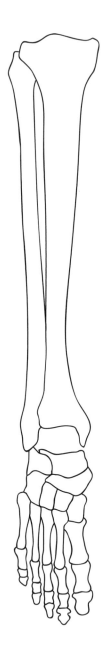

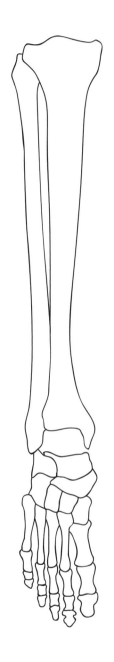

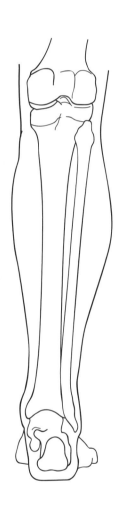

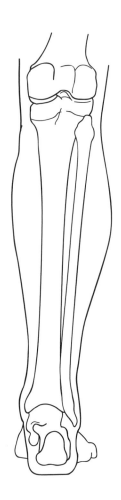

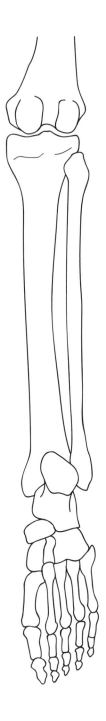

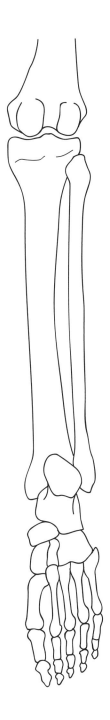

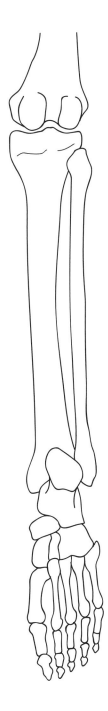

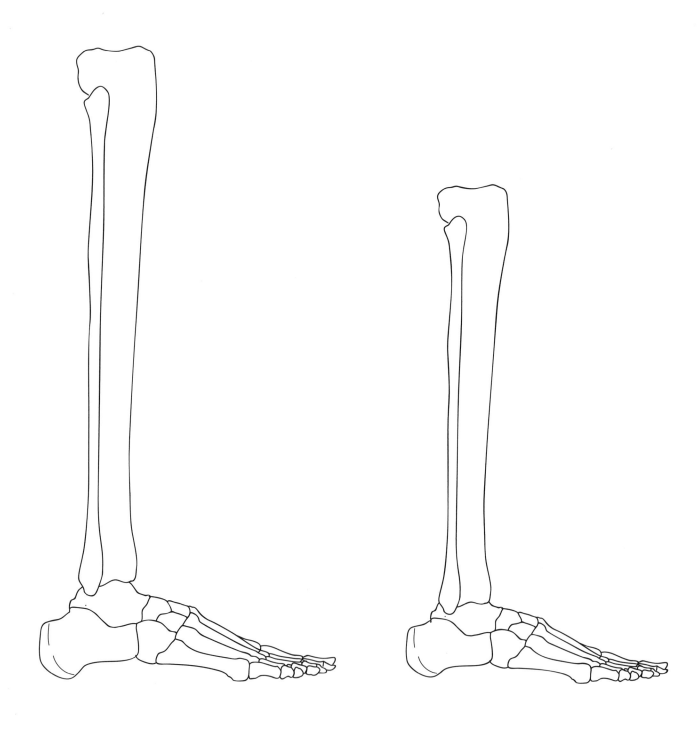

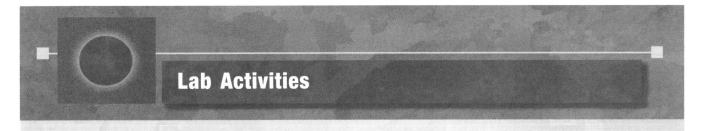

Lab Activities

Lab 15-1: Ankle Sprain

Objective: To provide a plan of treatment following an ankle sprain.

Equipment Needed: A lab partner, pen/pencil, paper

Step 1. Interview your partner about the injury.

Step 2. Explain and teach your partner about balance and the importance of the therapy.

Step 3. Teach your partner a progression of balance exercises for a client who is 2 weeks post injury. Think of a progression of at least eight different activities.

Step 4. Switch roles with your partner and repeat steps 1 through 3.

Lab 15-2: Achilles Rupture

Objective: To identify and assess a rupture to the Achilles tendon.

Equipment Needed: A lab partner, pen/pencil, paper

Step 1. Interview your partner about the injury.

Step 2. Demonstrate the Thompson's test on your partner.

Step 3. Design a strengthening program for a patient who is 6 months post surgery to repair the tendon.

Step 4. Teach your partner five ways to strengthen the tendon and a way to stretch it.

Step 5. Switch roles with your partner and repeat steps 1 through 4.

Lab 15-3: Amputation Drawing Lab

Objective: To become familiar with the varying types of L/E, specifically ankle/foot, orthoses.

Equipment Needed: A lab partner, L/E orthotics and prosthetics, resource books and catalogs, prosthetist as a guest lecturer, classroom space to try on orthoses, pencil and paper

Step 1. With a partner, try on the orthotics and prosthetics, with one of you assuming the role of the OTA, and the other of the client with a specific ankle/foot injury or disease.

Step 2. Assess each for movement or immobility, comfort, ease of putting the devices on and taking them off, and functional purpose.

Step 3. Determine price, availability, and recommended length of wear (in hours per day and total days per injury). Does the client need to be actively involved in putting the devices on and taking them off and wearing of the orthosis or prosthesis? What other considerations need to be addressed (e.g., shoes to be worn with the device, hygiene, preserving skin integrity, etc.)?

Step 4. Make a list of your findings to share with your classmates.

Chapter 16

GAIT

Key Words

double limb support	midstance	stance phase
foot drop gait	midswing	swing phase
initial contact	preswing	terminal stance
initial swing	quadriceps gait	terminal swing
load response	single limb support	Trendelenberg gait

INTRODUCTION

Human gait is a result of a complex interaction of muscles and joints of the lower extremities. The primary function of gait is to allow the body to be propelled through space. There are two phases of gait: the **swing phase** and the **stance phase**.

Through the phases of gait there are five primary joints acting in a variety of ways. The important joints during gait are the pelvis, hip, knee, ankle, and foot. The spine and upper limbs contribute to the gait cycle but are not as important as the lower extremities. The important muscles of gait are the gluteus maximus, gluteus medius, hamstrings, quadriceps, tibialis anterior, gastrocnemius/soleus, extensor digitorum longus and the extensor hallucis longus.

MAJOR PHASES OF GAIT

A gait cycle is the point of initial contact of one extremity and the point that that same extremity hits the ground again. The extremity goes through two phases: the stance phase and the swing phase. The stance phase begins when one extremity makes initial contact with the ground and continues as long as that same extremity remains in contact. The stance phase makes up approximately 60% of the gait cycle. During the swing phase the toe of the extremity leaves the ground and does not end until the heel of that same extremity hits the ground. The gait cycle includes two periods of **double-limb support** and one period of **single-limb support**.

Stance Phase

The stance phase of gait allows the lower leg to support the body and provides the stability so the body can be advanced over the supporting limb. The five stages of stance phase, shown in Figure 16-1 are:
Stages of stance

- **Initial contact** (heel strike)

- **Load response** (foot flat)

- **Midstance** (single leg stance)

- **Terminal stance** (heel off)

- **Preswing** (toe off)

Initial Contact Initial contact is the weight-loading portion of the stance phase. During this stage, one foot (the heel) is just contacting the ground while the other foot is accepting the weight of the body and providing shock absorption. Because both feet are in contact with the ground this is considered the first period of the double-limb stance.

Load Response and Midstance The next two stages of stance are load response and midstance. Load response occurs when the foot is flat on the ground. The midstance stage of gait is considered the single-limb support period. These two stages of gait exist when a single limb is able to accept the full weight of the body is able to balance on that leg. The other important requirements during these two stages are lateral hip stability and the tibia positioned over the fixed foot.

Terminal Stance and Preswing Terminal stance and preswing happen when the foot is preparing to leave the ground and the weight of the body is being transferred onto the other leg. When the weight shifts, the heel comes up off the ground. Preswing happens when the toe pushes off the ground, causing the leg to move forward and creating acceleration. This is where the second period of double-limb support occurs.

The Swing Phase

The swing phase occurs when the foot is not in contact with the ground (Figure 16-2). This phase is responsible for acceleration and deceleration of the gait cycle. There are three stages of the swing phase:

- **Initial Swing**

- **Midswing**

- **Terminal Swing**

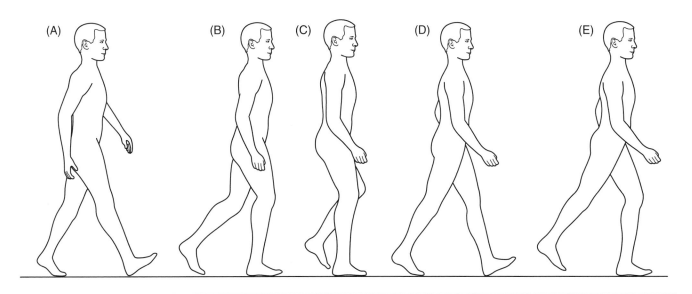

Figure 16-1 *Stance phases of gait (A) Initial Contact, (B) Load Response, (C) Midstance, (D) Terminal Stance, (E) Preswing*

During initial swing, acceleration of the leg occurs because of rapid knee flexion and dorsiflexion of the ankle. Midswing occurs when the swing leg is next to the weight-bearing leg of midstance. During terminal swing, the swing leg starts to slow down to prepare for weight loading. The deceleration occurs during the swing phase through extension of the knee.

OTA Perspective

Gait training is the physical therapist's responsibility as well as the issuing of ambulation aids (e.g., single-point cane, front-wheeled walker). However, functional mobility—what one *does* when ambulating, or the reason for walking—is within the OT domain. OT practitioners need to understand the typical childhood development of motor control, in which walking is the skill level of standing, normal gait patterns, and abnormal gait patterns due to injury or illness. OTs do more than serve as "reinforcers" of proper and safe ambulation during functional mobility tasks. To preserve meaning for the client, occupational performance needs to be addressed in its wholeness, and that includes walking. For example, what good is being able to walk if the client cannot choose when he wants to walk to the mailbox to retrieve a letter from his eldest granddaughter, carry it back to the house, open the front door, and sit at the dining room table where he can enjoy a cup of coffee and read her latest news?

Mobility is crucial not only for adults, but also for nonambulatory children. Typically, mobility devices augment an individual child's form of mobility. A child needs to be able to explore and access the environment, self-direct social experiences, and balance physical development with energy conservation in order to progress through "growth and development" stages.

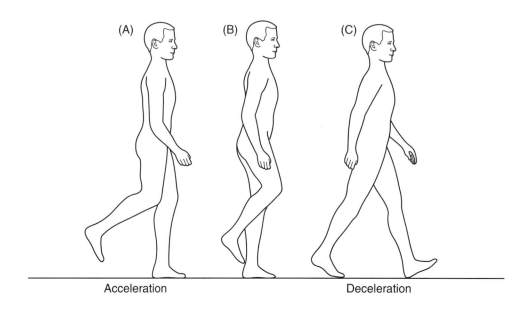

| Acceleration | Deceleration |

Figure 16-2   *Swing phases of gait*

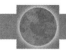 THE ACTION OF JOINTS DURING THE STANCE PHASE

The stance phase of gait is considered the closed chain portion of the gait cycle. Each joint is working to either bear weight or transfer weight. The foot is the fixed segment during the weight-bearing portion of stance. If alterations occur, the foot is the first joint to adapt, followed by the ankle, knee, hip, and pelvis.

Initial Contact

During initial contact (IC), the foot is in slight supination. The ankle is in 90 degrees of dorsiflexion and moving into plantar flexion. The knee is in full extension just before heel contact and begins to move into flexion as the heel hits the ground. The hip is in 20 to 40 degrees of flexion at heel strike and moves into extension. The pelvis is anteriorly rotated.

Load Response

Load response (LR) is defined as the period when the foot becomes flat and is in relative pronation while the ankle is in plantar flexion. The knee is in 20 degrees of flexion, moving into extension. The hip is moving into extension, adduction, and medial rotation. The pelvis continues to be anteriorly rotated.

Midstance

During the midstance (Midst) portion of gait, the foot is neutral and the ankle is in 3 degrees of dorsiflexion. The knee is in 15 degrees of extension, moving into flexion. The hip is in neutral, moving into extension. The pelvis, at this point, is rotating posteriorly.

Terminal Stance

During terminal stance (T St), also known as heel off, the foot moves into supination in order to become rigid. The ankle goes into plantar flexion. The knee is moving from slight flexion into extension. The hip is moving into 10 to 15 degrees of extension, abduction, and lateral rotation.

Preswing

Preswing (PS), or toe off, takes place when the foot is in supination and the ankle is in 20 degrees of plantar flexion. The knee is moving from full extension into about 40 degrees of flexion. The hip is moving into 10 degrees of extension and remains in abduction and lateral rotation.

 ## THE ACTION OF JOINTS DURING THE SWING PHASE

The swing phase is considered to be the open chain portion of the gait cycle. During the swing phase of the gait cycle, the joints are moving through their range of motion to accelerate and decelerate the limbs. The foot is not fixed, and any alterations occur from the spine down through the pelvis, hip, knee, ankle, and foot.

Initial Swing to Midswing

Initial swing to midswing (IS to Midsw) is the acceleration portion of the swing phase. The ankle and foot, through this portion of swing, are in 20 degrees of dorsiflexion and pronation, respectively. The knee is in 30 to 60 degrees of flexion. The hip moves from slight flexion (0 to 15 degrees) to 30 degrees of flexion and from lateral rotation to neutral. The pelvis is in posterior rotation.

Midswing to Terminal Swing

Midswing to terminal swing (Midsw to T Sw) is the deceleration part of the swing phase. The foot is in slight supination and the ankle is in neutral. The knee moves to full extension while the hip is in continued flexion of about 30 to 40 degrees. The pelvis moves into forward rotation. Table 16-1 summarizes the action of the joints during gait.

Table 16-1   *Joint Action during Gait*

	Initial Contact	Load Response	Midstance	Terminal Stance	Preswing	Initial Swing	Midswing	Terminal Swing
Pelvis	Anterior rotation	Anterior rotation	Posterior rotation	Posterior rotation	Anterior rotation	Posterior rotation	Posterior rotation	Anterior rotation
Hip	Flexion	Extension	Neutral to extension	Extension	Full extension	Flexion	Flexion	Flexion
Knee	Extension	Flexion moving into extension	Extension	Flexion moving into extension	Extension moving into full flexion	Flexion	Flexion	Flexion
Ankle	Dorsiflexion moving into plantar flexion	Plantar flexion	Slight dorsiflexion	Plantar flexion	Plantar flexion	Dorsiflexion	Dorsiflexion	Neutral
Foot	Supination	Pronation	Neutral	Supination	Supination	Pronation	Pronation	Supination

MUSCLE ACTION DURING THE STANCE PHASE

Initial Contact

The goal of initial contact is to position the foot and to begin deceleration. The ankle dorsiflexors (tibialis anterior) are contracting eccentrically to fight the force of gravity so the foot will not slap the ground. The knee flexors (hamstrings) start to contract so the knee will be ready to accept the weight. The hip extensors (gluteus maximus) contract to decrease hip flexion so the trunk is not thrown forward as the body moves forward.

Load Response

The load response goal is to accept weight, stabilize the pelvis, and decelerate mass. The ankle plantar flexors (gastrocnemius, soleus) are acting to slow down ankle dorsiflexion. The knee extensors (quadriceps) are firing eccentrically to slow down knee flexion. The gluteus medius is contracting to stabilize the pelvis so there is no lateral drop during load. Lateral drop of the pelvis occurs when the ilium of the stance leg shifts inferiorly relative to the ilium on the nonstance leg. The gluteus maximus and hamstrings are extending the hip to help transfer the weight of the body over the foot.

Midstance

At midstance, the knee is stabilized and momentum is preserved. The gastrocnemius and soleus are contracting (isometrically) to control the amount of dorsiflexion of the ankle over the fixed foot.

Terminal Stance

Acceleration of mass is the primary goal of terminal stance. The important muscles for this portion of gait are the gastrocnemius and soleus. These muscles contract concentrically so that the ankle goes into plantar flexion and allows for push-off from the toe to occur.

Preswing

During preswing, the goal is to prepare for swing. The hip flexors (iliopsoas, rectus femoris) are the primary muscle group that is active to move the hip into flexion for acceleration.

MUSCLE ACTION DURING THE SWING PHASE

Initial Swing

During initial swing (IS), the foot must clear the ground and the hips are moving through flexion, causing acceleration. The ankle dorsiflexors (tibialis anterior) are flexing the ankle. The rectus femoris and the iliopsoas are flexing the hip.

Midswing

Foot clearance is an important aspect of midswing (Midsw). The tibialis anterior is the primary muscle during this stage.

Terminal Swing

During terminal swing (T Sw), the goal is to decelerate the leg, preparing the foot for contact. The quadriceps are contracting concentrically to extend the knee, while the hamstrings are contracting eccentrically to manage deceleration of the knee. The gluteus maximus is contracting eccentrically to slow down hip flexion. Table 16-2 summarizes muscle movement during gait.

Table 16-2 *Muscle Action during Gait*

	Initial Contact	Load Response	Midstance	Terminal Stance	Preswing	Initial Swing	Midswing	Terminal Swing
Pelvis	Iliopsoas	Gluteus medius	Gluteus medius	Gluteus medius	—	—	—	—
Hip	Gluteus maximus	Gluteus maximus	Gluteus maximus	Gluteus maximus	Iliopsoas and rectus femoris	Iliopsoas and rectus femoris	Iliopsoas and rectus femoris	Gluteus maximus
Knee	Hamstrings	Quadriceps	Quadriceps and hamstrings	Quadriceps	Quadriceps	Hamstrings	Hamstrings	Quadriceps
Ankle	Tibialis anterior	Gastrocnemius and soleus	Gastrocnemius and soleus	Gastrocnemius and soleus	Gastrocnemius and soleus	Tibialis anterior	Tibialis anterior	Tibialis anterior

OTA PERSPECTIVE

So often we see patients who are many months down the road from a lower extremity injury or surgery but they still limp. Frequently, this is not related to weakness or lack of ROM or even balance but is purely a habit. They limped following surgery for these reasons and because of pain, but nobody had taken the time to correct the gait pattern. We become focused on the ROM and the strength, but the quicker the patient returns to a normal gait pattern, the quicker the ROM and the strength return.

There are many problems that can arise from the client walking with a chronic limp, such as degeneration of the joints, pain in the spine, and so on. The client may present with back pain but have an old injury that caused the limp, and unless a normal gait pattern is restored, it is difficult to treat the back pain.

 ABNORMAL GAIT

Abnormal gait occurs when any of the preceeding factors is not occurring or functioning appropriately. There can be many abnormal gait patterns caused by many muscular and neurogenic problems. The most common gait abnormalities caused by muscular weakness are **Trendelenberg gait**; **foot drop gait**, and **quadriceps gait**. Trendelenberg and quadriceps gaits occur during the stance phase of gait and foot drop gait can affect the swing phase.

Trendelenberg Gait

During normal gait the hip abductors (gluteus medius and gluteus minimus) are responsible for stabilizing the pelvis during the stance phase. If one or both muscles are weak, the pelvis will drop inferiorly on the swing side during the single-leg stance. The compensation for Trendelenberg is a lateral thrust of the pelvis. For example, if the right gluteus medius and gluteus minimus are weak, the left side of the pelvis will drop down when the right leg is in the stance phase of gait. A lateral thrust of the pelvis to the right will occur.

OTA Perspective

In the acute phase of treatment of a client with a neurological or orthopedic impairment, a (anti) footdrop splint may be indicated. The splint's main function is to maintain a dorsiflexed position necessary for ambulation; the splinting rationales also include preserving normal muscle tone and preventing further injury. The splint holds the foot in a static position perpendicular to the leg. Typically, these splints have some adjustability, are rigid with foam padding and strapping, and are commercially available. Clients tend to wear them until risk of contracture development has been eliminated owing to return of normal muscle tone, or it has been determined that ambulation is not a goal, or another device takes the place of the splint (e.g., ankle foot orthosis [AFO], high-top sneakers).

Footdrop Gait

Dorsiflexion is needed to help clear the toes during swing in order to fight gravity when the foot hits the ground. The tibialis anterior is the primary ankle dorsiflexor. When the tibialis anterior or any of the other dorsiflexors (extensor digitorum longus and extensor hallucis longus) is weak, the toes drag on the ground during midswing. The patient will compensate by trying to lift the knee higher. Also, because the dorsiflexors are weak, the foot cannot fight gravity and, thus, will slap the ground during initial contact.

Quadriceps Gait

The quadriceps need to contract during the stance phase of gait to extend the knee. If the quadriceps are weak and are not able to extend the knee, the compensation will be forward flexion of the trunk with strong plantar flexion of the ankle. This can result in hyperextension or genu recurvatum of the knee during stance.

 KEY CONCEPTS

- The purpose of gait analysis is to observe how the muscles and joints of the lower extremities function together to propel the body through space.
- There are two major phases of gait that must be understood. These include the swing phase, which characterizes the movement of the lower extremities through space during locomotion, and the stance phase, which is characterized by the actions that occur when the foot is on the ground during locomotion.
- The stance phase of gait includes five components: initial contact, load response, midstance, terminal stance, and preswing.
- The swing phase of gait includes three components: initial swing, midswing, and terminal swing.
- There are three abnormal gaits that are generally identified during gait analysis, including Trendelenberg gait, footdrop gait, and quadriceps gait. As a practitioner, it is important to know the characteristics of these different types of gait to understand the abnormalities that may exist between the muscles that contract during locomotion activities.

BIBLIOGRAPHY

Magee, D. J. (2002). *Orthopedic physical assessment* (4th ed.). Philadelphia: W. B. Saunders.

Norkin, C. C., & Levangie, P. K. (2001). *Joint structure and function* (3rd ed.). Philadelphia: F. A. Davis.

The Pathokinesiology Service and the Physical Therapy Department, Rancho Los Amigos Medical Center. (1996). *Observational gait analysis.* Downey, CA: Los Amigos Research and Education Institute, Inc.

 REVIEW QUESTIONS

Fill in the Blank

Provide the word(s) or phrase(s) that best completes the sentence.

1. The two phases of gait are the _____ and _____ phases.

2. _____ is a result of complex interactions of muscles and joints of the lower extremeties.

3. A _____ begins at the point of initial contact of one extremity and when that same extremity hits the ground again.

4. The stance phase makes up approximately _____ percent of the gait cycle.

5. The gait cycle includes two periods of _____ support and one period of _____ support.

6. Foot flat is a characteristic of _____ .

7. Toe off is a characteristic of _____ .

8. Heel off is a characteristic of _____ .

9. Heel strike is a characteristic of _____ .

10. Single leg stance is a characteristic of _____ .

Multiple Choice

Select the best answer to complete the following statements.

1. Abnormal gait can be caused by any of the following *except* _____ .
   a. muscular problems
   b. neurogenic problems
   c. joint weakness
   d. balanced muscle mass

2. A gait that is characterized by a lateral thrust of the pelvis is the _____ .
   a. Trendelenberg gait
   b. footdrop gait
   c. quadriceps gait
   d. normal gait

3. A gait that is characterized by the foot dragging through the midswing is the _____ .
   a. Trendelenberg gait
   b. footdrop gait
   c. quadriceps gait
   d. normal gait

4. A genu recuvatum of the knee is a characteristic of the _____ .
   a. Trendelenberg gait
   b. footdrop gait
   c. quadriceps gait
   d. normal gait

5. Muscles in proper proportions will cause _____ .
   a. Trendelenberg gait
   b. footdrop gait
   c. quadriceps gait
   d. normal gait

Matching

Match each of the following descriptions with the appropriate term.

_____ **1.** Heel off

_____ **2.** Heel strike

_____ **3.** Leg acceleration

_____ **4.** Leg next to load bearing

_____ **5.** Single leg stance

_____ **6.** Closed chain

_____ **7.** Foot flat

_____ **8.** Open chain

_____ **9.** Leg deceleration

_____ **10.** Toe off

A. Initial contact

B. Load response

C. Midstance

D. Terminal stance

E. Preswing

F. Initial swing

G. Midswing

H. Terminal swing

I. Stance phase

J. Swing phase

Critical Thinking

1. Recall what you know about cognition. Refer to Chapter 4 as necessary. Recall that cognitive processes include paying attention to tasks, following verbal and visual directions and cues, topographical orientation, problem solving, and avoiding errors. What other cognitive functions are necessary for walking around the house, the shopping mall, or exploring a newly opened park? For someone with significant cognitive impairments, "walking around" may not be automatic—most of us do not think about each step we take or each stage of the stance phase. If a client has a temporary physical decline (e.g., has become weak due to a hospitalization for pneumonia), should the therapist issue an ambulation device or address muscle strengthening? Recognizing that physical therapists are the ones responsible for gait training and issuing ambulation devices, what if the PT does the opposite of what you think is clinically best? What happens when a client with significant cognitive impairments has an orthopedic injury such as a joint replacement and is to be TTWB or PWB? (Review prior chapters if necessary.) Will that client be able to understand how to use a standard walker, maintain the appropriate weight-bearing status, and ambulate to the dining room? Will that client be safe consistently? What is the primary goal (safety, prevention of further injury)? What are other options for mobility? A joint replacement has a finite expected healing time; what if the new injury is more permanent (e.g., foot amputation)? Discussions such as this can assist with developing clinical reasoning, along with exploring role delineation and professional boundaries and personal and professional ethics.

2. Research the Trendelenberg test. Describe how the test is done and what denotes a positive test. Also describe the cause of a positive test and give five exercises to help correct it.

3. An 80-year-old woman fell and fractured her hip. She underwent surgery and is now in rehabilitation. The rehabilitation team is planning for discharge. As her therapist, describe all the situations that she might encounter at home and how you would make sure that she is able to accomplish them safely. She is ambulating with a walker independently.

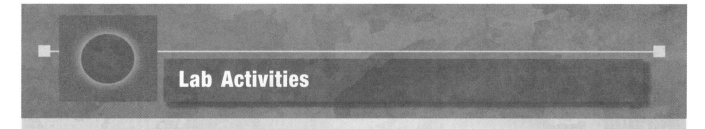

Lab Activities

Lab 16-1: Gait Patterns

Objective: To become familiar with various abnormal gait patterns.

Equipment Needed: An "open space"

Step 1.   Define the following abnormal gait patterns:

Trendelenberg gait

Footdrop gait

Quadriceps gait

Ataxic gait

Festinating gait

Gowers' sign

Step 2.   Choose three of the above gait patterns. Demonstrate the difference between the gait pattern and a normal gait pattern. Demonstrate Gowers' sign.

Lab 16-2: Gait Assessment

Objective: To accurately assess normal gaits at various paces.

Equipment Needed: A treadmill, small group, pen/pencil, paper

Step 1.   In groups of five, using a treadmill, assess each member of the group's gait. Use slow and fast walking and see if there is a difference. Assess either from the feet up or the spine down but look at all joints and stride length, and assess the different phases of the gait cycle.

Lab 16-3: Walking with Assistance

Objective: To properly teach a patient how to walk using assistve devices.

Equipment Needed: A lab partner, various assistive devices, pen/pencil, paper

Step 1.   Teach the following to your partner:

■ Non-weight bearing with crutches

■ Partial (50%) weight bearing with crutches

■ Partial weight bearing with a walker

■ Walking with a cane in one hand

In all the above examples, teach the correct pattern of gait as well as climbing up and down stairs and transfers out of a chair. Also adjust the crutches and the cane for the correct height for your partner.

Part IV
Muscles of the Superior Appendicular Skeleton

Chapters 17-22

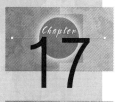

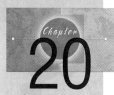

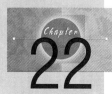

Chapter 17

THE SHOULDER GIRDLE

Key Words

acromioclavicular joint
acromioclavicular ligament
acromion process
conoid ligament
coracoclavicular ligaments
coracoid process
costoclavicular ligament
dorsal scapular nerve
glenoid
glenoid fossa

glenoid labrum
infraspinous fossa
interclavicular ligament
levator scapula
long thoracic nerve
median pectoral nerve
pectoralis minor
rhomboid
scapulohumoral rhythm
serratus anterior

shoulder girdle
spine of the scapula
sternoclavicular joint
sternoclavicular ligaments
subscapular fossa
supraspinous fossa
terminal nerves
trapezius
trapezoid ligament

INTRODUCTION

The structural attachment for the superior appendicular skeleton to the axial skeleton occurs at the **shoulder girdle** where the clavicle attaches to the sternum. There are five muscles located at the shoulder girdle that provide a stable base of support for the scapula as the muscles of the humerus contract through various planes and directions of movement. You may or may not have realized that the scapula and humerus have such an important role in movement. It is important to note that the shoulder girdle muscles attach on the scapula, clavicle, or vertebrae, not the humerus. In addition, shoulder girdle muscles do not provide any direct movements at the shoulder joint but rather complement the actions of the humerus by stabilizing the scapula.

MAJOR LANDMARKS OF THE SHOULDER GIRDLE

The shoulder girdle is located at the junctions between the sternum, clavicle, and scapula. Each bone is important for the stability, structure, and anchor for the muscles that move the shoulder girdle.

Sternum

The sternum can be found by palpating the middle of the chest (Figure 17-1). This bone has three distinct sections: the xiphoid process at the inferior portion; the body, which is a long bony plate found in the middle portion; and the manubrium, the superior portion that provides the attachment site for the clavicle. The sternum is the axial base for superior appendicular skeletal movements and provides a stable base for the contracting shoulder girdle, shoulder joint, and cervical muscles. When observing the sternum, notice that there are 16 individual costal cartilage sections with 16 individual attachments and 6 ribs that share one common cartilage attachment to the manubrium and body of the sternum. The remaining four ribs are false ribs and do not attach to the sternum. The costal cartilage allows for elevation and depression of the chest for respiration. The costae, in conjunction with the sternum and cartilage, provide protection for the vital organs of the circulatory and respiratory systems and the surface area for muscle attachment.

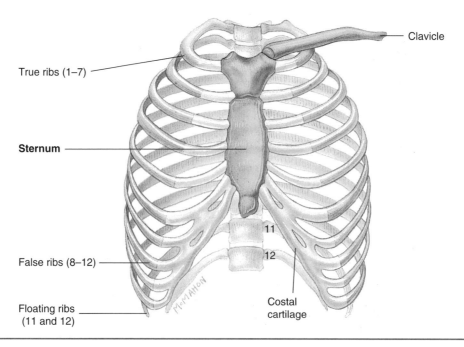

Figure 17-1 *Sternum*

Clavicle

The clavicle bone, which is connected to the sternum via the sternoclavicular ligament, is an S-shaped bone found in the superior shoulder region (Figure 17-2). The clavicle has a medial convex curve, which is distinctly named the sternal end because of its attachment to the sternum. Moving in the lateral direction, you will find the concave acromial end, which attaches to the acromion process of the scapula via the acromioclavicular ligament. Much like the sternum, the clavicle provides increased surface area for muscle attachment and provides further support for the muscles of the shoulder.

Scapula

Continuing in the lateral direction to the posterior superior shoulder is the scapula. This large upside-down triangular-shaped bone can be palpated between the second and seventh costal bones when the upper appendicular skeleton is in a resting position. The scapula is a large plate-like bone that provides a broad surface area for the origins and insertions of the shoulder girdle and shoulder joint muscles. (Figure 17-3)

The first structure on the posterior surface of the scapula is the **spine of the scapula**, which projects in the posterior direction. The spine increases the surface area of the scapula and provides a strong stable base for those muscles that have their attachments there. Moving in the lateral and anterior direction along the spine, observe a knob-like structure that projects from the lateral aspect of the spine. This structure is the **acromion process**.

The three sides of the scapular triangle make up distinct borders that provide significant landmarks, which are also important to the origin and insertion of the shoulder girdle and shoulder joint muscles. These borders are commonly referred to as the lateral (axillary) border, the medial (vertebral) border, and the superior border. Note that two large angles are formed on the medial surface of the scapula, with the lateral angle ending in a large fingerlike projection. The two angles of the scapula are the superior angle, connecting the medial border and superior border, and the inferior angle, which connects the medial border and the lateral border. The large projection on the anterior surface, where the lateral and superior borders meet, ends in the **coracoid process**, which provides additional surface area for shoulder girdle and shoulder joint muscle attachments.

Tracking of the medial border and inferior angle during shoulder girdle movement will become increasingly important as the actions of the muscles of the shoulder girdle are discussed. For example, locate the inferior angle on a partner and have him or her move the arms in a jumping jack motion. Track the inferior angle and note the mobility of the scapula in this movement.

The posterior and anterior surfaces of the scapula contain several deep plateaus that extenuate the surface area of the scapula. On the posterior surface of the scapula, anterior to the crest of the spine, are two large grooves (fossae) found superior and inferior to the spine that are important to muscle attachment. These structures are called the **supraspinous fossa** and the **infraspinous fossa**. Similarly, located on the anterior surface, is one continuous fossa that spans the entire surface of the anterior scapula, and is hence named the **subscapular fossa**. In a normal situation, one should not be able to palpate the subscapular fossa because the anterior surface of the scapula abuts the adjacent costal bones.

The section of the scapula that articulates with the humerus is called the **glenoid fossa**. The **glenoid** cavity is found on the lateral superior scapula and contains the **glenoid labrum**. The labrum is a rim of fibrocartilage that increases the depth of the joint cavity, providing additional support for the head of the humerus. The stability of the glenoid cavity and head of the humerus are discussed further in Chapter 18.

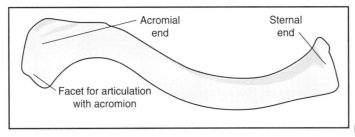

Figure 17-2 Clavicle

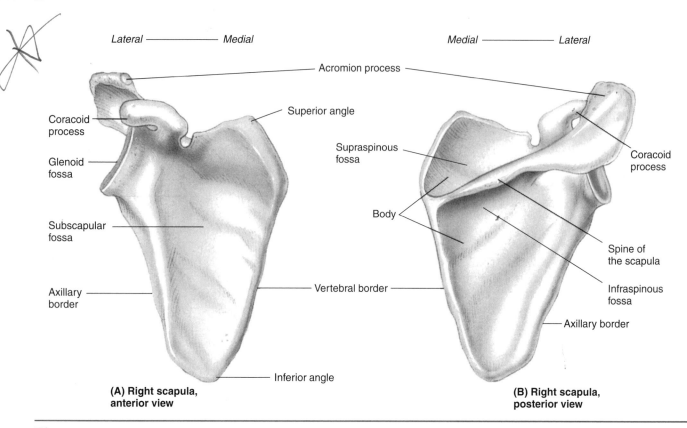

Figure 17-3 *Scapula*

BRACHIAL PLEXUS

Much like the lumbosacral plexus of the inferior appendicular skeleton, the brachial plexus is a group of nerves that stem from the ventral rami (singular, *ramus*) of the cervical nerves C5–T1 (Figure 17-4). However, the brachial plexus is much more complicated because it gives rise to rami, trunks, divisions, cords, and terminal nerves.

Ramus

Each nerve of the brachial plexus originates above its corresponding vertebra until the seventh cervical vertebrae. The eighth cervical nerve originates beneath C7. Moving in the inferior direction from the cervical vertebra C7 location, the nerves are

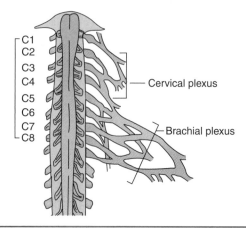

Figure 17-4 *Brachial Plexus*

identified by their origination inferior to the associated nerve. For example, cervical nerve C7 originates superior to the C7 vertebrae, and cervical nerve C8 originates inferior to the C8 vertebrae. Another example of this relationship shows that the T6 nerve originates inferior to the T6 vertebrae and so on.

Trunks

The ventral rami of the brachial plexus come together, forming a plexus in three given locations to provide a series of trunks. The first of these trunks is the superior trunk that forms a plexus by the junction between cervical nerves C5 and C6. A second trunk known as the middle trunk originates from cervical nerve C7. The third trunk is inferior and is, therefore, called the inferior trunk. The inferior trunk is formed from the junction between the cervical nerves C8 and T1 giving rise to a plexus. The most common terminal nerve associated with a trunk origin is the suprascapular nerve.

Divisions

Three nerve divisions are formed from the union between the different trunks in the upper extremity and do not provide terminals for any of the brachial plexus nerves. The plexus between the middle and superior trunk forms an anterior division of the brachial plexus. A second division is provided from the superior, middle, and inferior trunks, giving rise to the posterior division. The third division is formed by a continuation of the inferior trunk.

Cords

Each of the trunks ends in three different cords that provide the pathway for the terminal nerves that innervate the muscles of the arm, elbow, and wrist. From the divisions, the cords run laterally, posteriorly, and medially along the arm, elbow, and wrist.

Terminal Nerves

Eleven **terminal nerves** are identified from their extension from the cords. The most terminal nerves can be identified extending from the posterior cord. These nerves include the thoracodorsal, radial, and axillary nerves and two branches of the subscapular. Of these nerves, the axillary nerve branches from the radial nerve at the most lateral point on the second rib. The lateral cord provides two individual nerves, the lateral pectoral and musculocutaneous, and branches to form a junction, with the medial cord giving rise to the median nerve. The medial cord provides a pathway for the remaining three terminal nerves. These nerves include the medial pectoral, ulnar, and the union, with the lateral cord providing the median nerve. Note that a full discussion of the location of these nerves described in this section are provided as each region of the superior appendicular skeleton is discussed.

 ## NERVOUS INNERVATION

Four individual nerves innervate the muscles of the shoulder girdle: the accessory, dorsal scapular, median pectoral, and long thoracic nerves. Of these nerves, the accessory and dorsal scapular nerves innervate muscles located on the posterior surface, and the median pectoral and long thoracic nerves innervate muscles on the anterior surface of the back. Each nerve that innervates the shoulder girdle originates from the brachial plexus except the accessory nerve, which is one of three cranial nerves that provides innervation for the muscles in the human body.

Accessory Nerve

The accessory nerve is the 11th cranial nerve and originates at the inferior surface of the brain (Figure 17-5). The nerve tracks from an anterior to posterior direction, following the curve of the spine. The accessory nerve can be found deep to the digastric muscle and posterior to the sternocleidomastoid. As the nerve continues posteriorly, it runs deep to the trapezius muscle. Owing to its location, the accessory nerve innervates two muscles, the sternocleidomastoid and trapezius muscles of the shoulder girdle.

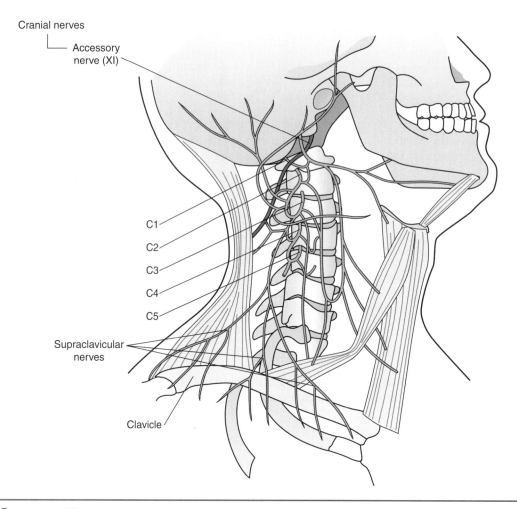

Figure 17-5 *Accessory Nerve*

Dorsal Scapular Nerve

The second nerve that innervates the posterior muscles of the shoulder girdle is the **dorsal scapular nerve** (Figure 17-6). The dorsal scapular nerve originates at the ventral ramus of C5 and tracks posteriorly through the scalene muscle group. From here, the nerve runs deep to the levator scapula muscle, following from the midpoint to its insertion on the superior angle of the scapula. Owing to the deep location of the dorsal scapular nerve, it innervates the rhomboids and levator scapula muscles of the shoulder girdle.

Median Pectoral Nerve

The **median pectoral nerve** has its origins on the medial cord of the brachial plexus, which branches from the ventral ramus of C8–T1 (see Figure 17-6). Tracking of the medial cord reveals that it continues down the forearm and terminates in the ulnar nerve and has a union with the lateral cord, forming the median nerve. These nerves are further discussed in later chapters.

The proximal section of the medial cord follows the axillary artery and can be found deep to the subclavian vein. Inferior to the first rib, the medial cord branches, giving rise to the median pectoral nerve. From the branch, the median nerve is found deep to the pectoralis minor muscle, which it innervates.

Long Thoracic Nerve

The last nerve of the shoulder girdle is the **long thoracic nerve** (see Figure 17-6). The nerve branches from the ventral rami of C5–C7. Much like the median pectoral nerve, the long thoracic nerve tracks inferiorly to the axillary artery and is deep to

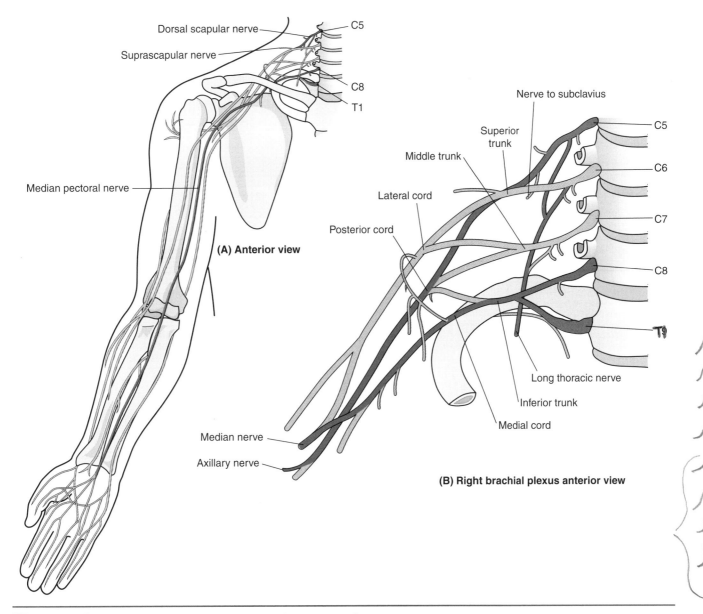

Figure 17-6 *Dorsal Scapular Nerve, Median Pectoral Nerve, Long Thoracic Nerve*

the subclavian vein. At the level of the first rib, the nerve tracks inferiorly to the pectoralis minor muscle. The nerve continues in the inferior direction and innervates the serratus anterior muscle. Table 17-1 summarizes the nerves in the shoulder girdle.

Table 17-1 *Nerves of the Shoulder Girdle*

Nerve	Affected Anterior Muscles	Affected Posterior Muscles
Accessory	None	Trapezius
Dorsal Scapular	None	Levator scapula Rhomboids
Long Thoracic	Serratus anterior	None
Median Pectoral	Pectoralis minor	None

MOVEMENT OF THE SHOULDER GIRDLE

Movement of the shoulder girdle only occurs around the sternoclavicular joint (SC joint). The SC joint allows for movements occurring mainly in the frontal and transverse planes with limited movement in the sagittal plane. When analyzing the movements of the shoulder girdle, track the motion of both the inferior angle and the medial border when deciding what movement is occurring. Palpation is an ideal way to learn the shoulder girdle movements. Furthermore, observe the motion of the scapula as it glides over the costal bones. Table 17-2 summarizes the movements that take place in the shoulder girdle.

Table 17-2   *Shoulder Girdle Movements*

Movement	Axis	Plane	Description
Protraction (Abduction)	Vertical	Transverse	Movement of the scapula away from the midline of the body
Retraction (Adduction)	Vertical	Transverse	Movement of the scapula toward the midline of the body
Upward Rotation	Sagittal	Frontal	Movement of the inferior angle in a lateral and superior direction
Downward Rotation	Sagittal	Frontal	Movement of the inferior angle in a medial and inferior direction
Elevation	Sagittal	Frontal	Movement of the scapula in the cranial or superior direction
Depression	Sagittal	Frontal	Movement of the scapula in a caudal or inferior direction
Scapular Tilt	Frontal	Sagittal	Movement of the inferior angle in the posterior direction

STABILITY OF THE SHOULDER GIRDLE

Stability at the shoulder girdle is paramount to the movements that occur elsewhere in the upper appendicular skeleton. Therefore, several ligaments can be found in the shoulder girdle that limit the amount of movement at the joint and stabilize the shoulder when the arm moves through a full range of motion.

Sternoclavicular Joint

The **sternoclavicular** (SC) **joint** is a triaxial diarthrodial joint found where the clavicle meets the sternum. Three ligaments can be found spanning the SC joint that stabilize, reinforce, and support the joint capsule. The three ligaments of the shoulder joint include the interclavicular, costoclavicular, and acromioclavicular.

Interclavicular Ligament

The **interclavicular ligament** connects the superior surface of the manubrium to the superior surface of the sternal end of the clavicles. This ligament limits the amount of depression, allowing for approximately 5 degrees of depression at the SC joint. A second pair of **sternoclavicular ligaments** provides anterior and posterior support for the SC joint. The anterior sternoclavicular ligament connects the anterolateral surface of the manubrium to the anterior surface of the sternal end of the clavicle. The anterior position of the anterior sternoclavicular ligament limits retraction movement of the scapula and allows 15 degrees of motion for the SC joint. Found immediately posterior to the SC joint is the posterior sternoclavicular ligament. This ligament spans the posterior surface of the SC joint, connecting the posterolateral manubrium to the posterior sternal end of the clavicle. The posterior position of the posterior sternoclavicular ligament allows for 15 degrees of protraction movement.

Costoclavicular Ligament

An accessory ligament, the **costoclavicular ligament**, supports the SC joint laterally to the joint capsule. The costoclavicular ligament connects the superior medial surface of the first costal bone to the inferior medial surface of the sternal end of

OTA Perspective

Both OT and PT test ROM via goniometry measurements, and muscle strength via the Manual Muscle Test (MMT). Both assessments are standardized, common evaluation tools used with clients with orthopedic or neurological diagnoses, or both, and with clients of all ages. Most facilities have created their own forms for documenting results. Once "service competency" has been assessed, OTAs and PTAs use goniometers and MMT to measure ROM and muscle strength, contributing to the evaluation and treatment plan.

Because these assessment tools measure physical capacities, they fall within the models of practice that treat impairments or deficits and restore function. When treating a client within those practice frameworks, it is imperative that the OTA and PTA understand a client's current physical limitations, along with goals and expectations, given the body's "normal functioning ability" and consequences of the medical diagnoses. Another reason why a study of kinesiology is important is that knowing what the body is capable of in terms of movement sets a foundation for designing a realistic client-centered OT or PT treatment plan.

the clavicle. Because of the movement demands of the shoulder joint for elevation, the ligament allows for 45 degrees of elevation movement. Although the costoclavicular ligament does not cross the SC joint, it provides a strong amount of stability for the SC joint.

Acromioclavicular Joint

The second joint of the shoulder girdle is found at the junction between the acromial end of the clavicle and the acromion process and is, hence, called the **acromioclavicular joint** (AC joint) (Figure 17-7). Motion at the AC joint is limited, allowing for small amounts of gliding and rotation during shoulder girdle movement.

OTA Perspective

As discussed in this chapter, upward rotation of the scapula describes the movement of the inferior angle of the scapula in a lateral and superior direction. This can also be described as the glenoid fossa facing anteriorly, laterally, and *superiorly*. Conversely, downward rotation of the scapula describes the movement of the inferior angle in a medial and inferior direction. This can be described as the glenoid fossa facing anteriorly, laterally, and *inferiorly*.

A downwardly rotated scapula decreases the subacromial space overlying the glenohumeral joint and predisposes the patient to an impingement syndrome and possible rotator cuff tear. Optimum positioning of the scapula is in an upwardly rotated position to minimize shoulder joint pathology.

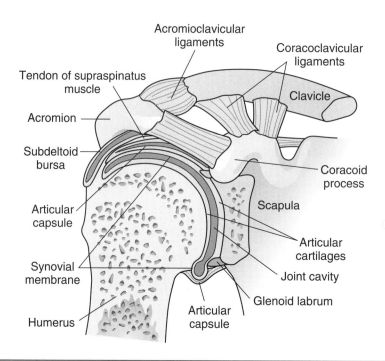

Figure 17-7 *The Acromioclavicular (AC) Joint and Associated Ligaments*

Three ligaments are found at the AC joint that limit the movement of the clavicle away from the acromion process and support the AC joint. The first of these ligaments is the **acromioclavicular ligament**, which holds the AC joint together. The acromioclavicular ligament spans the superior and inferior surfaces of the joint and prevents posterior movement of the clavicle. Quite often, the anatomical position of this ligament and extraneous stretching are the main cause of shoulder injuries around this joint. The **coracoclavicular ligaments**, **trapezoid ligament** and **conoid ligament**, are the two remaining AC joint ligaments that make up the AC joint. They are both known as accessory ligaments because neither connects the clavicle to the acromion process. However, both ligaments originate from the superior surface of the coracoid process and attach to the inferior surface of the acromial end of the clavicle. The purpose of the coracoclavicular ligaments is to stabilize the clavicle by preventing superior movement of the clavicle away from the scapula, thus limiting rotation.

 ## RELATED MOVEMENTS OF THE SHOULDER GIRDLE AND SHOULDER JOINT

The shoulder girdle consists of five muscles that cause movement around the SC joint. The stability that these muscles provide is based on the axial origin on the vertebral processes, occipital protuberance, nuchal ligament, costae, and the appendicular insertion on the scapular and clavicular landmarks. This arrangement allows the shoulder girdle muscles to stabilize the scapula as the humerus moves through a full range of motion around the shoulder joint; this is known as **scapulohumoral rhythm**. Hence, as the muscles of the shoulder joint contract, the shoulder girdle muscles also contract to extenuate the movement of the shoulder joint. Table 17-3 identifies the movements that occur around the shoulder joint and the ensuing movements that occur at the shoulder girdle. Reference Table 17-3 after reading Chapter 18 because the shoulder joint motions are discussed in that chapter in greater detail.

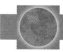 ## MUSCLES OF THE SHOULDER GIRDLE

The shoulder girdle consists of five muscles, some with multiple parts that cause many movements of the scapula around the SC joint. The shoulder girdle has two primary functions in human movement. These functions include stabilizing the shoulder girdle during static contractions and providing a strong base of support for shoulder joint movements. The stability pro-

Table 17-3 Relationship between Shoulder Joint Movements and the Shoulder Girdle Movements

Shoulder Joint Movement	Shoulder Girdle Movement
Sagittal Plane Movements at the Shoulder Joint:	
Flexion at the shoulder joint	Elevation, upward rotation, and protraction
Extension at the shoulder joint	Depression, downward rotation, and retraction
Hyperextension at the shoulder joint	Scapular tilt and downward rotation of the scapula
Frontal Plane Movements:	
Abduction at the shoulder joint	No movement until approximately 90 degrees then upward rotation and elevation of the scapula
Adduction at the shoulder joint	Downward rotation and depression of the scapula and no movement as the shoulder passes 90 degrees
Transverse Plane Movements:	
Horizontal adduction at the shoulder joint	Protraction of the scapula
Horizontal abduction at the shoulder joint	Retraction of the scapula
Internal rotation at the shoulder joint	Protraction of the scapula
External rotation at the shoulder joint	Retraction of the scapula
Nonplane Movements:	
Circumduction at the shoulder joint	Protraction and retraction of the scapula with abduction and adduction; elevation and depression and upward rotation and downward rotation of the scapula with flexion and extension

vided by these muscles is by a posterior or lateral axial skeleton origin, such as the costae, spine, or skull, and insertion into one of the landmarks on the scapula or clavicle. The muscles of the shoulder girdle are divided into anterior and posterior muscles. The anterior muscles are the **pectoralis minor** and **serratus anterior**. The posterior muscles include the **trapezius** (upper, middle, lower), **rhomboids** (major and minor), and **levator scapula**.

OTA Perspective

Tightness in the shoulder girdle—scapular immobility—affects the normal mobility or movement of the scapula and, therefore, normal shoulder movements (e.g., shoulder elevation). The scapula must be mobile before expecting U/E movements. Without the scapula "gliding" along with the U/E movement, joint trauma, muscle tearing, and pain may occur. Simplistically, scapular mobility is a treatment technique the therapist uses to passively move the client's muscle or muscle group through "normal" movements. With a client sitting in an upright position, and the therapist at his or her side, the therapist places both hands on the posterior and anterior aspects of the shoulder girdle, and then gently guides the muscle group through ROM (e.g., scapular protraction and retraction). This neurodevelopmental handling technique is commonly used when treating a client with a hemiplegic shoulder. The OTA or PTA student is encouraged to research neurodevelopmental theory and treatment techniques and relate them to the study of kinesiology.

Anterior Muscles of the Shoulder Girdle

The anterior muscles of the shoulder girdle provide elevation and protraction movements of the scapula when they contract. These muscles often work as antagonists to the posterior muscles of the region by limiting excessive retraction movements. The anterior muscles of the shoulder girdle include the pectoralis minor and serratus anterior.

Pectoralis Minor   The pectoralis minor is a triangle-shaped muscle located deep to the pectoralis major and deltoid muscle groups of the shoulder joint (Figure 17-8). The anterior position of the pectoralis minor with its insertion on the coracoid process of the scapula helps to provide anterior support for the shoulder girdle. During human movement, the pectoralis minor aids with depression, downward rotation, and protraction movements. Owing to the deep location of the pectoralis minor muscle, it is almost impossible to palpate accurately.

Name:	Pectoralis Minor
O:	Anterior and lateral position on ribs 3–5
I:	Coracoid process
A:	Depression, downward rotation, protraction, and scapular tilt
N:	Median pectoral nerve
P:	Deep to the pectoralis major

Serratus Anterior   The true multipennate muscle of the shoulder girdle is the serratus anterior muscle (Figure 17-9). The serratus anterior has its origin on the anterolateral surface of ribs 1–8 and spans to the anterior surface of the scapula, where it inserts to the vertebral border. When identifying this muscle, realize that the posterior portion is located deep to the scapula, which is truly the anterior surface of the scapula. Therefore, to palpate the majority of the posterior surface of the muscle is impossible. The role of the serratus anterior during human movement is to stabilize the shoulder girdle by limiting medial movements of the joint. The position of the serratus anterior makes it a strong antagonist to the rhomboid muscle.

To palpate the serratus anterior, abduct the humerus from the axilla. Move your fingers down the midaxillary line and locate the inferior jagged edges of the muscle on the anterior and lateral surfaces of the ribs. From this location palpate around the muscle and track the muscle in the posterior direction.

Name:	Serratus Anterior
O:	Anterior and lateral on ribs 2–8
I:	Medial border of the scapula
A:	Protraction and upward rotation
N:	Long thoracic nerve
P:	Anterolateral side of the thorax below ribs 5–6

Posterior Muscles of the Shoulder Girdle

The posterior muscles of the shoulder girdle provide elevation, depression, retraction, upward rotation, and downward rotation movements of the scapula when they contract. These muscles often work as antagonists to the anterior muscles of the region by limiting excessive protraction movements. The posterior muscles of the shoulder girdle include the trapezius, levator scapula, and rhomboid.

Trapezius   The trapezius muscle is the large diamond-shaped muscle located in the posterosuperior region of the shoulder girdle and posterior neck (Figure 17-10). On further study, understand that the muscle can be broken into three triangular regions: the upper, middle, and lower trapezius. The roles of the trapezius muscles depend on the direction of their fibers. For example, the fibers of the upper trapezius originate on the occipital protuberance and nuchal ligament and track diagonally to the insertion located on the acromion process of the scapula. The direction that these fibers run dictates that elevation and retraction movements occur when the trapezius muscle contracts.

The superior location of the trapezius muscle makes it simple to palpate. To palpate the muscle, locate the lateral segments of the cervical vertebrae through the thoracic vertebrae. Remember that the upper trapezius mainly occupies the space located in the cervical region. The other two sections are a little more difficult to separate from each other. The middle trapezius is mainly located medially to the spine of the scapula. When palpating these fibers, realize that the function of the trapezius is to stabilize the shoulder on the medial side of the scapula and limit the amounts of protraction movements of the scapula. Palpating efforts of the lower trapezius should begin with the hands at approximately T-4 and T-12, moving laterally toward the axillary border. When you palpate the trapezius, observe both sides of the muscle and look for equal muscle size.

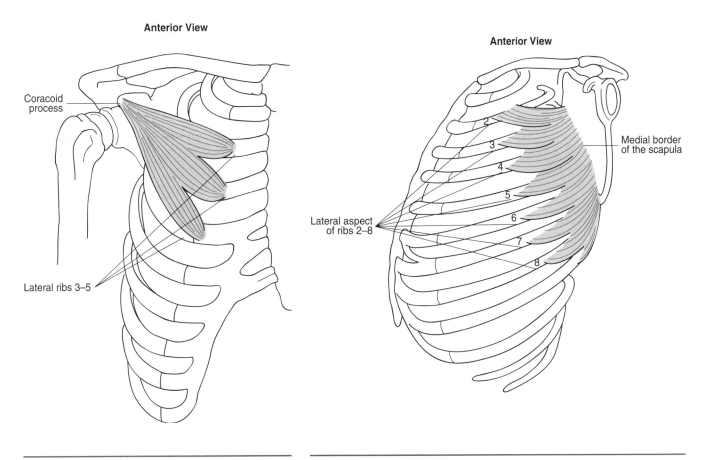

Figure 17-8 *Pectoralis Minor*

Figure 17-9 *Serratus Anterior*

Name: Upper Trapezius

O: Occipital protuberance and superior nuchal line (ligamentum nuchae) of the occipital bone

I: Acromion process of the scapula and lateral scapula

A: Elevation

N: Accessory nerve

P: Posterior side of the body from the base of the skull to the acromion process

Name: Middle Trapezius

O: Spinous processes of C7–T3

I: Acromion process of the scapula

A: Retraction

N: Accessory nerve

P: Posterior side of the body running across the thorax from scapula to scapula

Name: Lower Trapezius

O: Spinous processes of T4–T12

I: Superior position on the spine of the scapula

A: Depression

N: Accessory nerve

P: From the vertebral border of the scapula medially and inferiorly to 12th thoracic spine

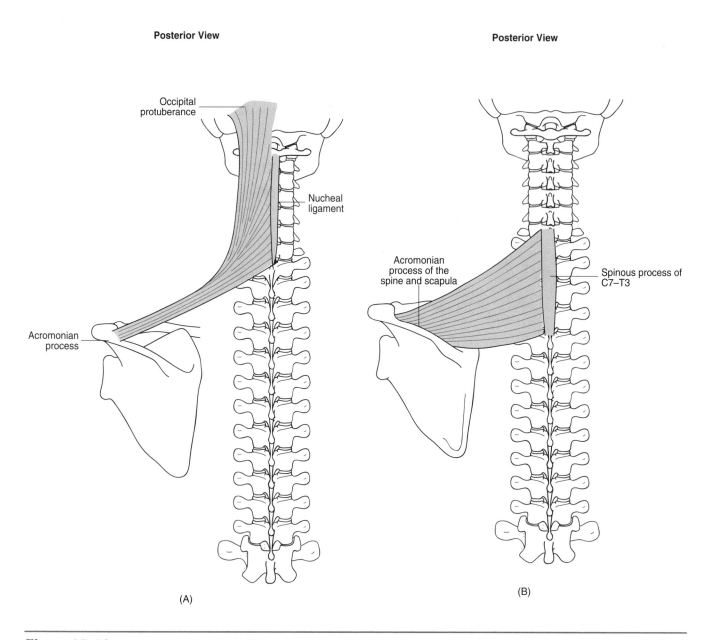

Posterior View

Posterior View

Occipital protuberance

Nucheal ligament

Acromonian process of the spine and scapula

Spinous process of C7–T3

Acromonian process

(A)

(B)

Figure 17-10 *Trapezius: (A) Upper; (B) Middle*

Levator Scapula

As the term *levator* indicates, the levator scapula muscle elevates the scapula (Figure 17-11). The muscle is located superior to the superior angle of the scapula. When the muscle contracts, the scapula elevates. On muscle identification of the levator scapula it is revealed to be a strap muscle located deep to the upper trapezius in the cervical region. Owing to this location, the levator scapula is difficult to palpate.

     Name: Levator Scapula

     O: Transverse processes of C1–C4

     I: Superior angle of the scapula

     A: Elevation

     N: Dorsal scapular nerve

     P: Cannot be palpated

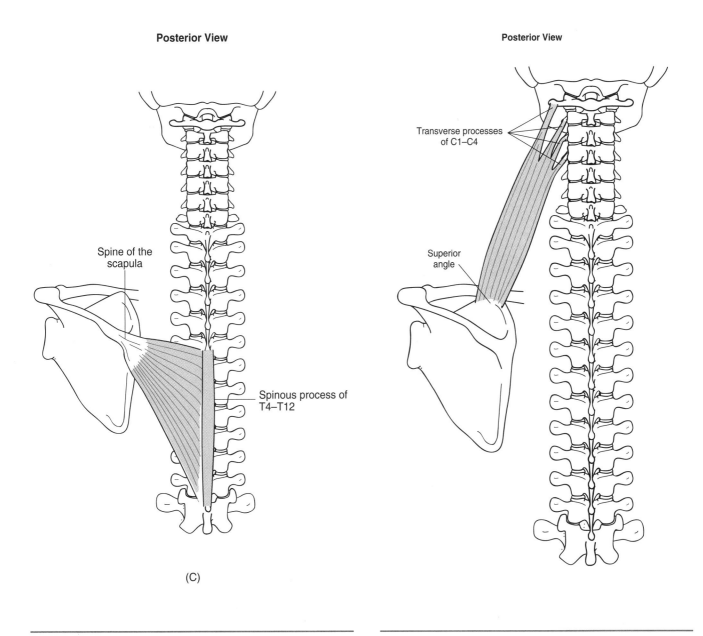

Posterior View

Spine of the
scapula

Spinous process of
T4–T12

(C)

Posterior View

Transverse processes
of C1–C4

Superior
angle

Figure 17-10 *Trapezius: (C) Lower Regions*

Figure 17-11 *Levator Scapula*

Rhomboids

The rhomboid muscle group is classified as rhomboid owing to its broad origin, which spans the distance from C7–T5, and an insertion, which covers the vertebral border of the scapula (Figure 17-12). The rhomboid muscle is broken into two components: the rhomboids major, which is the broader band located inferior to the thin and superiorly located rhomboids minor. During exercise movements that occur around the shoulder region, the rhomboid muscles stabilize the scapula against lateral movements of the shoulder girdle. When identifying this muscle group, realize that the rhomboid muscles are located deep to the trapezius muscles, which makes observing the body of the muscle difficult.

The rhomboid muscles can be difficult to palpate owing to the deep position of the muscle group. When you palpate the rhomboids, have an individual bring his or her arm to the posterior and then move the elbow joint into flexion. Then, with one hand on the arm and the other palpating medially to the vertebral border, have the individual resist against you with the arm. When palpating the muscle, begin on the medial border between the superior and inferior angles, moving diagonally in the direction toward the vertebrae, and note both sides.

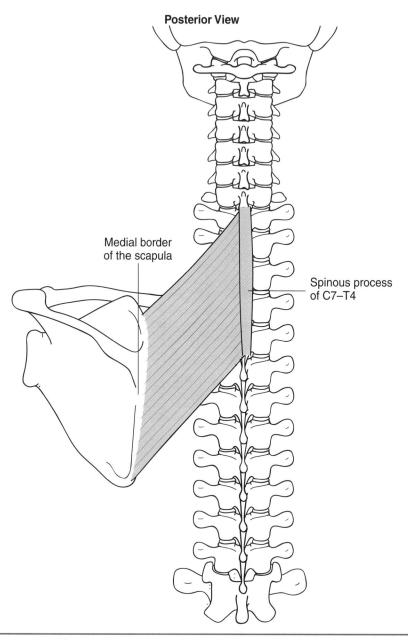

Posterior View

Medial border
of the scapula

Spinous process
of C7–T4

Figure 17-12   *Rhomboids*

Name:	Rhomboid Major
O:	Spinous processes of C7–T4
I:	Medial border of the scapula
A:	Retraction
N:	Dorsal scapular nerve
P:	Cannot be palpated
Name:	Rhomboid Minor
O:	Spinous process of C7
I:	Medial border of the scapula at the spine of the scapula
A:	Retraction
N:	Dorsal scapular nerve
P:	Cannot be palpated

KEY CONCEPTS

■ The major bones that provide surface area for the muscles of the shoulder girdle include the scapula, clavicle, and sternum. The scapula provides the largest surface area for muscles to attach to.

■ The ligaments of the shoulder girdle provide strong support for stabilizing the superior appendicular schedule through numerous joint movements. The major ligaments of the shoulder girdle include the sternoclavicular, costoclavicular, and acromioclavicular ligaments.

■ The major movements of the shoulder girdle can be tracked by observing the scapula during various movements. Included in these movements are stabilization, upward/downward rotation, protraction/retraction, and elevation/depression.

■ The nerves that innervate the muscles of the shoulder girdle have roots from both the cranial nerves and brachial plexus. These include the median pectoral, long thoracic, accessory, and dorsal scapular nerves.

BIBLIOGRAPHY

Hoppenfeld, S. (1976). *Physical examination of the spine and extremities*. London: Prentice Hall International.

Thompson, C. W., & Floyd, R. T. (2001). *Manual of structural kinesiology* (14th ed.). St. Louis, MO: Mosby

REVIEW QUESTIONS

Fill in the Blank

Provide the word(s) or phrase(s) that best completes the sentence.

1. The movement that occurs when the scapula moves in the lateral direction is called _____.

2. The muscle that moves the scapula in the superior direction has the name _____ _____.

3. A muscle that provides anterior support and has its insertion on the coracoid process of the scapula is called the _____ _____ .

4. A muscle of the shoulder girdle that has three heads is named the _____ _____.

5. The _____ of the muscle fibers in the different trapezius regions dictates the movement that occurs in a given area.

Multiple Choice

Select the best answer to complete the following statements.

1. The Rhomboid muscle group is classified as a _____ muscle group.
   a. multipennate
   b. strap
   c. unipennate
   d. rhomboid

2. The serratus anterior is classified as a _____ muscle because of the numerous heads that insert into one common tendon.
   a. multipennate
   b. strap
   c. unipennate
   d. rhomboid

3. A muscle that originates on the anterolateral surface of the chest and inserts on the anterior surface of the vertebral border is named the _____ muscle.
   a. upper trapezius
   b. levator scapula
   c. serratus anterior
   d. rhomboid

4. The _____ and _____ muscles provide elevation movements of the scapula.
   a. upper trapezius
   b. levator scapula
   c. serratus anterior
   d. rhomboid

5. The _____ muscle provides retraction of the scapula during human movement.
   a. upper trapezius
   b. levator scapula
   c. serratus anterior
   d. rhomboid

Matching

Match each of the following decriptions with the appropriate term.

_____ **1.** Medial edge of the scapula

_____ **2.** Angle that sits on the top of the scapula

_____ **3.** Deep groove under the scapular spine

_____ **4.** Deep groove above the scapular spine

_____ **5.** Deep groove on the anterior scapula

_____ **6.** Finger-like projection of the scapula

_____ **7.** Articulates with the clavicle, forming the AC joint

_____ **8.** Muscle with an insertion on the coracoid process

_____ **9.** Muscle with an origin on the nuchal ligament

_____ **10.** Muscle with an insertion on the superior angle of the scapula

A. Infraspinous fossa

B. Coracoid process

C. Acromion process

D. Subscapular fossa

E. Superior angle

F. Levator scapula

G. Upper trapezius

H. Supraspinous fossa

I. Medial border

J. Pectoralis minor

Critical Thinking

1. Imagine a person making a jump shot in basketball. Describe what is happening to the scapula (motions) from setup to release. Next list each muscle that is providing force to cause these motions (force coupling).

2. Describe how you would strengthen each of the muscles involved in number 1 above.

3. Define the term *idiopathic*. Plan a progressive strengthening program for a patient who is recovering from a long thoracic nerve palsy. Describe the care in the early stages as well as three exercises for the recovering muscle.

4. Draw a picture of the scapula in the space below. On the drawing, include the following landmarks:

   ■ Medial border

   ■ Lateral border

   ■ Superior border

   ■ Inferior Angle

   ■ Superior border

   ■ Spine of the scapula

   ■ Acromion process

   ■ Coracoid process

   ■ Infraspinous fossa

   ■ Supraspinous fossa

(continues)

Critical Thinking *(continued)*

5. Draw the following muscles of the shoulder girdle in the figures provided on the following pages:

   ■ Pectoralis minor

   ■ Serratus anterior

   ■ Levator scapula

   ■ Trapezius

   ■ Rhomboids

6. On the drawings from number 5 above, label the origin, insertion, action, and innervation for each of the above muscles.

7. If physical therapists and PTAs and occupational therapists and OTAs assess ROM and strength, within their respective scopes of practice, is this a redundant service? A duplicating of skilled services? How should documentation reflect the skilled service? This is an example of the importance of communication with team members. What happens when it is not clear which discipline is responsible for what tasks? Each facility is likely to have a protocol for identifying who does what (specifically regarding assessment responsibility). If there is not one, is it apparent why that might be necessary? Or do protocols like that place a limit on the practitioner's skills? Discuss situations in which use of these assessment tools would be and would not be another opportunity to acquire aspects of clinical reasoning.

8. Comprehending clear directions, and being able to follow those directions, is necessary on the client's part for the therapist to be able to accurately measure ROM and strength. Discuss measuring scapular mobility in an infant or small child. Brainstorm methods for assessing movements, including developmental aspects to consider. An example of assessing scapular abduction might be (1) in the supine position, reaching for a toy, (2) in the prone position, propped on the elbows (which is also assessing strength), and (3) "wheelbarrow walk." Considerations to rule out may include (1) visual field deficit or disinterest in the toy, (2) head and neck strength limitation, and (3) decreased forearm strength. A guided discussion such as this one may contribute to a development of clinical reasoning.

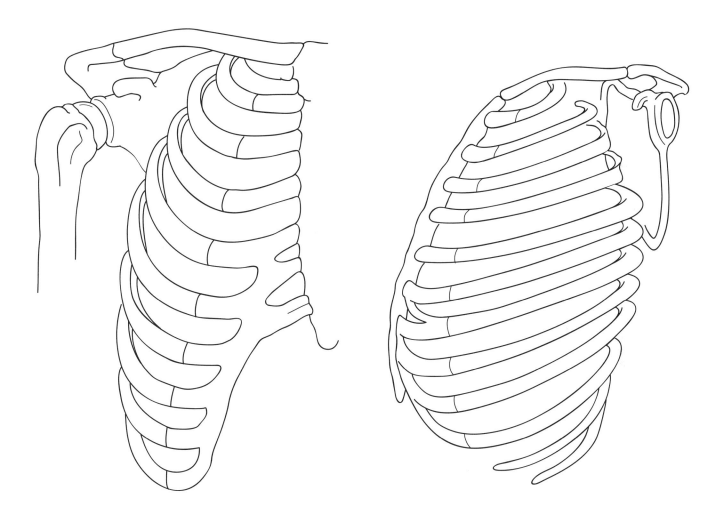

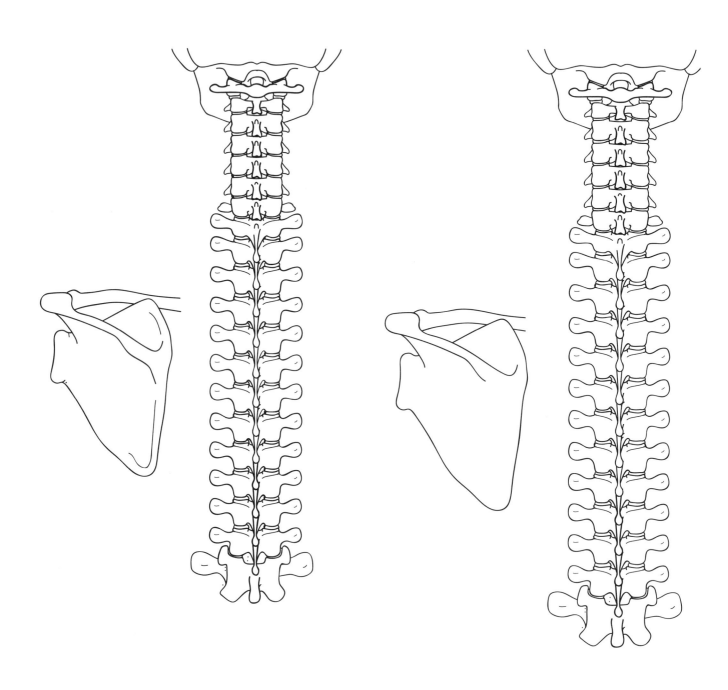

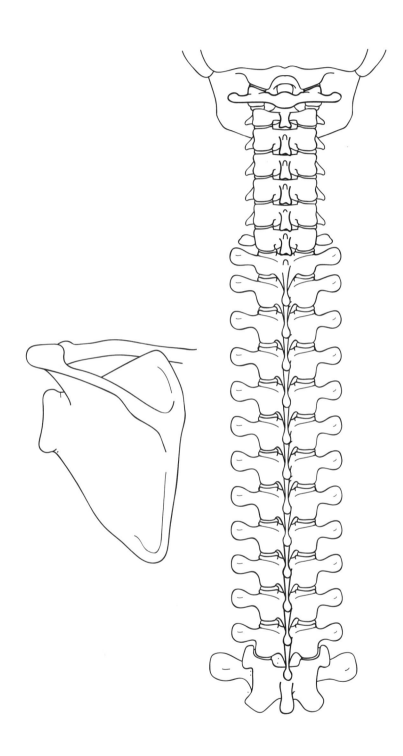

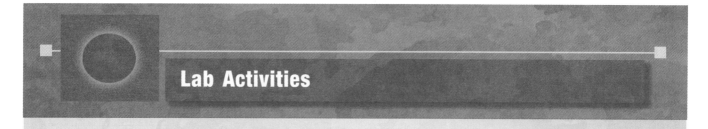

Lab Activities

Lab 17-1: Definitions Lab

Objective: To define several commonly used terms and concepts.

Equipment Needed: Medical dictionary, resource books on MMT and goniometry, pen and paper

Step 1.   Define the following terms and concepts:
Service competency
Evaluation vs. assessment
Scapular "winging"
Substitution movements; how to identify; how to eliminate

Lab 17-2: Shoulder Girdle Movement Identification

Objective: To visualize and palpate shoulder girdle movements. (If you are familiar with MMT and ROM measuring using the goniometer, use those assessment tools to measure shoulder girdle movement and strength.)

Equipment Needed: A lab partner, Tables 17-2 and 17-3, appropriate dress (e.g., sleeveless t-shirt), a goniometer, paper and pen for documenting findings, and resource manuals as necessary for directions on MMT and goniometry measurements

Step 1.   Visualize and palpate shoulder girdle movements according to Table 17-2. Use clear directions when giving movement commands to your partner. Do you feel the identified bones, joints, and muscles of the shoulder girdle?

Step 2.   Measure the ROM and strength of the shoulder girdle muscles. Document and compare to norms.

Lab 17-3: Assessment of Scapular Movement

Objective: To properly assess and evaluate movement of the scapula.

Equipment Needed: A lab partner, pen/pencil, paper

Step 1.   Assess your partner's static scapula positioning. Check for winging, a protracted or retracted position of the scapula compared to the other side, and the upward vs. downward rotation position.

Step 2.   Assess your partner's scapulohumeral rhythm. Good visibility of the scapula is essential, so dress appropriately.

Step 3.   Stand behind your partner and monitor motions of the scapula in both shoulder flexion and shoulder abduction. No motion of the inferior angle of the scapula should occur until 90 degrees of flexion. No motion of the inferior angle should occur until 60 degrees of abduction.

Step 4.   Observe the eccentric control also as your partner returns his or her arm to neutral.

Step 5.   List the muscles that perform upward rotation of the scapula.

Step 6.   List the muscles that perform downward rotation of the scapula.

Step 7.   Describe two exercises for each muscle that performs upward rotation. Teach these exercises to your partner.

Step 8.   The levator scapulae and the pectoralis minor muscles are downward rotators of the scapula and frequently need to be stretched, not strengthened. Teach your partner a stretch for these muscles and include instructions regarding the length to hold the stretch and the number of repetitions.

Chapter 18

THE SHOULDER JOINT

Key Words

capitulum	glenohumeral ligament	supraspinatus
coracoacromial ligament	infraspinatus	teres major
coracobrachialis	intertubercular groove	teres minor
coracohumeral ligament	latissimus dorsi	trochlea
deltoid	pectoralis major	
deltoid tuberosity	subscapularis	

INTRODUCTION

Imagine the freedom and multitude of movements that the upper extremity allows us. Humans can reach up in the cabinet to retrieve a dish, hold a child in our arms, and even throw a baseball at more than 90 miles per hour, to name a few. The shoulder joint, or glenohumeral joint, provides the space for articulation between the head of the humerus and the glenoid fossa of the scapula. The shoulder joint provides a large range of motion and, therefore, a variety of hand placements. As stated in Chapter 17, the humerus and scapula articulate with one another in a smooth fashion, causing smooth movements of the scapula. For instance, as the arm is abducted greater than 90 degrees the scapula rotates in an upward direction. When the arm returns from an abducted position (adduction) the scapula rotates downward.

Owing to the triaxial arrangement, the shoulder joint produces a large range of motion, and it sacrifices stability for mobility. As previously discussed, there are numerous joints throughout the body with each having its specific purpose or function. In short, the more stable a joint is, the less mobile it is. For example, remember that the fibrous joints of the skull (sutures) have little, if any, motion available but they are very stable. On the other hand, the shoulder joint is a synovial joint with a large amount of mobility but provides less stability. This "trade-off" is partially responsible for the numerous amounts of injuries that the shoulder joint incurs. Keep this trade-off in mind when reading this chapter.

LANDMARKS OF THE SHOULDER JOINT

The important landmarks of the scapula were identified in Chapter 17, so they will be listed here but not identified. Take some time to review any of the landmarks you are unfamiliar with. The major landmarks of the scapula that are important to the movements of the shoulder joint are the acromion process, coracoid process, glenoid fossa, supraspinous fossa, infraspinous fossa, subscapular fossa, vertebral border, and the axillary border.

Humerus

The humerus has numerous important landmarks that need to be identified (Figure 18-1). The humerus is a long bone structure that provides landmarks for the attachment of the shoulder, elbow, and wrist muscles. The landmarks of the humerus are often used as anatomical pulleys, which increase the mechanical effects of the muscle contractions of this region. When identifying the landmarks of the humerus, group them into the proximal, middle, and distal humerus.

Proximal Humerus The proximal region of the humerus is comprised of four anatomical structures that increase the efficiency of the forces applied to the region, and increase the surface area for shoulder joint muscle attachment. On a skeleton, or using the figures provided in this book, locate the structures of the humerus. Beginning on the rounded head of the humerus, locate its smooth articulating surface. This structure provides a smooth surface area that aids in the glide, spin, and roll movements of the humerus over the glenoid fossa of the scapula.

Moving laterally from the head, note two large projections with a groove separating these structures into anterior and posterior portions. These projections are named the greater and lesser tubercles. Of these structures, the lesser tubercle is located more anteriorly and the greater tubercle more posteriorly and laterally. Located between the two individual tubercles lies the bicipital groove (**intertubercular groove**). All three landmarks increase the surface area for the attachments of shoulder joint muscles and allow for a strong anatomical pulley relationship.

Middle Humerus Moving in the inferior direction along the lateral surface of the humerus, locate the **deltoid tuberosity** about one-half the distance of the humerus. The deltoid tuberosity is the insertion point for the deltoid muscle.

Distal Humerus Continuing along the lateral border of the humerus in the distal direction, locate the protruding lateral supracondylar ridge that projects laterally, forming the lateral edge of the epiphysis. From this location locate the lateral epicondyle. Although these structures are not important landmarks for the muscles of the shoulder joint, they are extremely important structures for the muscles of the forearm, wrist, and hand.

From the lateral epicondyle, locate the distal articulating surface of the humerus and observe the two rounded projections that articulate with the radius and ulna. The first of these rounded structures is located laterally and is called the **capitulum**. During movements of the elbow joint, the convex shape of the capitulum allows the concave head of the radius to roll in the sagittal plane. Additionally, during movements of the radioulnar joint, the radial head rotates over the capitulum.

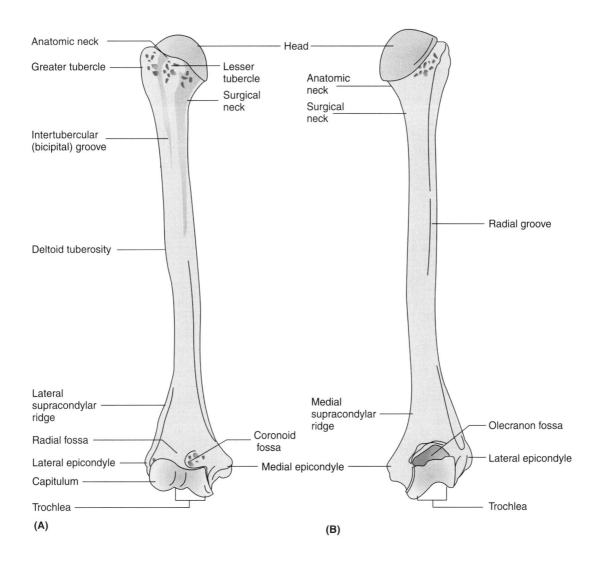

Figure 18-1 *Humerus*

Moving in the medial direction, locate the second rounded convex structure called the **trochlea**, which attaches to the concave olecranon process of the ulna. When these two structures articulate, they provide a large amount of stability for the elbow region and limit the amount of movement in the frontal and transverse planes.

Located on the posterior surface of the distal humerus is the olecranon fossa. This deep impression into the bone increases the ability of the ulna to roll over the trochlea by increasing the distance through which the ulna can move. If the olecranon fossa did not exist, the functional ability would be limited because the ulna would roll over the olecranon fossa.

Moving in the medial direction from the trochlea, locate the medial epicondyle of the distal humerus. Much like the lateral epicondyle, the medial epicondyle is an important anatomical structure of the wrist and forearm muscles.

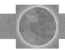

NERVOUS INNERVATION

Six separate nerves innervate the muscles that cause actions around the shoulder joint. Each of the six nerves originates at the brachial plexus and runs distally down the arm and to the hand. The nerves of the shoulder joint include the axillary, musculocutaneous, suprascapular, lower and upper subscapular, thoracodorsal, and lateral pectoral.

OTA PERSPECTIVE

The shoulder is the most commonly dislocated major joint in the body owing to its inherent large amount of motion and little stability. This dislocation most commonly occurs in an anterior direction with the humeral head coming forward; however, the shoulder can dislocate posteriorly and some patients experience multidirectional instability.

The most common position to dislocate the shoulder is with the arm at 90 degrees of abduction and externally rotated. This is common in climbing, kayaking, and throwing motions.

Axillary Nerve

The axillary nerve is a terminal nerve of the posterior cord of the brachial plexus and, therefore, originates from the ventral rami of C5–T1 (Figure 18-2). The posterior cord tracks in the distal and inferior directions from the rami to the level of the second rib at the armpit. At this location, the posterior cord branches into the upper subscapular, thoracodorsal, lower subscapular, radial, and axillary nerves. As the axillary nerve branches from the posterior cord, it tracks posteriorly behind the proximal region of the humerus then branches and innervates the deltoid and teres minor muscles. From the branching, the nerve continues in the distal direction and innervates more muscles.

Musculocutaneous Nerve

The musculocutaneous nerve is a terminal nerve of the lateral cord of the brachial plexus and, therefore, originates from the ventral rami of C5–C7 (see Figure 18-2). Much like the posterior cord, the lateral cord tracks in the distal and inferior directions from the rami of C5–C7 to the level of the second rib at the armpit. At this location the musculocutaneous nerve tracks along the anterior surface of the humerus along the biceps brachii muscle. The nerve actually tracks through the biceps brachii as it tracks toward the skin. As the nerve tracks in the distal direction, it innervates the coracobrachialis more proximal to the biceps brachii and brachialis muscles of the elbow joint.

Suprascapular Nerve

The suprascapular nerve is a terminal nerve extending from the superior trunk and originates from ventral rami of C5 and C6 (see Figure 18-2). Inferior to the acromial end of the clavicle, the suprascapular nerve tracks in the posterior direction and is found superficial to the posterior surface of the scapula. This position allows the suprascapular nerve to easily innervate the supraspinatus and infraspinatus muscles.

Upper and Lower Subscapular Nerves

Both the upper and lower subscapular nerves are branches of the posterior cord (see Figure 18-2). At the armpit, approximately the level of the second rib, the upper subscapular nerve is the first of the terminal nerves that branches from the posterior cord. As the upper subscapular nerve branches, it tracks deep to the subscapularis muscle and innervates the muscle there. Much like the upper subscapular nerve, the lower subscapular nerve tracks in the posterior direction. This posterior track allows the lower subscapular nerve to innervate the teres major muscle on the posterior surface of the superior lateral back.

Thoracodorsal Nerve

Located between the upper and lower subscapular nerve lies the thoracodorsal nerve, which is also a terminal nerve of the posterior cord (see Figure 18-2). The thoracodorsal nerve extends posteriorly to innervate the latissimus dorsi muscle of the back.

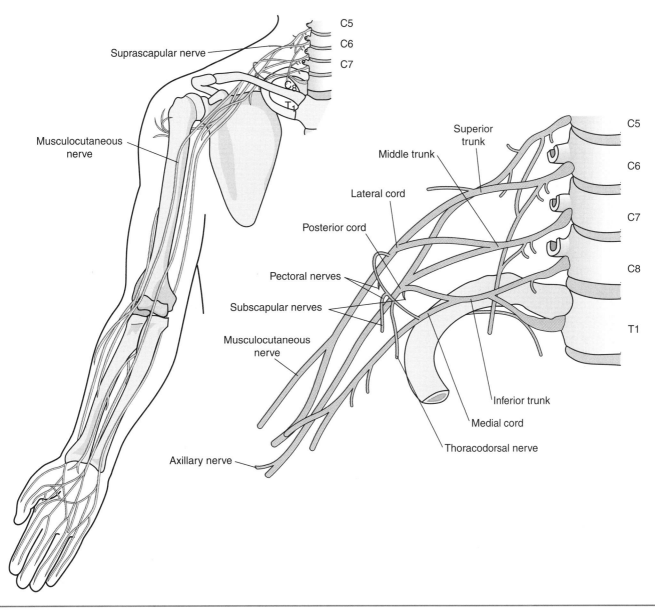

Figure 18-2 *Nerves of the Shoulder Joint*

Lateral Pectoral Nerve

The final nerve that innervates the muscles that cause actions around the shoulder joint is the lateral pectoral nerve (see Figure 18-2). The lateral pectoral nerve stems from the lateral cord, which originates from the ventral rami of C5–C7. At the level of the coracoid process of the scapula, the nerve tracks in the anterior direction toward the chest. As it tracks in the anterior direction, it terminates at the pectoralis major, which this nerve innervates. Table 18-1 summarizes the nerves in the shoulder joint and the areas they affect.

 MOVEMENTS AROUND THE SHOULDER JOINT

The shoulder joint is a triaxial joint that allows motions in all three planes. An analysis of the movements in the region reveals that there are four general movements that can occur at the shoulder joint. Of the movements, flexion, extension, and hyperextension occur in the sagittal plane around a frontal axis. Both abduction and adduction occur in the frontal plane around a sagittal axis. Finally, medial and lateral rotation, horizontal abduction, and horizontal adduction all occur in

Table 18-1 *Nerves of the Shoulder Joint*

Nerve	Affected Anterior Muscles	Affected Lateral Muscles	Affected Posterior Muscles
Axillary	Anterior deltoid	Middle deltoid	Posterior deltoid, teres minor
Suprascapular	None	Supraspinatus	Infraspinatus
Subscapular	None	None	Teres major, subscapularis
Musculocutaneous	Coracobrachialis	None	None
Pectoral	Pectoralis major	None	None
Thoracodorsal	None	None	Latissimus dorsi

the transverse plane around a vertical axis. When studying the movements of the shoulder girdle, practice the activities that allow the shoulder to move through a full range of motion to help you learn their functions. Table 18-2 summarizes the movements of the shoulder joint.

Owing to the large range of motion allowed at this joint, it can be susceptible to injuries. It should be obvious that the shoulder joint is an extremely versatile and quite functional joint for most athletic movements and ADL.

Table 18-2 *Movements of the Shoulder Joint*

Movement	Plane	Axis
Flexion	Sagittal	Frontal
Extension	Sagittal	Frontal
Hyperextension	Sagittal	Frontal
Abduction	Frontal	Sagittal
Adduction	Frontal	Sagittal
Rotation	Transverse	Vertical
Horizontal Abduction	Transverse	Vertical
Horizontal Adduction	Transverse	Vertical

 STABILITY OF THE SHOULDER JOINT

Several ligaments hold the head of the humerus in place with the glenoid fossa to provide the stability of the shoulder joint. In addition to the ligament structures, the shoulder joint relies on the rotator cuff, which is a combination of four tendons of muscles that cross the joint and which provides anterior, lateral, and posterior support for it.

The glenohumeral joint is a synovial joint that allows a great deal of motion, but because of this mobility, its stability is compromised. In spite of this large range of motion, there are ligaments and structures that aid in providing integrity to the joint.

As with all synovial joints, the glenohumeral joint is encompassed by a joint capsule. The fibrous portion of the joint capsule attaches at the glenoid fossa and inserts on the head of the humerus. Because of the need for excessive range of motion, the joint capsule is fairly lax.

Ligaments

The superior, middle, and inferior **glenohumeral ligaments** provide anterior support for the joint (Figure 18-3). These three ligaments are usually described as thickenings or "pleats" in the joint capsule. They are not distinctly defined. The **coracohumeral ligament** provides support from the superior direction. It originates on the coracoid process and joins with

OTA Perspective

In the *Occupational Therapy Practice Framework* language, shoulder ROM movements are *body functions*, a broad term within the *client factors* context. This underlying factor—ROM—affects what a client *does*: occupational performance both as a *motor skill* (e.g., reaching) and as a *performance in areas of occupation* (e.g., PADL, play). A comprehension of shoulder movements, specifically the stability and mobility aspects, is necessary whether treating clients from a top-down approach or a bottom-up approach.

the superior portion of the joint capsule and supraspinatus tendon, inserting on the greater tubercle. The **coracoacromial ligament**, although not directly related to the glenohumeral joint, also provides superior support.

The Rotator Cuff

The rotator cuff is mainly comprised of the tendon insertions of the supraspinatus, infraspinatus, and teres minor muscles on the posterosuperior aspect of the humerus (Figure 18-4). These tendons blend with the joint capsule to form the cuff. In addition, the distal end of the subscapularis forms the anterior aspect of the rotator cuff. The combination of these muscles make up the SITS muscle group. Respectively, the SITS muscles are the *S*upraspinatus, *I*nfraspiantus, *T*eres minor, and *S*ubscapularis. Although all small muscles, the rotator cuff has enormous responsibility in upper extremity movement. First, these muscles provide stability to the glenohumeral joint. That is, they confine the head of the humerus into the glenoid fossa of the scapula. This first function of stability leads to the second function of the rotator cuff—rotation. The head of the humerus is allowed to rotate internally and externally to provide even greater range of motion and variety of movement at this joint. Pitching a baseball is an example of a functional activity utilizing both internal and external rotation of the shoulder joint.

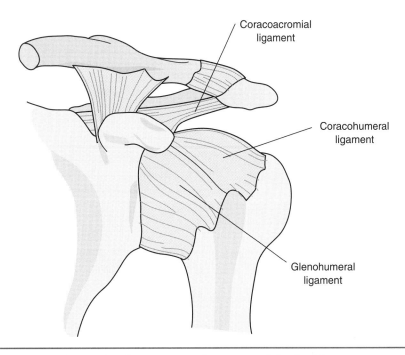

Figure 18-3 *Glenohumeral, Coracohumeral, and Coracoacromial Ligaments of the Shoulder Joint*

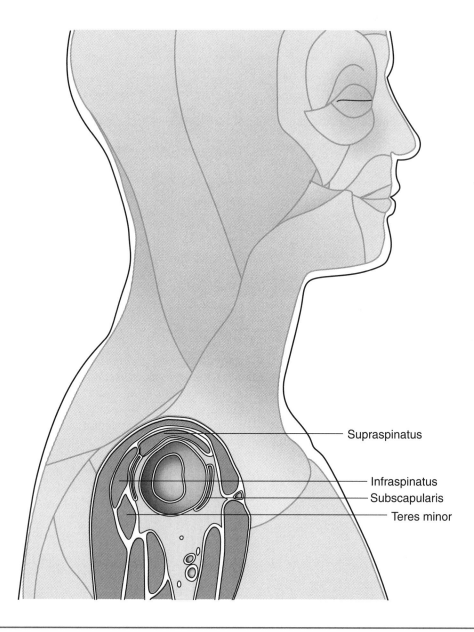

Figure 18-4 *Rotator Cuff*

Because of its small muscle size and possible lack of strength, the rotator cuff is where some people experience a high incidence of injury. Increasing strength and endurance of these muscles is critical to pain-free and injury-free motion at the shoulder joint. All of the muscles acting on the shoulder joint are discussed next in order from anterior to posterior location.

 MUSCLES OF THE SHOULDER JOINT

Nine muscles cause motions at the shoulder joint. Some of the larger and more powerful ones are located superficially, whereas the smaller and weaker rotator cuff muscles are located deep. The superficial muscles are the pectoralis major, latissimus dorsi, deltoid (anterior, middle, posterior), and teres major.

OTA Perspective

Frozen shoulder is clinically known as adhesive capsulitis. This pathology is a unique situation that only occurs in the shoulder and involves an inflammatory response and then a contracture of the joint capsule. The joint becomes painful and then progressively stiffer in a consistent pattern of loss of ROM. The characteristic pattern is a loss of external rotation, abduction, and internal rotation. The cause is often unknown but it can also be secondary to a traumatic injury to the upper extremity and following a period of immobilization. Clients often notice a gradual decrease in their ability to do their ADL. The clients are frequently women 40–50 years old and it often affects those with diabeties.

Treatment consists of stretching exercises, joint mobilizations, and ROM exercises. The treatment may help but the condition spontaneously resolves within 2 years in the majority of cases, with only occasional residual stiffness.

Pectoralis Major

The **pectoralis major** is a large triangular-shaped muscle spanning the anterior superior region of the chest (Figure 18-5 A and B). Originating on the clavicle and sternum, the pectoralis major converges into its insertion on the bicipital groove of the humerus. Owing to the variety of muscle fiber directions of this muscle, it is a powerful shoulder flexor and also performs adduction, horizontal adduction, and internal rotation.

The pectoralis major can be palpated in the anterior and superior regions of the chest. To locate the muscle, first palpate the lateral portion of the sternum. Note the origin of the muscle stemming from the lateral border of the body and manubrium of the sternum and the medial third of the sternal end of the clavicle. Follow the triangle shape of the muscle in the lateral direction toward the armpit. The pectoralis major muscle is superficial, which makes it simple to palpate.

Name:	Pectoralis Major
O:	Lateral border of the body and manubrium of the sternum and the medial third of the clavicle
I:	Bicipital groove of the humerus
N:	Pectoral nerve
A:	Horizontal adduction, flexion, internal rotation, and adduction
P:	Anterosuperior chest

Coracobrachialis ~~No~~

The **coracobrachialis** is a small muscle located deep to the deltoid and biceps brachii (Figure 18-6). It mainly assists with shoulder flexion movements. Because of its location, the coracobrachialis is difficult to palpate.

Name:	Coracobrachialis
O:	Lateral portion of the coracoid process
I:	Anteromedial humerus at approximately half the distance
N:	Musculocutaneous nerve
A:	Shoulder flexion
P:	Difficult to palpate

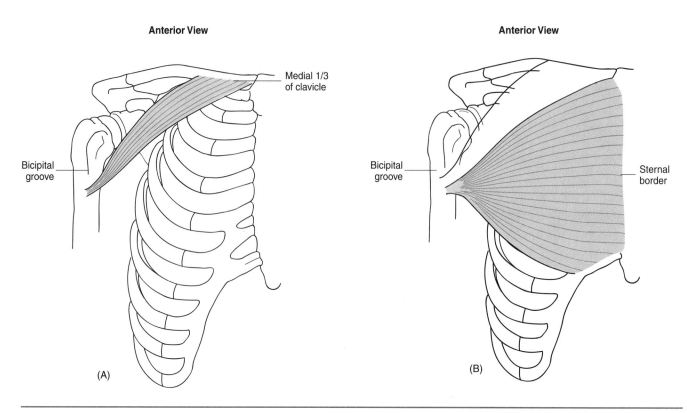

Anterior View

Medial 1/3
of clavicle

Bicipital
groove

(A)

Anterior View

Bicipital
groove

Sternal
border

(B)

Figure 18-5 A and B *Pectoralis Major*

Anterior Deltoid

The entire **deltoid** muscle is shaped like an upside-down triangle (Figure 18-7). If you divided the triangle into thirds, you would essentially divide the three heads of the deltoid. The anterior deltoid is part of a multipennate muscle located at the anterior region of the shoulder. Suprisingly, this small muscle is a powerful shoulder flexor and also assists in shoulder abduction, internal rotation, and horizontal adduction. It can be palpated on the anterosuperior side of the humerus.

Name:	Anterior Deltoid
O:	The lateral third of the clavicle
I:	Deltoid tuberosity
N:	Axillary nerve
A:	Abduction, shoulder flexion, horizontal adduction, and internal rotation
P:	Anterolateral shoulder

Middle Deltoid

The middle head of the deltoid is located on the lateral aspect of the superior humerus (Figure 18-8). The middle deltoid is part of the multipennate muscle and performs true abduction of the shoulder. It can be palpated laterally from the acromion process to the deltoid tuberosity of the humerus.

Name:	Middle Deltoid
O:	Acromion process
I:	Deltoid tuberosity
N:	Axillary nerve
A:	True abduction
P:	Lateral shoulder

Posterior Deltoid

The posterior deltoid muscle is the final third of the multipennate deltoid muscle (Figure 18-9). The muscle is located on the posterosuperior aspect of the humerus. This small muscle contributes to shoulder abduction, shoulder extension, horizontal abduction, and external rotation. Often this muscle is much weaker than its anterior counterpart and contributes to muscle imbalance at the glenohumeral joint. It can be palpated on the posterosuperior aspect of the humerus.

Name: Posterior Deltoid

O: Lateral half of the spine of the scapula

I: Deltoid tuberosity

N: Axillary nerve

A: Abduction, shoulder extension, horizontal abduction, and external rotation

P: Posterolateral shoulder

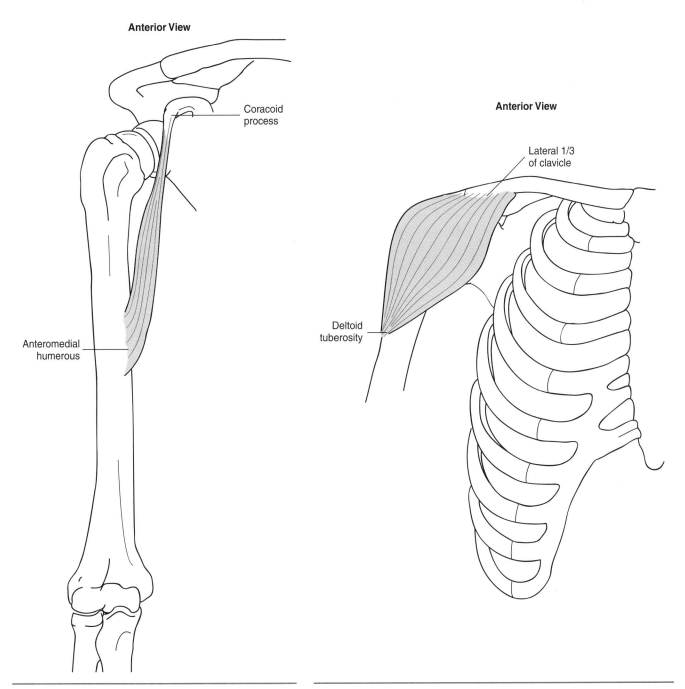

Figure 18-6 *Coracobrachialis*   **Figure 18-7**   *Anterior Deltoid*

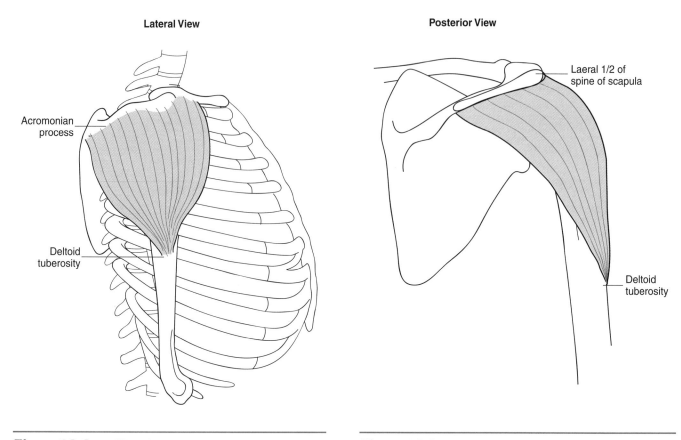

Lateral View

Acromonian process

Deltoid tuberosity

Posterior View

Laeral 1/2 of spine of scapula

Deltoid tuberosity

Figure 18-8 *Middle Deltoid*

Figure 18-9 *Posterior Deltoid*

All three portions of the deltoid muscle are superficial to other regions of the shoulder, which makes them easy to palpate. To locate the three regions of the deltoid muscle, begin by palpating the large bulk of the anterior deltoid at the acromial end of the clavicle distal to the concavity. Moving in the superolateral direction, find the middle deltoid. From this location, trace the muscle in the posterior direction to find the posterior deltoid. Locate the acromion process in the divot formed by the combination of the three individual sections.

Latissimus Dorsi

The **latissimus dorsi** muscle is a large superficial muscle spanning the inferior and lateral regions of the back (Figure 18-10). The latissimus dorsi is a powerful adductor of the shoulder and also aids in internal rotation, horizontal adduction, and shoulder extension. Owing to its superficial location, the latissimus dorsi can be palpated on the lower, lateral portion of the back and, superiorly underneath the arm.

When attempting to palpate the latissimus dorsi muscle, realize once again that this is an extremely large muscle taking up the major portion of the surface area of the back. Begin to palpate the latissimus dorsi muscle by locating the broad origin. From here the muscle fibers track toward the glenhumoral joint. The bulk of the muscle, however, can be located on a line from approximately T6 and inferior to the inferior angle of the scapula.

Name:	Latissimus Dorsi
O:	Spinous processes of T7–L5, the sacrum, and the medial portion of the ischium
I:	Bicipital groove of the humerus
N:	Thoracodorsal nerve
A:	Internal rotation, adduction, horizontal abduction, and extension
P:	Posteroinferior region of the thorax, moving superiorly and laterally toward the armpit

Posterior View

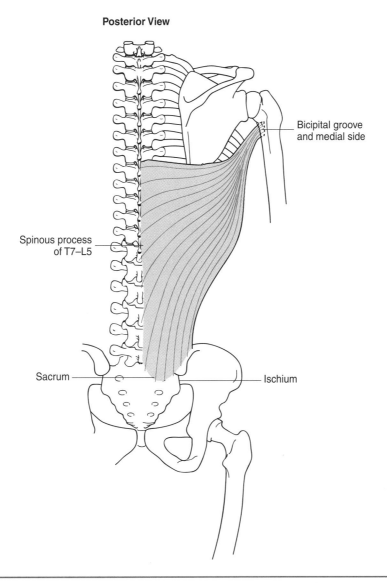

Bicipital groove
and medial side

Spinous process
of T7–L5

Sacrum

Ischium

Figure 18-10 *Latissimus Dorsi*

Teres Major

The **teres major** muscle is often referred to as the "little latissimus dorsi" because they have the same insertion and movements (Figure 18-11). The teres major muscle is located in a position spanning from the inferior angle of the scapula and moving laterally to the lesser tubercle. Essentially, the muscle movements are the same as those of the latissimus dorsi.

To palpate the teres major muscle, first locate the inferior angle of the scapula. The belly of the muscle can be traced from this location, moving in the superior and lateral directions superior to the latissimus dorsi muscle.

Name:	Teres Major
O:	Inferior angle of the scapula
I:	Lesser tubercle
N:	Suprascapular nerve
A:	Internal rotation, adduction, horizontal abduction, and extension
P:	Posterior surface of the thorax, moving diagonally upward from the inferior angle of the scapula

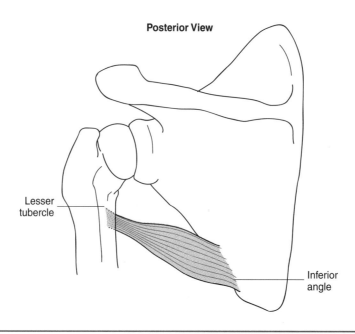

Figure 18-11   *Teres Major*

Teres Minor

Located just superior to the teres major, the **teres minor** is a small rotator cuff muscle (Figure 18-12). As with all rotator cuff muscles, it stabilizes the head of the humerus in the glenoid fossa and assists in shoulder adduction and external rotation. It can be palpated between the lateral border of the scapula and the posterior deltoid.

    Name: Teres Minor

    O: Middle third of the lateral scapular border

    I: Greater tubercle

    N: Suprascapular nerve

    A   Adduction and external rotation

    P: Between the lateral border of the scapula and posterior deltoid

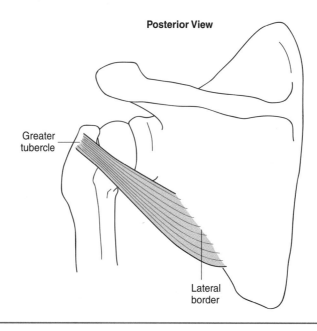

Figure 18-12   *Teres Minor*

Infraspinatus

The **infraspinatus** muscle is a small rotator cuff muscle that originates from within the infraspinous fossa (Figure 18-13). The muscle is active during horizontal abduction and external rotation. It can be palpated directly below the spine of the scapula.

    Name: Infraspinatus

      O: Infraspinous fossa

       I: Posterosuperior greater tubercle

      N: Suprascapular nerve

      A: Horizontal abduction and external rotation

      P: Directly below the spine of the scapula

Supraspinatus

The **supraspinatus** muscle is a small muscle that originates directly from the supraspinous fossa of the scapula (Figure 18-14). As with all rotator cuff muscles, it stabilizes the humerus and aids in abduction of the shoulder. It can be palpated inferior to the spine of the scapula.

    Name: Supraspinatus

      O: Supraspinous fossa

       I: Superior aspect of the greater tubercle

      N: Suprascapular nerve

      A: Abduction

      P: Inferior to the spine of the scapula

Subscapularis

The **subscapularis** muscle is found on the anterior side of the scapula in the subscapular fossa (Figure 18-15). Its tendon contributes to the rotator cuff, which stabilizes the anterior surface of the humerus. It mainly acts as an internal rotator. Owing to its anterior location on the scapula, this muscle may be difficult to palpate.

    Name: Subscapularis

      O: Subscapular fossa

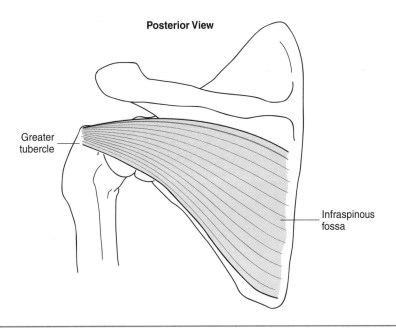

Figure 18-13 *Infraspinatus*

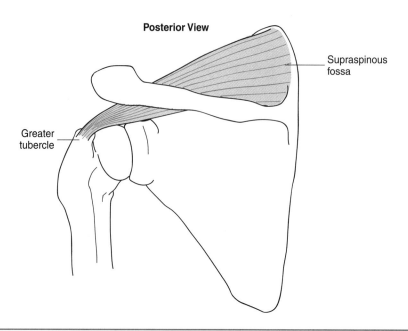

Figure 18-14 *Supraspinatus*

I:	Lesser tubercle of the humerus
N:	Upper and lower subscapular nerve
A:	Internal rotation
P:	Difficult to palpate

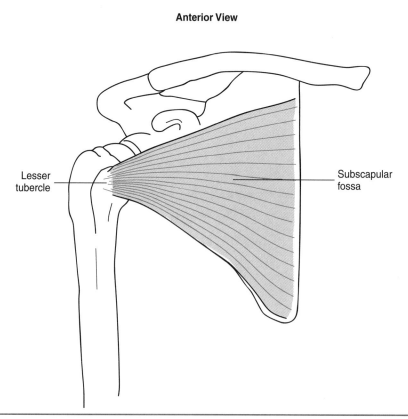

Figure 18-15 *Subscapularis*

OTA Perspective

The musculoskeletal makeup of the shoulder makes it a complex structure. The "hemiplegic shoulder" adds to that complexity. A study of kinesiology lays a foundation for understanding what is "normal." This knowledge is necessary for treating a client with a shoulder impairment such as hemiplegia because it forms a basis for which to compare assessment results and, subsequently, plan treatment and realistic goals. Pain, spasticity or flaccidity, and shoulder subluxation or dislocation may be complications arising from a hemiplegic shoulder diagnosis. Review what you know about a hemiplegic diagnosis (resulting from a CVA or TBI), along with researching theory and treatment techniques (e.g., neurodevelopmental models). This will assist an OTA student in understanding the importance of studying kinesiology.

KEY CONCEPTS

- The shoulder joint is a triaxial joint located between the glenoid fossa of the scapula and the head of the humerus. The joint allows for nine separate movements, including flexion/extension, horizontal adduction/horizontal abduction, internal rotation/external rotation, abduction/adduction, and circumduction.

- The rotator cuff is comprised of four muscles that provide the stability of the shoulder joint. These muscles provide stability for the joint on the anterior, superior and posterior regions of the muscle. The SITS rotator cuff muscles include the infraspinatus, supraspinatus, teres minor, and subscapularis.

- The muscles of the shoulder girdle and shoulder joint work in unison to provide movements of the superior appendicular region. Whereas the shoulder joint muscles move the arm through a full range of motion, the shoulder joint provides a strong base for the shoulder joint movements to act around.

BIBLIOGRAPHY

Hall-Craggs, E. C. B. (1990). *Anatomy as a basis for clinical medicine* (2nd ed.). Baltimore: Urban and Schwarzenberg.

Norkin, C. C., & Levangie, P. K. (2001). *Joint structure and function: A comprehensive analysis* (3rd ed.). Philadelphia: F. A. Davis.

Thompson, C. W., & Floyd, R. T. (2001). *Manual of structural kinesiology* (14th ed.). St. Louis, MO: Mosby.

WEB RESOURCES

- For more information and resources on the shoulder, visit www.shoulder1.com.

(This Web address was current as of September 2003.)

REVIEW QUESTIONS

Fill in the Blank

Provide the word(s) or phrase(s) that best completes the sentence.

1. The deltoid (all three heads) is innervated by the _____ nerve.

2. Horizontal abduction and adduction occur in the _____ plane.

3. The rotator cuff consists of tendons from four muscles—the _____, _____, _____, and _____.

4. The teres major has similar actions to _____.

5. A jumping jack activity occurs in the _____ plane.

Multiple Choice

Select the best answer to complete the following statements.

1. The most powerful adductor of the shoulder is the _____ muscle.
  a. pectoralis major
  b. infraspinatus
  c. deltoid
  d. latissimus dorsi

2. The major action of the subscapularis is _____ .
  a. external rotation
  b. abduction
  c. internal rotation
  d. horizontal adduction

3. Reaching up in a cabinet requires the action of the _____ muscle.
  a. latissimus dorsi
  b. anterior deltoid
  c. infraspinatus
  d. posterior deltoid

4. The latissimus dorsi is innervated by the _____ nerve.
  a. thoracodorsal
  b. dorsal scapular
  c. axillary
  d. musculocutaneous

5. Performing a push-up exercise involves the _____ muscles.
  a. latissimus dorsi, middle deltoid
  b. pectoralis major, anterior deltoid
  c. subscapularis, infraspinatus
  d. coracobrachialis, latissimus dorsi

Matching

Match each of the following descriptions with the appropriate term.

_____ **1.** Frontal plane movement, bringing arms to the side

_____ **2.** Subscapularis

_____ **3.** Attachment for the deltoid

_____ **4.** Movement of the hands toward the midline

_____ **5.** Intertubercular groove

A. Deltoid tuberosity

B. Rotator cuff muscle

C. Horizontal adduction

D. Bicipital groove

E. Adduction

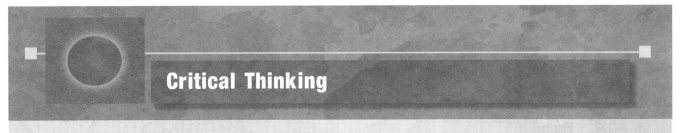

Critical Thinking

1. List the actions of the rotator cuff muscles. Describe how you would strengthen each of the muscles. Imagine a person throwing a baseball. After the ball has left the hand, describe the action or function of the rotator cuff muscles to slow the arm down or decelerate.

2. Imagine ADL, the actions we perform, and the muscles involved at the shoulder while performing these actions. Now imagine a person performing a general strength-training routine. Again, think of the movements performed and the muscles involved causing these movements. Which part of the shoulder joint may be stronger or used more frequently? What should you as a health care professional address or target to prevent muscle imbalances?

3. Draw a picture of the humerus in the space below. On your drawing, include and label the following landmarks:

   ■ Head of the humerus

   ■ Greater tubercle

   ■ Lesser tubercle

   ■ Bicipital groove

   ■ Deltoid tuberosity

   ■ Lateral epicondyle

   ■ Medial epicondyle

   ■ Olecranon fossa

   ■ Capitulum

   ■ Trochlea

(continues)

Critical Thinking *(continued)*

4. On the figures provided on the following pages, draw the nine muscles of the shoulder joint, including:

- Pectoralis major
- Anterior deltoid
- Middle deltoid
- Posterior deltoid
- Coracobrachialis
- Latissimus dorsi

- Teres major
- Teres minor
- Infraspinatus
- Supraspinatus
- Subscapularis

5. On the drawings from number 4, label the origin, insertion, action, and innervation for each of the muscles.

6. Following are examples of stress placed on a developing shoulder. Discuss how these and similar activities are beneficial for growth and development, and how an injury might hinder that growth and development and occupational performance. For the student who is interested in learning more, research and discuss prevention techniques and restorative interventions should an injury occur.

- Children holding onto both parents' hands while swinging in-between them
- Adolescents on a swim team, competitively swimming the butterfly stroke
- Young adults pitching in a fast-pitch baseball game

7. Define the following terms:

- Dislocation
- Subluxation
- Reduction

In the case of the recurrent dislocation of the shoulder, describe the muscles that should be strengthened to prevent dislocation and also other treatments that should be done.

8. During an anterior dislocation of the shoulder, nerve damage can occur. Based on your anatomical knowledge, what nerve would be involved? Describe the signs and symptoms involved with injury to this nerve. Describe three other complications of a shoulder dislocation.

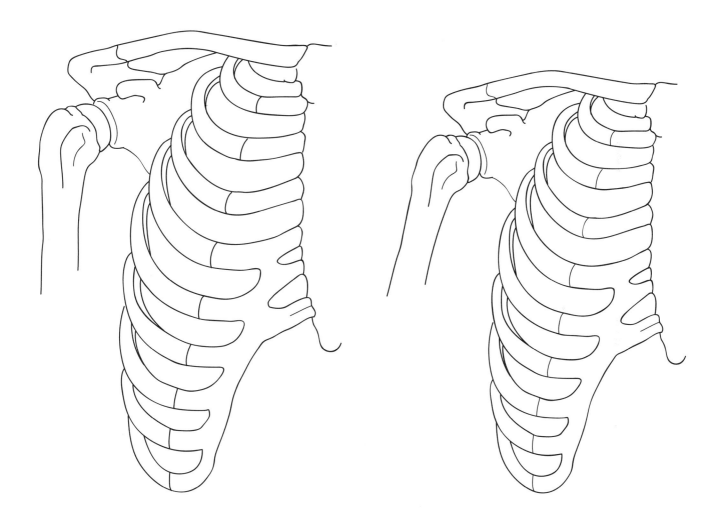

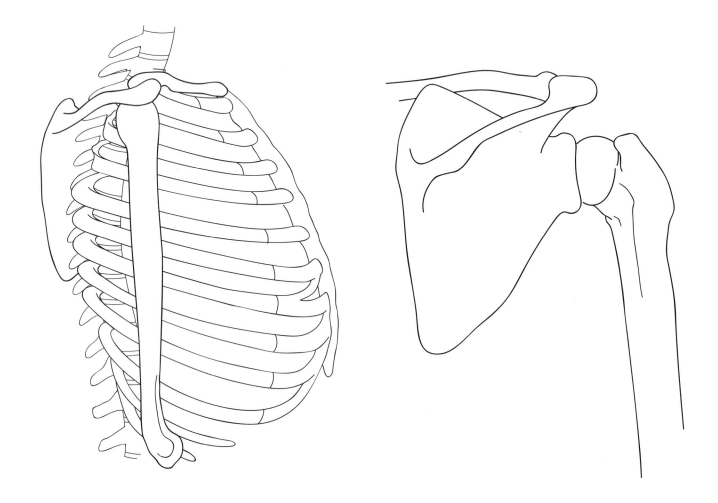

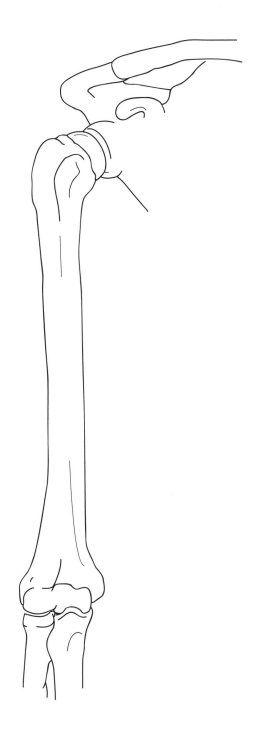

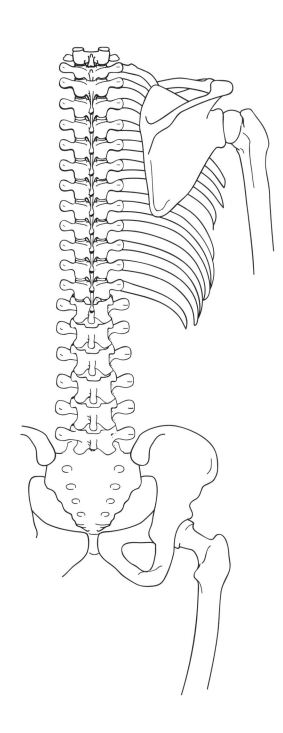

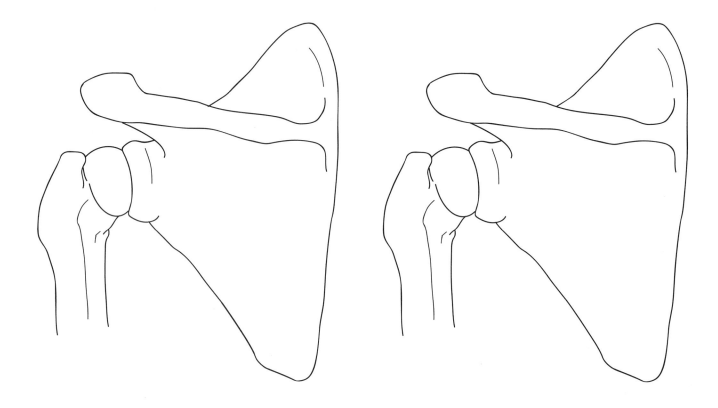

Anterior View

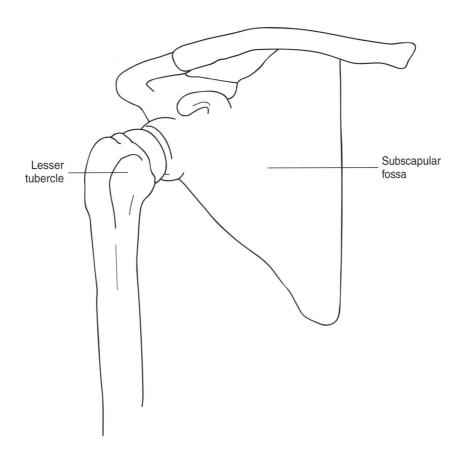

Lesser
tubercle

Subscapular
fossa

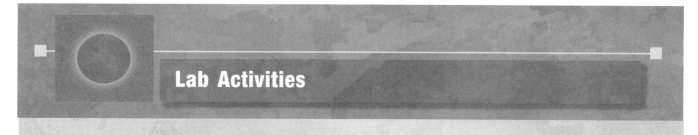

Lab Activities

Lab 18-1: Shoulder Movement and ADL

Objective: To relate ADL to shoulder movements

Equipment Needed: Pen and paper if ideas are to be written down

Step 1.   For each movement listed in Chapter 17, Table 17-3, identify an ADL.

Lab 18-2: Shoulder Stability/Mobility Lab

Objective: To compare and contrast stability/mobility movements within common ADL and to perform an activity analysis.

Equipment Needed: Pen and paper if ideas are to be written down.

Step 1.   Identify three ADL that rely on shoulder joint stability more than on shoulder joint mobility.

Step 2.   Identify three ADL that rely on shoulder joint mobility more than on shoulder joint stability.

Step 3.   Recall open and closed kinetic chains from Chapter 7. Identify the six ADL movements in steps 1 and 2 as either open or closed kinetic chains.

Step 4.   Choose one of the above and compete an activity analysis of that ADL, focusing on the physical aspects of the task.

Lab 18-3: Bicipital Tendonitis

Objective: To assess and plan treatment for bicipital tendonitis.

Equipment Needed: A lab partner, pen/pencil, paper, appropriate dress

Step 1.   Interview your partner who is presenting with bicipital tendonitis in the bicipital groove.

Step 2.   Palpate the biceps tendon on your partner and perform a transverse friction massage.

Step 3.   Research the depth and time for the treatment and explain to your partner the effects of the treatment and what they should feel.

Step 4.   Switch roles and repeat steps 1 through 3.

Lab 18-4: Frozen Shoulder

Objective: To assess and plan therapy for the client with a frozen shoulder.

Equipment Needed: A lab partner, pen/pencil, paper, proper dress

Step 1.   One partner should role-play a 55-year-old female client presenting with a right frozen shoulder. It has been present for several months and her major complaint at this time is stiffness rather than pain. The other partner should interview the patient about her injury.

Step 2.   Measure and record the available ROM of the shoulder.

Step 3.   Teach the client four home exercises to maintain and increase the ROM using three different pieces of apparatus.

Step 4.   Switch roles and repeat steps 1 through 3.

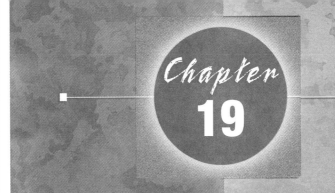

THE ELBOW AND RADIOULNAR JOINTS

Upon completion of this chapter, the reader should be able to:

- Describe the movements of the elbow and radioulnar joints.

- Locate and identify the major landmarks of ligaments of the elbow and radioulnar joints.

- Identify and discuss the joints involved in the elbow and radioulnar joints.

- Name the major muscles associated with the elbow and radioulnar joints.

- Describe the general origin, insertion, action, and innervation of the muscles of the elbow and radioulnar joints.

- Describe the cooperative function of the muscles discussed in this chapter.

anconeus
annular ligament
biceps brachii
brachialis
brachioradialis
coranoid process

lateral collateral ligament
medial collateral ligament
olecranon fossa
olecranon process
pronator quadratus
pronator teres

radial notch
radial tuberosity
styloid process
triceps brachii
trochlear notch
ulnar tuberosity

INTRODUCTION

The elbow joint consists of three bones: the humerus, radius, and ulna. The scapula also plays an important role owing to the fact that muscles of the elbow complex originate there. The diverse function of the elbow joint makes ADL and many athletic movements possible. The muscles and joints of the elbow are designed to assist the hand during various tasks. For instance, the elbow joint and accompanying muscles allow us to lift a bag of groceries, brush our teeth, or throw a baseball.

MAJOR LANDMARKS OF THE ELBOW AND RADIOULNAR JOINTS

The following bones have landmarks that are important to the function of the elbow and radioulnar joints.

Scapula

The importance of the scapula to the movement at the elbow joint cannot be overlooked (Figure 19-1). The main landmarks of importance to the elbow joint that are not discussed in Chapters 17 and 18 include the supraglenoid tubercle, infraglenoid tubercle, and coracoid process. The supraglenoid tubercle is a small bump, just superior to the glenoid fossa. This is the origin for the long head of the biceps brachii. The infraglenoid tubercle is a small bump, just inferior to the glenoid fossa. It is the origin for the long head of the triceps brachii muscle. Because the biceps brachii and triceps brachii each have an origin on the scapula, they also have minor influences on motions at the scapula. The coracoid process is a hook-shaped landmark on the anterior surface of the scapula and is the origin for the short head of the biceps brachii muscle.

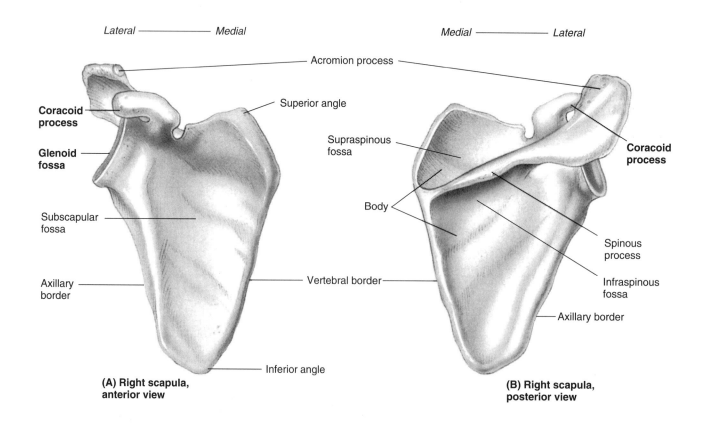

Figure 19-1 *The Scapula*

OTA Perspective

The bursa located over the olecranon can become inflamed or infected. It can be caused by trauma or in patients with rheumatoid arthritis. The patient will present with a large, localized egg-like swelling on the posterior tip of the elbow. Treatment may involve excision, if the bursa becomes infected, or anti-inflammatories.

Humerus

The humerus contains many important landmarks that affect muscle involvement at the elbow (Figure 19-2). The medial epicondyle is a bony projection located on the medial side of the humerus at the distal end. It is an attachment point for the pronator teres muscle. The lateral epicondyle is a bony projection located on the lateral end of the distal humerus. It is an attachment point for the supinator and anconeus muscles. The lateral supracondylar ridge, often confused with the lateral epicondyle, is located superior to the lateral epicondyle and provides attachment for the brachioradialis. The trochlea is a rounded bony area located on the medial side at the distal anterior end of the humerus. The trochlea articulates with the ulna. Just lateral to the trochlea is the capitulum. This bony area articulates with the head of the radius. The olecranon fossa is a large groove located on the posterior side of the humerus that articulates with the **olecranon process** of the ulna.

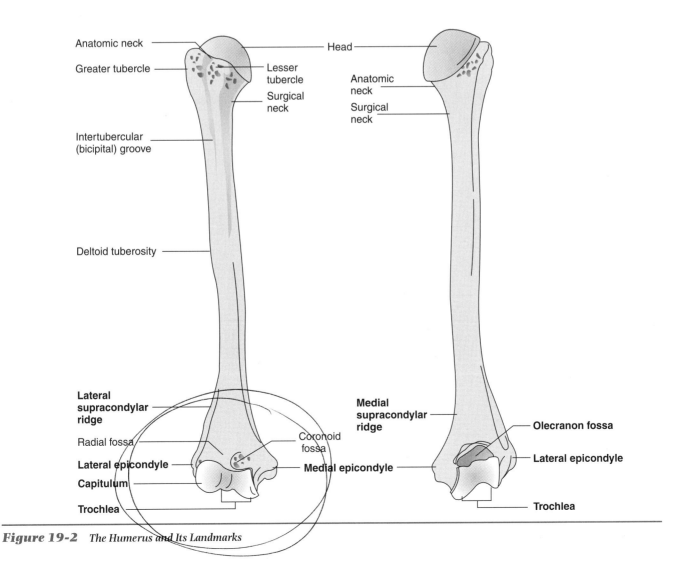

Figure 19-2 *The Humerus and Its Landmarks*

Radius

In the anatomical position, the radius is considered to be the lateral bone of the forearm and is located on the thumb side (Figure 19-3). The articulation between the capitulum of the humerus and the proximal radial tuberosity provide the humeroradial joint. At this location the radial tuberosity spins around the humerus.

    The radius, like other bones, provides important landmarks for the muscles of the elbow to attach to. The **radial tuberosity** is a large, rough area located on the proximal end on the medial surface. The radial tuberosity provides an attachment point for the biceps brachii. The **styloid process** is the pointed distal end on the lateral side of the radius. It is the attachment point for the brachioradialis muscle. On the proximal radius is a round structure known as the radial head. The radial head articulates with the radial notch of the ulna, which provides the articulation between the radius and ulna and the subsequent radioulnar joint.

Ulna

In the anatomical position, the ulna is the bone located on the medial side of the forearm. The curved, hook-shaped proximal end is called the olecranon process and articulates with the **olecranon fossa** of the humerus. The olecranon fossa is the attachment point for the triceps brachii muscle. The **trochlear notch** forms the anterior surface of the proximal ulna. As the name implies, it articulates with the trochlea of the humerus. Just distal to the trochlear notch on the lateral side is the **radial notch**, which articulates with the radius bone. The **coranoid process** lies just below the trochlear notch and is one attachment point for the brachialis muscle. Just distal to the coranoid process is a small, rough area called the **ulnar**

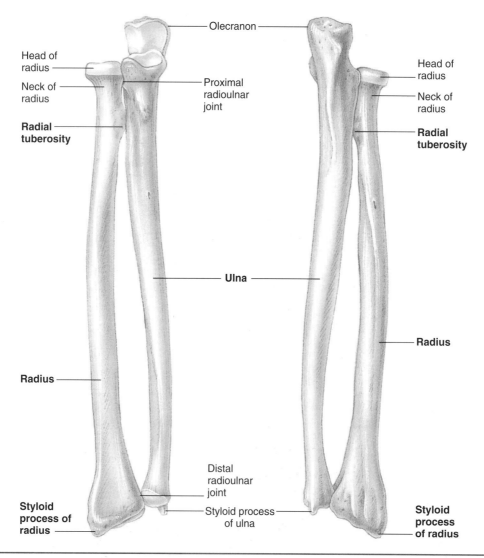

Figure 19-3 *The Radius and Ulna*

OTA Perspective

Tennis elbow is also called lateral epicondylitis. Pain is located over the lateral epicondyle and may radiate into the foramen extensor muscles. Pain is present with palpation and also reproduced with gripping exercises and resisted wrist and finger extension. Patients complain of pain when shaking hands and gripping and lifting objects. Tennis elbow is somewhat of a misnomer because only a small percentage of the sufferers actually play tennis!

The cause of the symptoms may be acute inflammation or degenerative changes in the connective tissue or overuse of the wrist extensor muscles that attach there. OT treatment consists of modalities to decrease the inflammation, strengthening exercises, and stretches. The patients' activities should also be analyzed to see if there is a causative factor, for example, a repetitive work activity that can be adapted, or a change in tennis racket grip size or technique. Sometimes, an injection by the physician is needed.

Pain on the medial side of the elbow reproduced by resisted wrist flexion is termed golfer's elbow.

tuberosity, which provides another attachment point for the brachialis muscle. The styloid process of the ulna is the pointed distal end of the medial ulna. Finally, the head of the ulna is a concave area located on the proximal end of the bone.

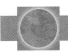 ## NERVOUS INNERVATION

As the nerves of the brachial plexus pass the final branches at the armpit and second rib, identification of the major nerves that innervate the muscles of the distal appendicular skeleton becomes more simplified. The more important aspects to understand after the nerves branch are the directions that the nerve fibers travel along the humerus, forearm, and hand regions. Therefore, this section on nervous innervation focuses primarily on the three nerves that extend to the distal regions of the superior appendicular skeleton. These three nerves are the radial, median, and ulnar nerves. However, the musculocutaneous nerve is reviewed first to describe its relationship to several muscles of the radioulnar joint.

Musculocutaneous Nerve

The musculocutaneous nerve is a terminal nerve of the lateral cord of the brachial plexus and, therefore, originates from the ventral rami of C5–C7 (Figure 19-4). Much like the posterior cord, the lateral cord tracks in the inferior and lateral direction from the rami of C5–C7 to the level of the second rib at the armpit. At this location, the musculocutaneous nerve tracks in the anterior direction along the biceps brachii muscle. The nerve actually tracks through the biceps brachii in the superficial direction. As the nerve tracks in the distal direction, it innervates the coracobrachialis muscle located proximal to the biceps brachii and brachialis muscle of the elbow joint.

Proximal Radial Nerve

The radial nerve is a branch of the posterior cord and originates from the ventral rami of C6–T1 (see Figure 19-4). The radial nerve branches from the posterior cord at the armpit at the level of the second rib. From this location, the radial nerve tracks anteriorly to the insertion of the latissimus dorsi muscle on the proximal humerus. From this location, the radial nerve

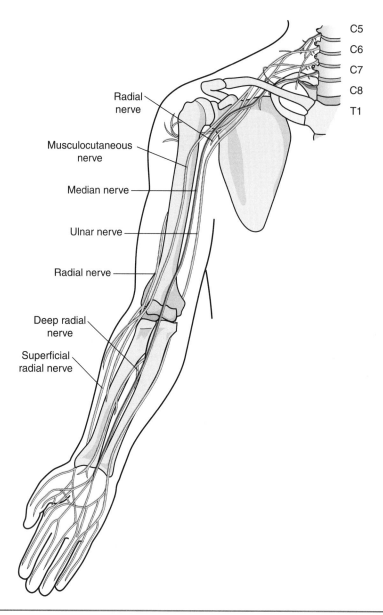

Figure 19-4 *Nerves of the Elbow and Forearm*

tracks along the posterior surface of the humerus. Along the posterior surface of the humerus, the radial nerve innervates the triceps brachii muscle and brachioradialis muscle as it tracks anteriorly to the lateral epicondyle of the humerus. From the anterior position, the radial nerve innervates the supinator and anconeus muscle located in the elbow. The lateral location also allows the radioulnar nerve to innervate the extensors of the wrist joint, including the extensor carpi radialis longus, extensor carpi radialis brevis, and extensor carpi ulnaris.

Distal Radial Nerve

After the radial nerve crosses the radioulnar joint, it branches into a deep branch and superficial branch. The deep branch crosses back to the posterior surface of the hand, tracking past the head of the radius along the interosseus membrane. From here, the deep nerve branches several times, terminating at the muscles that innervate the hand muscles. The superficial branch of the radial nerve, however, tracks along the anterior surface of the radius to the distal regions of the forearm and hand, terminating in the distal cutaneous branches.

Proximal Median Nerve

The median nerve is a branch from both the lateral and medial cords and, therefore, originates from the ventral rami of C6–T1 (see Figure 19-4). Much like the majority of terminal nerves, the median nerve branches at the armpit at the level of the second rib. From the branch, the nerve tracks distally along the medial aspect of the humerus and anteriorly to the trochlea of the humerus. This anterior orientation allows the nerve to innervate the pronator teres muscle located at the radioulnar joint and two of the wrist muscles, the palmaris longus and flexor carpi ulnaris.

Distal Median Nerve

After the median nerve crosses the elbow joint, it tracks distally along the center of the forearm, bisecting the radius and ulna. As the nerve extends to the distal reaches of the hand, it tracks inferiorly to the flexor retinaculum of the hand, innervating the fine motor movement muscles of the hand.

Proximal Ulnar Nerve

The ulnar nerve is a terminal nerve arising from the medial cord of the brachial plexus and originating at the ventral rami of C8 and T1 (see Figure 19-4). In the armpit region, at approximately the level of the second rib, the ulnar nerve branches from the medial cord and tracks down the medial surface of the humerus posteriorly to the ulnar nerve, and tracks posteriorly to the medial epicondyle of the humerus. The humeral segment of the proximal ulnar nerve does not innervate any of the muscles of the elbow and radioulnar joints.

Distal Ulnar Nerve

Tracking of the distal ulnar nerve reveals that, as the nerve crosses the elbow joint, it innervates the flexor carpi ulnaris muscle that causes flexion at the wrist joint. Further distal tracking reveals that the distal ulnar nerve travels on the ulnar side of the forearm toward the distal region of the hand. In this location, the ulnar nerve also innervates the fine motor muscles of the hand. Table 19-1 summarizes the innervation of the elbow.

Table 19-1   *Nerves of the Elbow and Forearm*

Nerve	Affected Anterior Muscle	Affected Posterior Muscle
Musculocutaneous	Biceps brachii, brachialis	None
Radial	Brachioradialis, supinator	Triceps brachii, anconeous
Median	Pronator quadratus	Pronator teres

MOVEMENTS OF THE ELBOW AND RADIOULNAR JOINTS

There are actually quite a few articulations that are involved in the elbow complex. First, the elbow joint consists of the humeroulnar and humeroradial joints. More specifically, the humeroulnar joint has two separate articulations. The trochlea of the humerus articulates with the trochlear notch of the ulna, and as the joint reaches full extension, the olecranon process of the ulna unites with the olecranon fossa of the humerus. The humeroradial joint consists of the radius, which articulates with the capitulum of the humerus. The elbow joint is uniaxial and only allows motions in the sagittal plane.

In addition to the elbow joint, there is an articulation located between the radius and ulna. Although there are both proximal and distal radioulnar joints, this joint is usually considered a pivot joint because it allows motions in the transverse plane.

At the radioulnar joint, supination and pronation are the prominent movements. These movements were described in more detail in Chapter 1. Because the ulna is a stable bone (it does not move), the radius rotates around it during supination and pronation. Therefore, from a kinesiology perspective, a muscle must attach on the radius to cause supination or pronation.

OTA Perspective

The brachial plexus (BP) consists of spinal nerves C5–C8 and T1 and supplies motor movement to the shoulder, wrist, and hand. Located on the right and left sides of the neck, inferior to the clavicle, brachial plexus injuries (BPIs) manifest themselves in an upper extremity (U/E) weakness or total paralysis. Erb's palsy (C5–6±7) is thought to result from a stretching or avulsion of the BP by extreme traction. C5 spinal root injury leads to weakness of the biceps brachii; this muscle flexes the elbow and is a powerful supinator. Symptoms may include a limp or paralyzed arm, lack of muscle control, and possible decreased sensation in the arm and hand.

Further research is suggested to better understand the diagnosis, along with a review of this textbook—specifically Chapters 8, 17, and 18—with regard to how the elbow joint interacts within the U/E musculature.

 ## STABILITY OF THE ELBOW AND RADIOULNAR JOINTS

The elbow joint contains three ligaments: the medial collateral (ulnar collateral), the lateral collateral (radial collateral), and the annular ligament (Figure 19-5). All of these ligaments add stability to the joint.

Medial (Ulnar) Collateral Ligament

The **medial (ulnar) collateral ligament** is triangular shaped and is found on the medial side of the elbow. It attaches on the medial epicondyle of the humerus and runs diagonally to the medial sides of the coranoid and olecranon processes of the ulna. The function of the medial collateral ligament is to provide medial reinforcement.

Lateral (Radial) Collateral Ligament

The **lateral (radial) collateral ligament** is a triangular-shaped ligament. It attaches on the lateral epicondyle of the humerus and inserts on the annular ligament and lateral side of the ulna. The function of this ligament is to provide lateral stability to the elbow joint.

Annular Ligament

The **annular ligament** holds the radius close to the ulna and stabilizes the joint during supination and pronation movements. It attaches on the radial notch of the ulna running anterior to posterior.

Joint Capsule

The joint capsule is a thin layer surrounding the joint being protected by muscles on the anterior and posterior sides. On the medial and lateral sides, the joint is protected by the medial collateral, lateral collateral, and annular ligaments. Lastly, the interosseus membrane is a thin connective tissue situated between the radius and ulna that holds the bones together and is a source for muscle attachment.

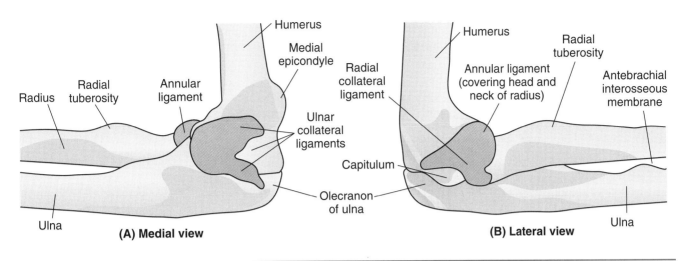

Figure 19-5 *Ligaments of the Elbow*

 MUSCLES OF THE ELBOW AND RADIOULNAR JOINTS

This section provides diagrams, descriptions, and relevant information regarding the muscles of the elbow complex and radioulnar joints. Students sometimes find it easier to learn muscles in terms of location. Table 19-2 can assist you in learning these relationships.

Table 19-2 *Muscles of the Elbow*

Location	Elbow Joint	Radioulnar Joint
Anterior Arm	Biceps Brachii Brachialis	Pronator quadratus Pronator teres
Posterior Arm	Triceps brachii Aconeus	None
Lateral Arm	Brachioradialis	Supinator

Elbow Flexors

The tendons of the muscles that cause flexion of the elbow joint cross the joint on the anterior surface. These muscles are associated with the strong contractions that allow for stability and power.

Biceps Brachii The **biceps brachii** is a fusiform-shaped muscle located on the anterior aspect of the upper humerus (Figure 19-6). This is a powerful elbow flexor and assists in supination. It can be palpated on the anterior portion of the upper humerus. The biceps brachii muscle has two muscle bellies: a short head and long head. The long head is located laterally and contains the bicipital tendon that runs through the intertubercular groove. The short head is located on the medial side.

Name: Biceps Brachii

O: Short head: coracoid process of the scapula

              Long head: supraglenoid tubercle

  I: Radial tuberosity of the radius and bicipital aponeurosis

N: Musculocutaneous nerve

A: Elbow flexion, supination of the forearm, weak shoulder flexion at the shoulder joint

P: Anterior portion of the upper arm, lateral to medial

Brachialis The **brachialis** muscle is another fusiform-shaped muscle located just deep and distal to the biceps brachii (Figure 19-7). The brachialis muscle acts as an elbow flexor but inserts on the coranoid process of the ulna so it is not affected by the position of the radioulnar joint. The brachialis muscle can be palpated deep to the biceps brachii on the lateral side of the humerus.

Name:	Brachialis
O:	Distal third of the anterior humerus
I:	Ulnar tuberosity of the ulna
N:	Musculocutaneous nerve
A:	Elbow flexion
P:	Distal end of the humerus on the lateral side, deep to the biceps brachii

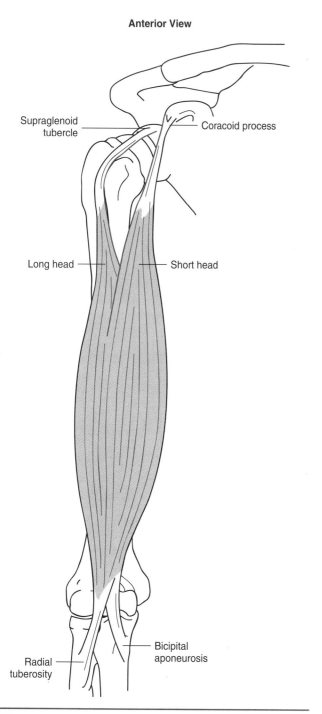

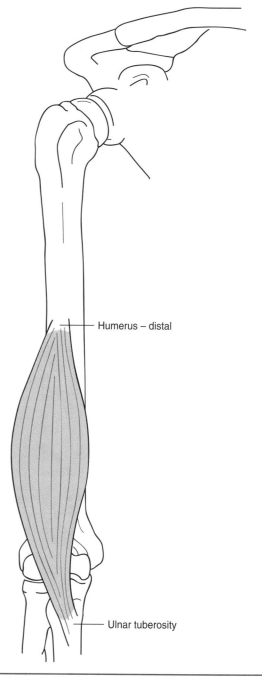

Figure 19-6 *Biceps Brachii*

Figure 19-7 *Brachialis*

Brachioradialis The **brachioradialis** muscle is a long strap muscle that runs from the lateral supracondylar ridge to the styloid process located at the distal radius (Figure 19-8). The brachioradialis is located on the anterolateral side of the forearm. This muscle can be a strong flexor of the forearm when the forearm is in a semipronated position between supination and pronation. The brachioradialis can be palpated easily on the anterolateral side of the forearm.

Name:	Brachioradialis
O:	Supracondylar ridge of the humerus
I:	Styloid process of the radius
N:	Radial nerve
A:	Elbow flexion (especially when the radioulnar joint is in a position midway between supination and pronation)
P:	Anterolateral aspect of the forearm, running from the elbow to the wrist

Elbow Extensors

The muscles that cause extension of the elbow joint are located on its posterior surface. These muscles are associated with the strong contractions that allow for stability and power. The posterior elbow joint muscles include the three heads of the triceps brachii muscle and the anconeus.

Triceps Brachii The **triceps brachii** is a powerful muscle with three heads, thus the prefix "tri" (Figure 19-9). It is located on the posterosuperior humerus, spanning from the upper humerus and scapula to the olecranon process. Because the long head of the triceps crosses the shoulder joint and attaches on the infraglenoid tubercle, it has the ability to assist in shoulder extension. In addition, its main action is extension of the elbow.

To palpate the triceps brachii muscle, extend your elbow against static resistance. Notice the large muscle that protrudes on the posterior surface of the humerus. Palpate the triceps brachii beginning just inferior to the acromion process of the scapula on the posterior surface of the humerus. Follow the muscle belly in the distal direction on the olecranon process of the ulna. Note the bulk of the muscle and you will understand that the triceps brachii muscle provides powerful elbow extension movements.

Name:	Triceps Brachii
O:	Lateral head: approximately halfway down the humerus on the posterior surface
	Long head: infraglenoid tubercle on the lateral border of the scapula
	Medial head: distal two-thirds of the posterior and medial humerus
I:	All heads insert via a central tendon on the olecranon process of the ulna
N:	All heads are innervated by the radial nerve
A:	Elbow extension, extension of the shoulder joint (long head only)
P:	Posterior aspect of the upper arm

Anconeus The **anconeus** is a small muscle located on the posterior surface of the olecranon process of the ulna (Figure 19-10). It assists in elbow extension at best. It can be palpated on the posterolateral aspect of the ulna.

Name:	Anconeus
O:	Posterior surface of the lateral epicondyle of the humerus
I:	Medial surface of the the posterior ulna and olecranon process
N:	Radial nerve
A:	Assists in elbow extension
P:	Posterolateral aspect of the ulna

Supinators and Pronators

The pronator and supinator muscles of the elbow joint work solely around the superior and inferior radioulnar joints. These muscles include the supinator, pronator teres, and pronator quadratus muscles.

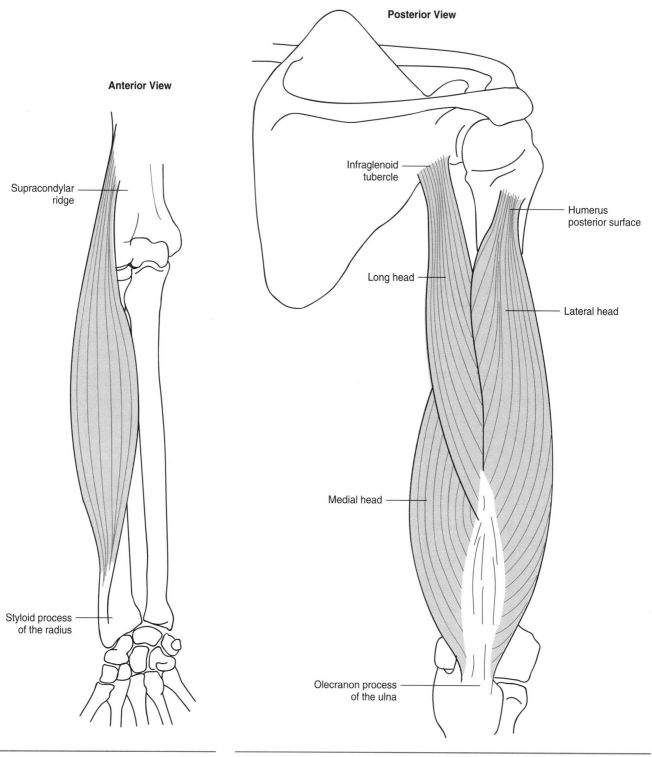

Figure 19-8 *Brachioradialis*

Figure 19-9 *Triceps Brachii*

Supinator The supinator muscle is located between the lateral humerus on the distal portion and the posterior aspect of the superior ulna (Figure 19-11). As the name implies, this muscle supinates, but, more specifically, it supinates when supination and extension of the elbow are both needed. This muscle cannot be palpated.

Name:	Supinator
O:	Lateral epicondyle of the humerus and supinator crest of the ulna
I:	Proximal end of the radius on the lateral surface

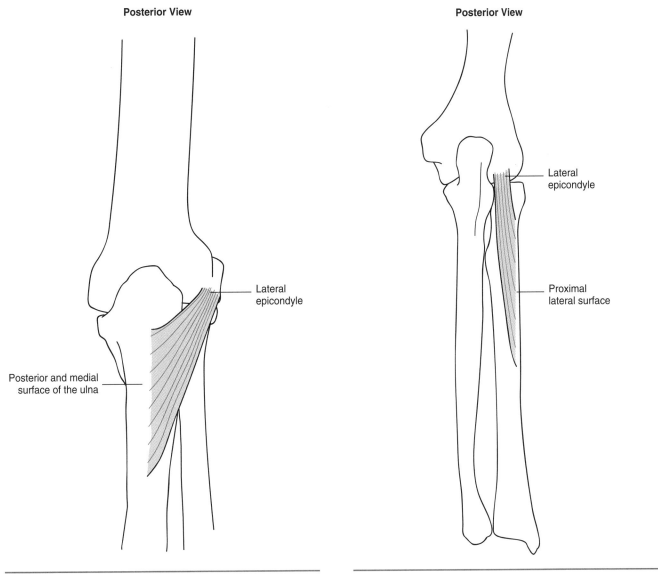

Posterior View   **Posterior View**

Lateral
epicondyle

Proximal
lateral surface

Lateral
epicondyle

Posterior and medial
surface of the ulna

Figure 19-10   *Anconeus*   ***Figure 19-11***   *Supinator*

N:	Radial nerve
A:	Supination of the forearm
P:	Cannot be palpated

Pronator Teres   The **pronator teres** muscle tracks medial to lateral from the medial epicondyle of the humerus to the distal surface of the ulna (Figure 19-12). As the name implies, this muscle pronates but, more specifically, when elbow flexion and pronation are both required. It can be palpated on the anteromedial surface of the forearm.

Name:	Pronator Teres
O:	Medial epicondyle of the humerus and medial side of the ulna
I:	Lateral surface of the radius
N:	Median nerve
A:	Pronation of the forearm, weak elbow flexion
P:	Anteromedial surface of the forearm

Pronator Quadratus The **pronator quadratus** muscle is a flat, four-sided muscle located deep on the distal anterior forearm (Figure 19-13). It acts as a pronator of the forearm. Owing to the deepness of this muscle, it cannot be palpated.

Name: Pronator Quadratus

O: Distal end of the anterior ulna

I: Distal end of the anterior radius

N: Median nerve

A: Pronation of the forearm

P: Cannot be palpated

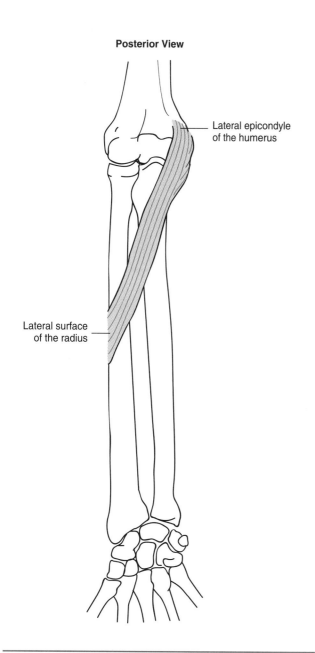

Figure 19-12 *Pronator Teres*

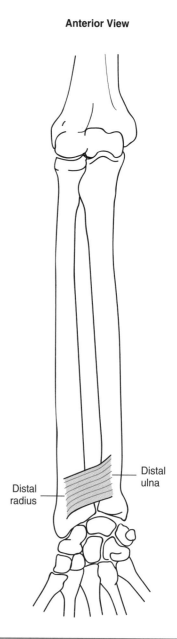

Figure 19-13 *Pronator Quadratus*

KEY CONCEPTS

■ The elbow and radioulnar joints are two separate joints located at the junction between the arm and forearm. The elbow joint provides movement in the sagittal plane, allowing for flexion and extension. The radioulnar joint provides movement in the transverse plane, including pronation and supination.

■ The muscles of the elbow joint cross on the anterior surface. These muscles are powerful flexors and extensors. The elbow flexors include the biceps brachii, brachialis, and brachioradialis. The extensors cross on the posterior surface of the elbow joint and include the triceps brachii and anconeus muscles.

■ The muscles of the radioulnar joint cause pronation and supination movements. These muscles include the pronator teres, pronator quadratus, and supinator.

BIBLIOGRAPHY

Arnheim, D. D. & Prentice, W. E. (2002). *Principles of athletic training* (11th ed.). St. Louis, MO: Mosby.

Jenkins, P. B. (2002). *Hollingshead's functional anatomy of the limbs and back* (8th ed.). Philadelphia: W. B. Saunders.

Thompson, C. W. & Floyd, R. T. (2001). *Manual of structural kinesiology* (14th ed.). St. Louis, MO: Mosby.

WEB RESOURCES

• For the student who is interested in learning more, research Erb's palsy, related surgeries, use of E-Stimulation, and predicted outcomes and prognosis. A helpful resource and Web site is the National Brachial Plexus/Erb's Palsy Association at www.nbpepa.org.

• Go to www.tenniselbow.net, a site that features treatment, orthopedic surgery, and physical therapy techniques to treat tennis elbow.

• The site www.ortho-u.net/o2/128.htm features injuries that occur to the radius. It also includes diagnostic exams that highlight radial head disorders.

(These Web addresses were current as of February 2004.)

REVIEW QUESTIONS

Fill in the Blank

Provide the word(s) or phrase(s) that best completes the sentence.

1. The biceps brachii muscle causes _____ at the elbow joint and _____ at the radioulnar joint.

2. Supination and pronation occur at the _____ joint.

3. The biceps brachii and brachialis are innervated by the _____ nerve.

4. The medial head of the triceps is innervated by the _____ nerve.

5. The brachialis inserts on the _____; therefore it is not affected by forearm position.

Multiple Choice

Select the best answer to complete the following statements.

1. The biceps brachii muscle group inserts on the _____ of the radius.
   a. coranoid process
   b. olecranon fossa
   c. radial tuberosity
   d. styloid process

2. The correct actions of the triceps brachii are _____ .
   a. elbow flexion
   b. shoulder extension/hyperextension
   c. elbow extension
   d. shoulder extension/hyperextension and elbow extension

3. The brachioradialis is innervated by the _____ nerve.
   a. radial
   b. median
   c. ulnar
   d. musculocutaneous

4. The long head of the biceps brachii is located on the _____ side of the arm.
   a. posterior
   b. lateral
   c. medial
   d. inferior

5. The ligament of the elbow that holds the radius and ulna together is the _____ .
   a. ulnar collateral
   b. radial collateral
   c. annular
   d. anterior cruciate

Critical Thinking

1. Imagine a person using a screwdriver to screw together two objects. Identify the joints, joint movements, and muscles involved in this motion.

2. Picture a person performing a "pull-up" exercise. This movement can be performed two ways—with the forearm supinated and pronated. Compare this motion with both hand positions. What (if any) muscles would be affected by changing forearm position. Which method do you think is most efficient?

3. On the figures provided, label the structures of the humerus, radius, ulna, and carpals. On the drawing and a skeleton, locate and label the following landmarks:

   - Supracondylar ridge
   - Lateral epicondyle
   - Capitulum
   - Trochlea
   - Medial epicondyle
   - Radial tuberosity
   - Radial notch
   - Ulnar tuberosity
   - Olecranon fossa
   - Olecranon process
   - Interosseous membrane

   - Radial head
   - Styloid process of the radius
   - Styloid process of the ulna
   - Scaphoid
   - Lunate
   - Triquetrum
   - Pisiform
   - Trapezium
   - Trapezoid
   - Capitate
   - Hamate

4. On the figures provided on the following pages, draw the following major muscles of the elbow and radioulnar joint:

   - Biceps brachii
   - Brachioradialis
   - Brachialis
   - Triceps brachii

   - Supinator
   - Pronator teres
   - Pronator quadratus
   - Anconeus

5. On the drawings from number 4, label the origin, insertion, action, and innervation for each of the muscles.

(continues)

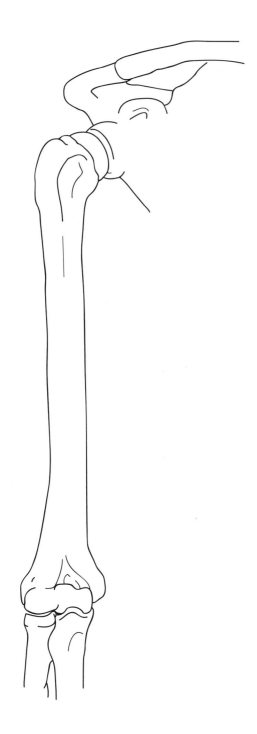

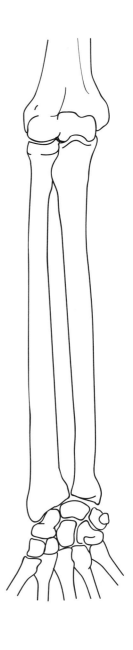

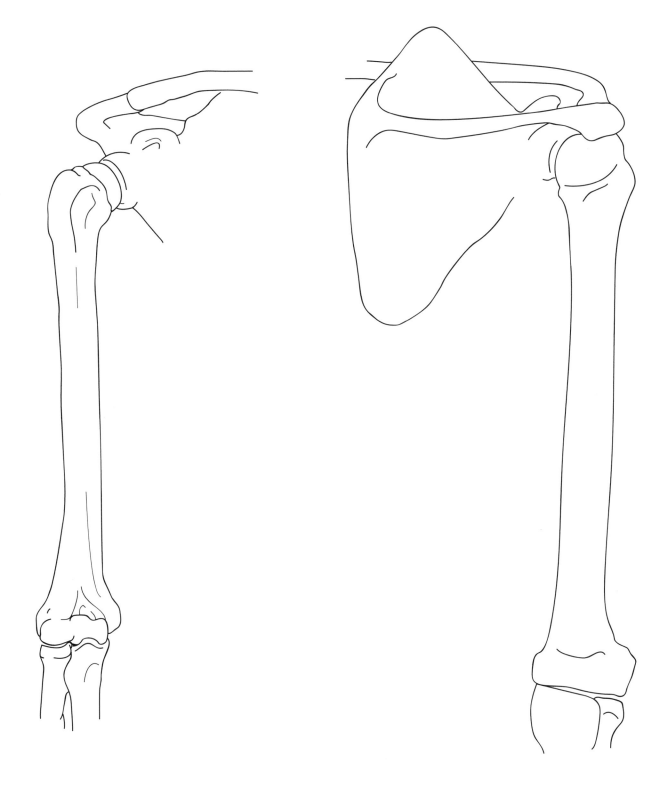

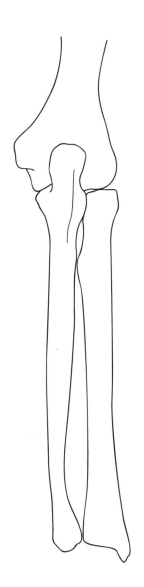

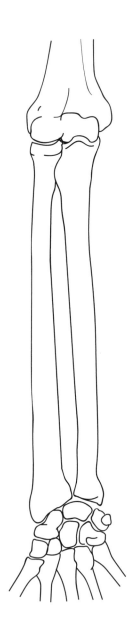

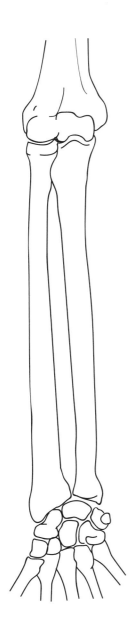

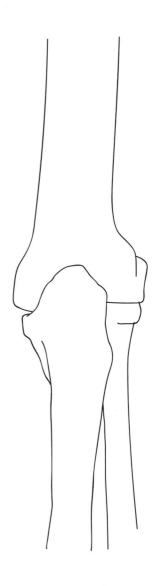

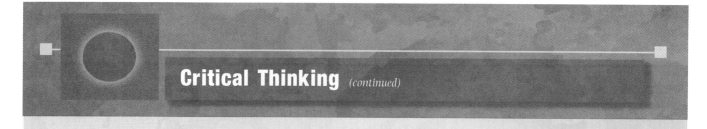

Critical Thinking *(continued)*

6. Define *inflammation*. List four modalities used in OT to decrease inflammation. For each one list three contraindications.

7. Define the role of a bursa. Name three bursae in the body (other than the olecranon bursa) that can become inflamed. Pick one of these and describe the signs, symptoms, and the etiology of the injury.

8. Emma was born with a birth complication diagnosis of Erb's palsy (vaginal delivery, 10 pounds plus birth weight). This BPI affects 1 or 2 infants per 1,000 live births. No other deficits or complications were present at birth. The pediatric neurologist ordered OT to train the mother in PROM and infant development activities. Emma is the youngest of four healthy, active, and bright siblings and the daughter of intelligent parents (lawyer, physician). Activities will include defining terms, supplying resources to the parents and siblings, assessment tools, and treatment ideas. Be prepared to conduct some research to assist you in working with this case study.

Case Study

Erb's Palsy is a relatively rare diagnosis and can be a highly emotional situation for the parents. The uncertainty of the extent of the recovery and resulting impairments, along with possible treatment interventions, including surgery, and limited concrete information about what "will" happen vs. what "may" happen, can contribute to creating this emotional situation. As an OTA, at what point, if at all, do you think you should be therapeutically involved? Why? Would you have a conversation with the pediatric neurologist or pediatric surgeon? What would you say or ask? Imagine a situation in which you are competently and confidently treating the infant (e.g., performing U/E PROM) and the parents walk in and begin to ask you questions to which you do not know the answers. What will your responses be? What will you report to or request from the supervising OT? You see the infant as your client. Are the parents also your clients? How might you document this situation? In this particular case study, the parents are highly educated and experienced in parenting. Anticipate that you react differently to these parents vs. a single parent of a low socioeconomic and educational status, and this infant is a first-born child. Why is that? Is it ethical? Is it in the infant's best interest? Once you have completed the activities and read the "epilogue," would you change any of your perceptions, parental/sibling involvement, or treatment suggestions?

a. What nerves does the BP consist of?

b. In terms of BP, define: Avulsion

                                   Rupture

                                   Praxis/Stretch

                                   Neuroma

c. What neurological features may be present with Erb's palsy? Respectfully mimic this posture and compensatory movements.

d. An evaluation might include assessing infant reflexes and (B) U/E AROM, PROM. What might treatment consist of? To what goal(s)?

e. As the child ages, with improving "spontaneous" recovery (as expected per diagnosis/research), what activities might you recommend to maintain available ROM and strength?

f. In what might a child with 85% recovery *not* be able to excel? Respectfully mimic the movements with minimal residual deficits, and identify compensatory movements to accomplish the task.

(continues)

Critical Thinking *(continued)*

Epilogue

Emma is now 10 years old, excels in soccer, loves math and science, enjoys water slalom skiing (one leg on the single ski and holding onto the ski rope with the other foot!, and performing this "trick" in tandem with her sister!), plays the piano, and wants you to know that she has positive self-esteem and "can do whatever I want to!" Her complications from Erb's palsy were not an issue for Emma and her parents because they did not impact activities she was involved in; therefore, her parents did not initiate a discussion with Emma regarding her left arm movements. Emma did not realize that she had any movement limitations until she was 7 years old. In music class, when asked to perform the movements to the children's song "head, shoulders, knees, and toes," she realized that she could not touch her left shoulder with her left hand as she was able to do so on the right side of her body.

Emma's carrying angle is slightly greater on the left than on the right. Left supination and external rotation are limited, for which she compensates by abducting her shoulder and flexing her elbow in order to complete activities that require left forearm supination (e.g., drinking from a glass held with both hands). Emma was not splinted and received very little therapy because her mother demonstrated extreme competence in carrying out a home program of ROM and developmental activities. All developmental milestones were met with the mother's time line expectations based on the three older children's experiences. Emma was encouraged to crawl (including up the stairs) and, therefore, did not walk until she was a year old, and was encouraged to "keep up with her siblings," both as natural ways to increase and maintain AROM and U/E strength.

Both of Emma's parents were extremely anxious the first few months of her life. She was fussy and appeared to be only comforted when she was held and cuddled; she slept best when held and had great difficulty with comforting herself. This behavior might have indicated some amount of discomfort, again, adding to the parents' anxiety and concern regarding the extent of her BPI. When she was about 3 months old, during bath time, she "sculled" the water with both hands, enjoying her bath time. Her mother then realized that her discomfort was fading, and spontaneous movement was returning.

Both parents wished they had been able to tap into more resources rather than adopt the prevailing attitude of "wait and see." The availability of specialty medical knowledge has increased at significant rates. The Internet sites listed in this chapter did not exist 10 years ago, nor did other research study results. Emma's parents yearned for concrete information and outcome predictions based on empirical science. Not all parents may want such information. This is up to the parents and the OT practitioner and the treatment team should follow the parents' lead in providing information.

Emma is a strong, emotionally stable, vibrant, bright child. Her personality and disposition, including her persistence, has fostered a risk-taking and adventurous attitude and a sense of independence in Emma. She loves her siblings, who readily include her in their activities (by the way, she does a pretty good job of keeping up with them!). Her parents are looking forward to Emma, along with the rest of the children, continuing to thrive in whatever she desires to accomplish.

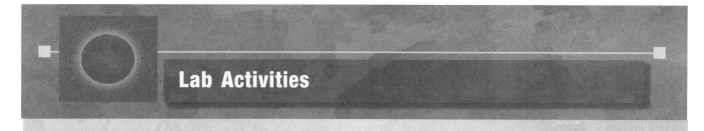

Lab Activities

Lab 19-1: Elbow Fracture

Objectives: To implement a rehabilitation plan for the client with an elbow fracture.

Equipment Needed: A group of three people, pen/pencil, paper, proper clothing

A 10-year-old girl sustains an elbow fracture and her arm is immobilized for 6 weeks. Following the removal of the cast, she presents to OT with her mother. She has a stiff elbow and wrist following immobilization and is reluctant to move her arm. She lives a long way from the clinic and will only be able to attend sporadically for treatment.

Step 1.   Pick one of the characters to role-play, the child, the mother, or the therapist.

Step 2.   Simulate the treatment of the girl with the mother present. The therapist assesses and measures the available ROM of the affected joints.

Step 3.   Demonstrate passive motion of the elbow, radioulnar joints, and wrist to the mother. Explain why you are doing them, the goals of treatment, and recommended frequency of treatment. Make sure the mother is proficient in the treatment.

Step 4.   Switch roles and repeat steps 1 through 3.

Step 5.   Switch roles once again and repeat steps 1 through 3. All members of the group should have the opportunity to role-play each character.

Lab 19-2: Tennis Elbow

Objective: To develop a treatment plan for tennis elbow.

Equipment Needed: A lab partner, pen/pencil, paper, proper clothing

Step 1.   Interview the client presenting with lateral epicondylitis.

Step 2.   Develop a strengthening program for the forearm and elbow muscles.

Step 3.   Teach your partner a strengthening program using different forms of resistance that includes concentric and eccentric activities.

Step 4.   Switch roles and repeat steps 1 through 3.

Chapter 20

THE FOREARM AND WRIST

Key Words

INTRODUCTION

Imagine the multitude of movements that the upper extremity allows us to perform. More specifically, imagine the specific movements, both athletic and functional, that the wrist allows us to perform. The wrist allows us to perform gross motor movements like hitting a tennis ball and throwing a baseball. Conversely, the wrist allows us to perform fine motor movements like typing on a keyboard and sewing a button on a shirt. The complete upper extremity works together to allow movement of the wrist and hand. For example, the shoulder girdle stabilizes the scapula, which, in turn, allows the shoulder joint and elbow to place the arm in a desired position. Once the arm is in a desired position, the wrist allows us stability and even greater hand placement.

Many people feel intimidated by the complexity of the muscles and nerves of the wrist. The aim of this chapter is to simplify some of this complex material and provide an understandable way to learn the muscles, structures and functions of this critical region.

MAJOR LANDMARKS OF THE FOREARM AND WRIST

The wrist consists of the distal ends of the radius proximally and the carpal bones distally. Remember, the ulna is not considered directly a part of the radiocarpal joint but is discussed in this section owing to its relevance to joint stability.

First, the distal radius and ulna provide the concave region for the carpal bones to "fit into" (Figure 20-1). The radius is the shorter bone of the forearm and contains a somewhat pointed structure on the lateral and distal end (assuming anatomic position) called the styloid process. The ulna also contains a styloid process on the distal and medial side assuming anatomical position. Palpate each of these bony prominences on yourself.

To some, the wrist is considered an extremely complex joint. In reality the wrist joint actually is considered as two joints: the **radiocarpal** and the **midcarpal** joints (Figure 20-2). The radiocarpal joint is composed of the distal end of the radius and radioulnar disk proximally and the **scaphoid**, **lunate**, and **triquetrum** bones distally. This synovial joint is further classified as a condyloid joint, with the radius and radioulnar disk forming the concave region and the scaphoid, lunate, and triquetrum bones forming the convex region. This convex-concave relationship allows the individual carpals and the radius and radioulnar disk to slide over the carpals during wrist movement. Notice that the ulna is not considered part of this joint. This is because an articular disk is located between the ulna and proximal row of carpals.

The eight carpal bones provide the convex region of the wrist complex. These eight bones are situated on two rows of four to form the wrist. In the anatomical position, the proximal row of carpals (lateral to medial) contains the scaphoid, lunate, triquetrum, and **pisiform** bones. Interestingly, the scaphoid, lunate, and triquetrum bones have the ability to vary their collective shape to meet the demands of the space between the forearm and hand. The pisiform, though, acts as a sesamoid bone, increasing the mechanical advantage of the tendon of the flexor carpi ulnaris. The distal row of carpals (lateral to medial) contains the **trapezium**, **trapezoid**, **capitate**, and **hamate**. These irregular-shaped bones glide past one another to provide movement at the wrist.

OTA Perspective

Colles' fracture was first described by Abraham Colles in the 19th century and is possibly the most common fracture seen by orthopedic surgeons. The most common cause is a fall on the outstretched hand (FOOSH), especially in elderly women. The fracture involves the radius (and frequently the ulna) just proximal to the wrist joint. The classic presentation is the "dinner fork deformity," with dorsal angulation of the radius. Treatment may involve internal fixation with surgery, or if the displacement is not severe, immobilization for 6 to 8 weeks. Therapy is almost always indicated, once movement is allowed.

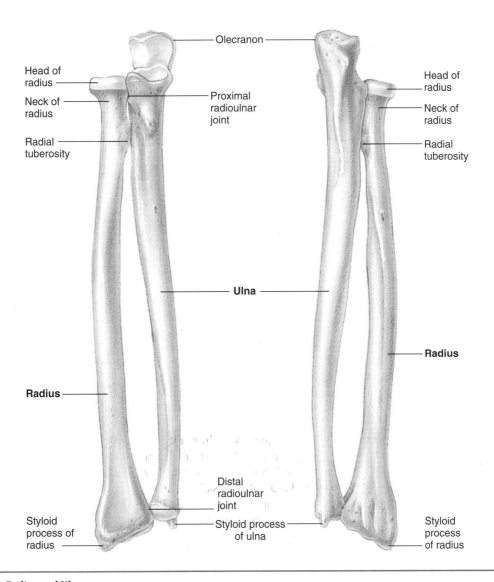

Figure 20-1 *Radius and Ulna*

 NERVOUS INNERVATION

The nerves that innervate the wrist and hand are the terminal branches of the brachial plexus and include the radial, median, and ulnar nerves. Like their names suggest, these nerves track along the radius and ulna specifically with the median nerve tracking superiorly to the **interosseous membrane**. The interosseous membrane is a tough, thin membrane connecting the radius and ulna. The radial nerve branches distally from the posterior cord, the median from the lateral and medial cord, and the ulnar nerve from the medial cord (Figure 20-3). Table 20-1 summarizes the nerves of the wrist and hand.

Table 20-1 *Innervation of the Wrist and Hand*

Nerve	Affected Anterior Muscles	Affected Posterior Muscles
Median	Flexor carpi radialis, palmaris longus	None
Ulnar	Flexor carpi ulnaris	None
Radial	None	Extensor carpi radialis longus, extensor carpi radialis brevis, extensor carpi ulnaris

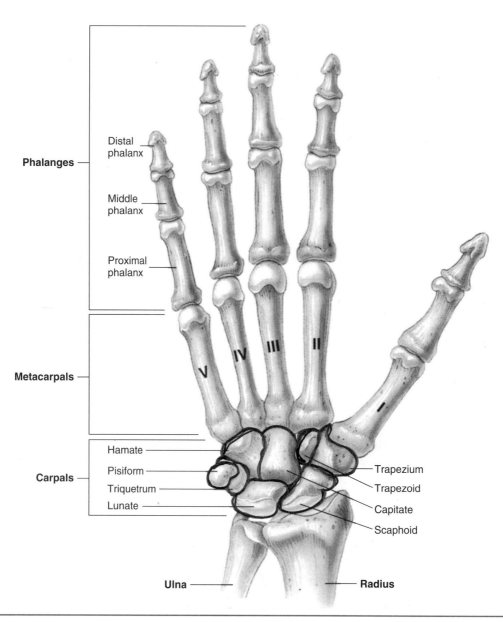

Phalanges
- Distal phalanx
- Middle phalanx
- Proximal phalanx

Metacarpals

Carpals
- Hamate
- Pisiform
- Triquetrum
- Lunate

- Trapezium
- Trapezoid
- Capitate
- Scaphoid

Ulna   **Radius**

Figure 20-2   *Carpal Bones*

MOVEMENT OF THE WRIST

The midcarpal or **intercarpal joint** is composed of the proximal and distal rows of carpal bones. Although these small bones only glide over one another, the joint structures as a whole are essential for the wrist movements.

There are four distinct movements that can occur at the wrist joint. These are wrist flexion, wrist extension that occurs in the sagittal plane around an X-axis, ulnar deviation (adduction), and radial deviation (abduction) occurring in the frontal plane around a sagittal axis. The amount of movement that occurs at the radiocarpal and midcarpal joints during flexion and extension is debated. According to Brunnstrom, the majority of wrist flexion occurs at the radiocarpal joint with a lesser contribution coming from the midcarpal joint (Smith, Weiss, & Lehmkuh, 1996). During wrist extension, Brunstrom claims that most movement occurs at the midcarpal joint with a smaller contribution at the radiocarpal joint. During ulnar deviation, movement mainly occurs at the radiocarpal joint, and during radial deviation, movement mainly occurs at the midcarpal joint. Regardless of the debate, the wrist allows us four extremely important movements. Refer to Table 20-2 to describe the movements, planes, and axis of wrist motion.

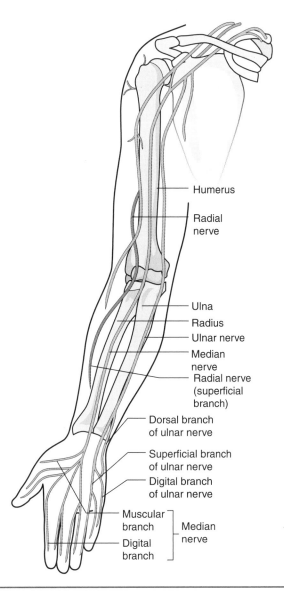

Figure 20-3 *Nerves of the Hand and Wrist*

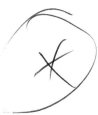

Table 20-2 *Movements of the Wrist*

Motion	Plane	Axis	Description
Flexion	Sagittal	Frontal	Movement of the wrist in the anterior direction
Extension	Sagittal	Frontal	Movement of the wrist in the posterior direction
Radial Deviation	Frontal	Sagittal	Lateral movement of the hand
Ulnar Deviation	Frontal	Sagittal	Medial movement of the hand

STABILITY OF THE WRIST

There are four main ligaments that add stability to the wrist or radiocarpal joint: the **radial** and **ulnar collateral ligaments** and the **palmar** and **dorsal radiocarpal ligaments**.

OTA Perspective

Carpal tunnel syndrome is caused by the compression of the medial nerve as it enters the hand. The median nerve passes under the fibrous flexor retinaculum along with nine tendons, all covered with synovium. Any situation that causes swelling in the tunnel results in compression of the nerve. These situations include pregnancy and repetitive overuse of the flexor tendons. Symptoms include parathesia, and eventually pain, in the median nerve distribution of the palmar aspect of the thumb, index, middle, and possibly half of the ring finger. The patient may also complain of weakness in the fingers and hand. Treatment is aimed at reducing the swelling, maintaining nerve mobility, and preventing recurrence of the condition.

Radiocarpal and Ulnar Collateral Ligaments

The radial collateral ligament (RCL) originates on the radius and inserts on the scaphoid, trapezium, and first metacarpal. The ulnar collateral ligament (UCL) originates on the ulna and passes to the pisiform and triquetrum, where it inserts. The RCL and UCL provide medial and lateral support, respectively.

Palmar and Dorsal Radiocarpal Ligaments

The only major ligament on the posterior side of the wrist is the dorsal radiocarpal ligament. It attaches from the styloid process of the radius to the lunate and triquetrum carpal bones. Although weaker and looser than the palmar radiocarpal ligament, this ligament limits the amount of flexion allowed at the wrist

The palmar radiocarpal ligament is perhaps the most important ligament to wrist stability and function. This strong ligament limits wrist extension and attaches from the anterior portion of the distal radius and ulna to the anterior surface of the scaphoid, lunate, and triquetrum carpal bones. Because many activities occur when the wrist is extended, it has a greater probability of being sprained or injured.

OTA Perspective

As you know, the four wrist movements are flexion and extension, both in the sagittal plane around a frontal axis, and ulnar deviation (adduction) and radial deviation (abduction), both in the frontal plane around a sagittal axis. Another wrist action is "wrist tenodesis," which is the reciprocal motion of the wrist and digits that occurs during active or passive wrist flexion and extension. While the wrist is being extended, the fingers flex; when the wrist is moving into flexion, the fingers extend. In part, this occurs because the intrinsic finger muscles and tendon units have a fixed resting length. It is important to keep this tenodesis action in mind when assisting with ROM and splinting with a client with a wrist injury. Try it: relax your fingers and flex your wrist, then extend your wrist. Did you notice the automatic extension and then flexion of your fingers?

Palmar Aponeurosis

The palmar fascia, or **palmar aponeurosis**, also has importance to wrist function. It is a somewhat thick band of fascia located superficially over the palmar side of the hand. From a muscular standpoint, the palmar aponeurosis is the distal attachment of the palmaris longus muscle. In addition, this fascia covers the tendons of the extrinsic wrist muscles and provides some protection to the deeper structures of the hand.

 MUSCLES OF THE FOREARM AND WRIST

Once again, consider the variety of movements that our hand allows us to accomplish. We can grasp a barbell with a variety of resistances, snap our fingers to the beat of a song, and even thread a needle. Interestingly, many of the muscles that provide function to our wrist and fingers are located proximal to the wrist joint. These muscles are called extrinsic muscles. By definition, extrinsic muscles have their origin proximal to the wrist, cross the wrist, and may even have an action at the fingers. Consider the importance of this arrangement. If all of the muscles that operate the wrist and fingers originated intrinsically, or distal to the wrist, we would have enormous muscle mass within our hand. This would be counterproductive for some of the fine motor movements that are essential to human movement. On the contrary, we have the bulk of muscle mass in the forearm region, and the muscle tendons operate our wrist and fingers like strings on a puppet.

This chapter discusses the specific muscles that exert their main action at the wrist. Although these muscles cross the elbow, their contribution to elbow flexion or extension is negligible. Before starting this discussion of the wrist muscles, it is imperative that students understand certain terminology pertaining to the wrist. By understanding the meaning of the following terms or prefixes, students seem to develop a better appreciation for learning the muscles of the wrist.

The following terms should be studied and memorized: **carpi**, **radi**, **ulnar**, longus, and brevis. Carpi is used to describe the wrist region (i.e., carpals). Radi is used to describe proximity or relation to the radius bone. Similarly, ulnar describes proximity or relation to the ulnar bone. Longus implies "long." Brevis implies "short." Comprehending these terms will assist you in the learning process of the wrist and hand muscles. Many times the name of a muscle can tell something about the muscle's location or action. For example, flexor carpi radialis is a wrist flexor that inserts near the radius side of the forearm.

Anterior Muscles of the Forearm

The anterior muscles of the forearm share a common origin on the medial epicondyle and track toward the hand along the anterior surface of the forearm. Additionally, the median nerve innervates the muscles. The muscles of the anterior forearm include the flexor carpi radialis, flexor carpi ulnaris, and palmaris longus.

OTA Perspective

Numerous injuries and illnesses may affect forearm and wrist function—strength, ROM, coordination, and participation in occupational performance (functional activities). These common diagnoses may include hemiparesis from a CVA or TBI; carpal tunnel syndrome (a median nerve injury at the wrist, which is a nerve compression syndrome of a cumulative trauma disorder); rheumatoid arthritis or osteoarthritis; Colles' fracture (a distal radius fracture); below elbow amputation (BEA); wrist drop (a common term for a radial nerve injury); or trauma (e.g., deep laceration).

Initial treatments may include surgery, immobilization through use of external fixators, casting, static or dynamic splinting, or prosthetic devices, followed up by restoration of physical capacities. Surgeons, physicians, and individual facilities may have policies and protocols for rehabilitation for the specific diagnosis.

Flexor Carpi Radialis The **flexor carpi radialis** tracks diagonally from the medial epicondyle to the base of the second and third metacarpals (Figure 20-4). It is located on the anterior side of the forearm. This muscle acts as an agonist for wrist flexion and radial deviation. As with all of the wrist muscles, it is easier to palpate the tendinous insertion rather than the origin. It can be palpated on the anterior side of the forearm in line with the second and third metacarpals.

Name:	Flexor Carpi Radialis
O:	Medial epicondyle of the humerus
I:	Second and third metacarpal bones
A:	Wrist flexion and radial deviation
N:	Median nerve
P:	In line with the second and third metacarpals, slightly lateral and on the anterior surface of the forearm

Flexor Carpi Ulnaris The **flexor carpi ulnaris** muscle lies on the anteromedial side adjacent to the ulna, as its name implies (Figure 20-5). It is an agonist in wrist flexion and is one of two muscles to cause ulnar deviation. This muscle can be palpated just inferior to the medial epicondyle and running distally toward the wrist.

Name:	Flexor Carpi Ulnaris
O:	Medial epicondyle of the humerus
I:	Pisiform, hamate, and fifth netacarpal bone
A:	Wrist flexion and ulnar deviation
N:	Ulnar nerve
P:	Anterior and medial surface of the forearm, just below the medial epicondyle, running distally to the wrist

Palmaris Longus Although the **palmaris longus** muscle originates medially, it runs centrally down the anterior side of the forearm (Figure 20-6). This muscle only performs wrist flexion. It can be palpated at the origin near the anteromedial aspect of the forearm and centrally near the insertion just proximal to the wrist.

Name:	Palmaris Longus
O:	Medial epicondyle of the humerus
I:	Third metacarpal bone and the palmar aponeurosis
A:	Wrist flexion
N:	Median nerve
P:	Anteromedial aspect of the forearm, running down the center of the wrist

Posterior Muscles of the Forearm

The posterior muscles of the forearm share a common origin on the lateral epicondyle and supracondylar ridge and track toward the hand along the anterior surface of the forearm. Additionally, the muscles are innervated by the radial nerve. The muscles of the posterior forearm include the extensor carpi radialis longus, extensor carpi radialis brevis, and extensor carpi ulnaris.

Extensor Carpi Radialis Longus The **extensor carpi radialis longus** muscle, as with all of the wrist extensors, is located on the posterior side of the forearm (Figure 20-7). It is a very powerful extensor of the wrist, especially when the forearm is pronated. It can be palpated on the posterior aspect of the forearm from the lateral epicondyle, running distally in line with the second metacarpal.

Name:	Extensor Carpi Radialis Longus
O:	Lateral epicondyle
I:	Second metacarpal bone (posterior surface)
A:	Wrist extension and radial deviation
N:	Radial nerve
P:	In line with the second metacarpal on the posterior aspect of the forearm

Extensor Carpi Radialis Brevis The **extensor carpi radialis brevis** muscle is located on the posterior side of the forearm (Figure 20-8). This muscle, in combination with extensor carpi radialis longus, makes up the majority of the wrist

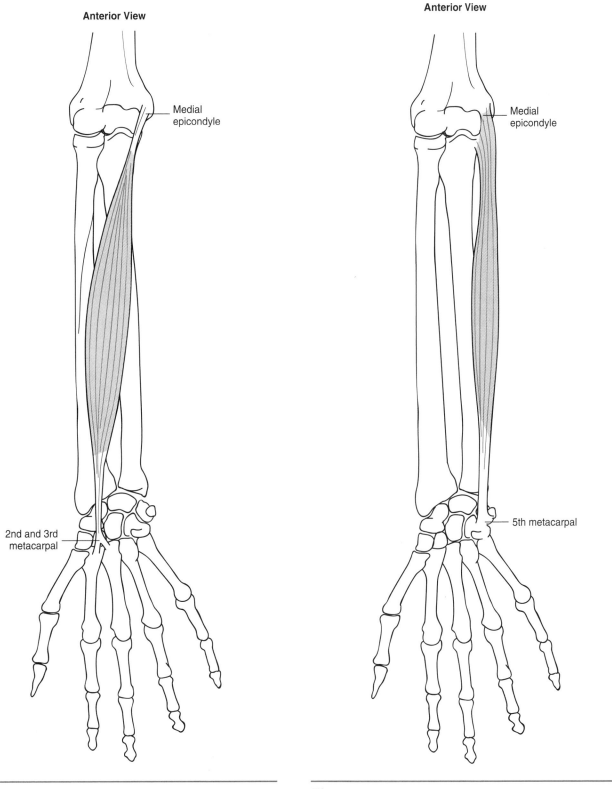

Figure 20-4 *Flexor Carpi Radialis*   **Figure 20-5** *Flexor Carpi Ulnaris*

extensor mass. It acts as an agonist for wrist extension, as its name implies. It also works concurrently with the extensor carpi radialis longus and flexor carpi radialis to cause radial deviation. The tendon of the extensor carpi radialis brevis is difficult to identify but may be palpated when the wrist is tightly closed, in line with the third metacarpal on the posterior surface of the hand.

Name: Extensor Carpi Radialis Brevis

O: Lateral epicondyle

I: Third metacarpal (posterior surface)

A: Wrist extension

N: Radial nerve

P: Difficult to palpate

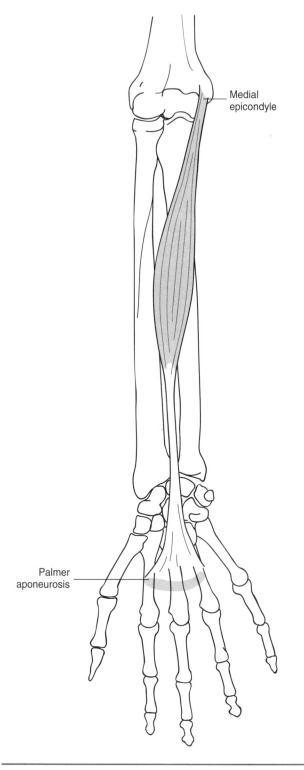

Figure 20-6 *Palmaris Longus*

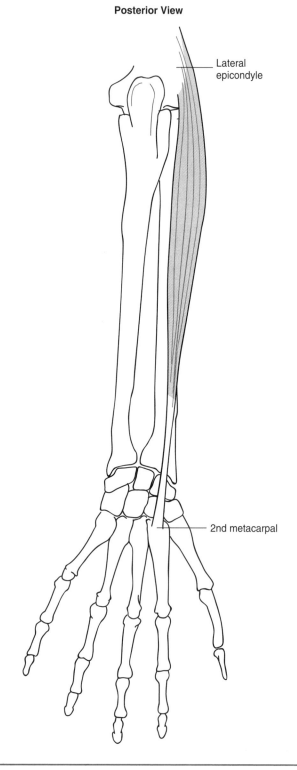

Figure 20-7 *Extensor Carpi Radialis Longus*

Extensor Carpi Ulnaris The **extensor carpi ulnaris** muscle crosses diagonally from the lateral epicondyle to the base of the fifth metacarpal bone (Figure 20-9). It causes extension of the wrist and works synergistically with the flexor carpi ulnaris to cause ulnar deviation. This muscle can be palpated about 2 inches inferior to the lateral epicondyle of the humerus. The tendon may then be followed distally toward the head of the ulna.

Name: Extensor Carpi Ulnaris

O: Lateral epicondyle

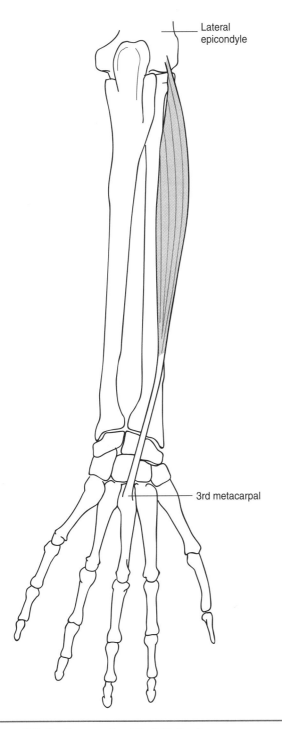

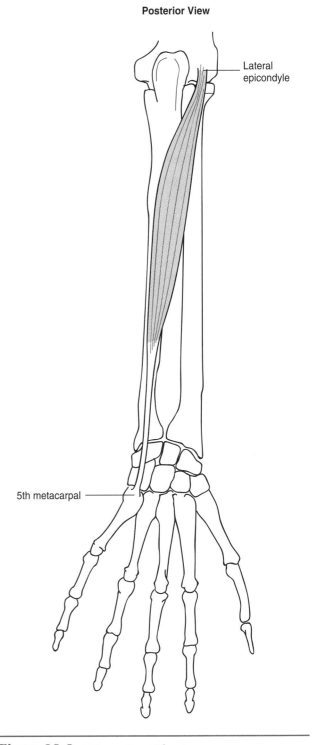

Figure 20-8 *Extensor Carpi Radialis Brevis*   **Figure 20-9** *Extensor Carpi Ulnaris*

I: Fifth metacarpal bone

A: Wrist extension and ulnar deviation

N: Radial nerve

P: Just inferior to the lateral epicondyle of the humerus

COMMON IDENTIFICATION COMPONENTS OF THE WRIST

Students often find it helpful to learn the similarities of various muscle groups. Let us look at the muscles of the wrist and identify some similarities. After studying the wrist muscles, we can make some general assumptions. First, all of the wrist flexors lie on the anterior side of the forearm and originate from the medial epicondyle of the humerus. The wrist flexors also all cause wrist flexion, with some providing assistance for radial or ulnar deviation.

The wrist extensors all lie on the posterior aspect of the forearm. In addition, they also originate from the lateral epicondyle of the humerus. All of the wrist extensors cause wrist extension, and some contribute to radial or ulnar deviation. Use Table 20-3 to assist in understanding these similarities.

Table 20-3 *Similarities in Muscles of the Wrist*

Muscle	Action	Origin	Nerve
Flexor Carpi Radialis	Wrist flexion, radial deviation	Medial epicondyle	Median
Flexor Carpi Ulnaris	Wrist flexion, ulnar deviation	Medial epicondyle	Ulnar
Palmaris Longus	Wrist flexion	Medial epicondyle	Median
Extensor Carpi Radialis Longus	Wrist extension, radial deviation	Lateral epicondyle	Radial
Extensor Carpi Radialis Brevis	Wrist extension	Lateral epicondyle	Radial
Extensor Carpi Ulnaris	Wrist extension, ulnar deviation	Lateral epicondyle	Radial

KEY CONCEPTS

■ Wrist flexion and extension and radial and ulnar deviation are the movements that can occur at the wrist. Students should be able to describe and demonstrate these motions.

■ The main joint of the wrist complex is the radiocarpal joint. The ulna is not considered part of this joint because the articular disk that adjoins the ulna and carpal bones interferes with the direct articulation of the ulna and carpals. The midcarpal joint also contributes to wrist movement, with the carpal bones gliding over one another. The major ligaments that comprise the wrist joint include the radial and ulnar collateral ligaments, the dorsal and palmar radiocarpal ligaments, and the palmar aponeurosis.

■ Use Table 20-3 to gain a deep understanding of the muscles that operate the wrist and forearm as well as their origins, insertions, actions, and innervations.

■ From an anatomical standpoint, the forearm musculature is conveniently divided. The wrist flexor musculature is on the anterior side of the forearm, whereas the wrist extensor musculature lies posteriorly. The anterior musculature originates on the medial epicondyle and is innervated by the median nerve. Conversely, the posterior musculature originates on the lateral epicondyle and is innervated by the radial nerve. Because the wrist muscles lie extrinsically, or proximal to the wrist, we have the ability to perform gross motor tasks as well as fine motor skills.

BIBLIOGRAPHY

Hall-Craggs, E. (1990). *Anatomy as a basis for clinical medicine* (2nd ed.). Baltimore: Urban and Schwarzenberg.

Norkin, C. C., & Levangie, P. K. (2001). *Joint structure and function: A comprehensive analysis* (3rd ed.). Philadelphia: F. A. Davis.

Smith, L. K., Weiss, E. L., & Lehmkuhl, L. (1996). *Brunnstrom's clinical kinesiology* (5th ed.). Philadelphia: F. A. Davis.

Thompson, C. W., & Floyd, R. T. (2001). *Manual of structural kinesiology* (14th ed.). St. Louis, MO: Mosby.

WEB RESOURCES

- Go to www.physsportsmed.com/issues/aug_96.gutierez.htm, a site that features an article about scaphoid fractures.
- The site www.wristfracture.co.uk/treatments.htm features the etiology, signs and symptoms, diagnostic tests, and treatment modalities for wrist fractures.
- Another site that features the etiology, signs and symptoms, diagnostic tests, and treatment modalities for wrist fractures is www.ctsplace.com.

(These Web addresses were current as of February 2004.)

REVIEW QUESTIONS

Fill in the Blank

Provide the word(s) or phrase(s) that best completes the sentence.

1. In general, the wrist flexors originate on the _____ epicondyle.

2. The _____ nerve innervates each of the wrist extensors.

3. The possible movements at the wrist include _____, _____, _____, and _____.

4. In general, the wrist extensors are located on the _____ side of the forearm.

5. The extensor carpi ulnaris performs _____ and _____.

Multiple Choice

Select the best answer to complete the following statements.

1. The palmar aponeurosis is the insertion point for the _____ muscle.
   a. extensor carpi radialis
   b. flexor carpi radialis
   c. palmaris longus
   d. flexor carpi ulnaris

2. The flexor carpi ulnaris is innervated by the _____ nerve.
   a. median
   b. ulnar
   c. radial
   d. musculocutaneous

3. From the anatomical position, radial deviation moves the wrist in the _____ direction.
   a. posterior
   b. anterior
   c. medial
   d. lateral

4. Of the following structures the _____ is quite often sprained.
   a. palmar radiocarpal ligament
   b. dorsal radiocarpal ligament
   c. ulnar collateral ligament
   d. radial collateral ligament

5. The wrist flexors are primarily innervated by the _____ nerve.
   a. radial
   b. median
   c. ulnar
   d. femoral

Matching

Match each of the following descriptions with the appropriate term.

_____ **1.** Also called the palmar fascia

_____ **2.** Generally innervates the posterior forearm muscles

_____ **3.** From the anatomical position, a lateral movement of the wrist

_____ **4.** Generally innervates the anterior forearm muscles

_____ **5.** From the anatomical position, a medial movement of the wrist

A. Ulnar deviation

B. Radial deviation

C. Median nerve

D. Radial nerve

E. Palmar aponeurosis

Critical Thinking

1. If your client had a damaged radial nerve, what actions of the elbow and radioulnar joints would be affected?

2. If your client had a damaged median nerve, what actions of the elbow and wrist joints would be affected?

3. Research the following tests related to carpal tunnel:

   a. Tinel's test

   b. Phalen's test

   Your patient is a 40-year-old female whose job involves data entry on the computer and who has been recently diagnosed with carpal tunnel syndrome. Describe the advice you would give her to minimize her symptoms. Research the correct ergonomic position that she should use at her desk when using her computer or the telephone.

4. The treatment of carpal tunnel includes reducing the swelling at the radiocarpal joint. List the modalities that you would use and justify their use and their effects.

5. Research four possible complications of a Colles' fracture, listing signs or symptoms for each of these.

6. A typical OT evaluation includes a chart review and an interview. The OT is searching for information that may assist in choosing which assessments to use, what the appropriate goals may be, what the "prior (to the injury, to the hospitalization, or to the OT evaluation) functional status" was, who the client's support system is, and what the discharge plans are. It might be obvious in the case of an elderly client who is living alone and was just diagnosed with hemiplegia, that a more thorough chart review and interview are indicated. Is this the case with other wrist/forearm diagnoses? What information might be necessary for a 40-year-old with a cumulative trauma diagnosis that is likely not necessary for a 10-year-old with a Colles' fracture? Besides the primary diagnosis, what other information seems necessary? And what information might be secondary? Quickly being able to assess the situation, ruling in and out what is pertinent, is vital given the "business of health care" and funding constraints. Learning how to do this, through practice and discussion or reflection with an experienced practitioner, contributes to the process of developing clinical reasoning.

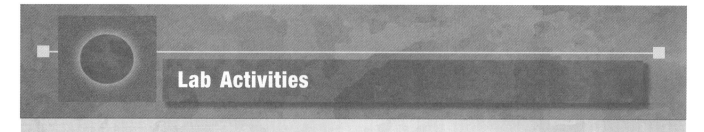

Lab Activities

Lab 20-1: Strengthening the Wrist

Objective: To develop treatment plans and therapies for strengthening the wrist.

Equipment Needed: A lab partner, preferably an OT lab, some hand weights, pencil and paper

Step 1.   Demonstrate various ways to strengthen the wrist extensors and flexors using a variety of methods and equipment.

Step 2.   Record these methods and keep in an accessible place to use for your repertoire of strengthening and rehabilitation exercises.

Lab 20-2: Assessment of Wrist Function

Objective: To evaluate and assess wrist function.

Equipment Needed: A lab partner, pencil and paper

Step 1.   Identify two tasks of daily living that involve the wrist or forearm (e.g., writing a note, typing, etc.).

Step 2.   have your partner mimic the motion to the best of his or her ability.

Step 3.   Identify the specific muscles being utilized during these activities and what actions they are performing.

Step 4.   Have your partner perform a different activity and repeat the process with you identifying the muscles being used and the muscle actions (wrist extension, wrist flexion, radial or ulnar deviation) involved.

Lab 20-3: Colles' Fracture

Objective: To properly assess and prepare an exercise program for an individual recovering from a Colles' fracture.

Equipment Needed: A lab partner, pen/pencil, paper

Your partner sustained a Colles' fracture 6 weeks ago and had the cast removed yesterday.

Step 1.   Describe the condition of the forearm.

Step 2.   Measure ROM of the wrist, hand, and elbow.

Step 3.   Prescribe an exercise program for this stage of the rehabilitation. Also instruct your partner in ways to help with the swelling, pain, and skin condition at home.

Your partner is now 4 weeks post cast removal.

Step 4.   Test the strength of the forearm and hand.

Step 5.   Prescribe and demonstrate an exercise program of at least six exercises for this stage of the rehabilitation. Include functional activities that the patient can do at home.

Step 6.   Switch roles and repeat steps 1 through 5.

Lab 20-4: Forearm/Wrist Immobilization

Objective: To compare and contrast functional abilities with and without a wrist injury; and to gain empathy for clients with a wrist injury by role-playing the ADL with an imagined injury.

Equipment Needed: A lab partner; pen and paper for writing reaction paper; ace wrap, casting materials, or long forearm cock-up splint for immobilization

Step 1.   Have your partner assist you to immobilize the dominant forearm/wrist.

Step 2.   Proceed with several daily ADL (e.g., writing, typing on a keyboard, using a key to unlock the door, drying dishes, etc.), receiving assistance from the partner as necessary.

(continues)

Lab Activities *(continued)*

Step 3. Write a reaction paper, answering the following questions. Keep in mind that the only change was immobilization (pain and strength were not contributing factors in the students' experiences). Did you choose relatively easy ADL? Those you were accustomed to doing, or those you only participate in occasionally? How did you compensate? Did "success" with the task require a "trial-and-error" method? What compensatory method(s) was effective, but not efficient, or potentially unsafe? Was there a task that you could not independently complete? How might this experience assist you in treating clients with forearm/wrist injuries?

Lab 20-5: Forearm/Wrist Injury

Objective: To increase a comprehensive understanding of a forearm/wrist injury, incorporating research, assessments, and treatment ideas, within a role-play situation.

Equipment Needed: A lab partner; resource books; pen and paper for writing a case study and reaction paper; common ADL equipment

Step 1. With a partner, choose one of the diagnoses mentioned in the OTA Perspective boxes. Research the diagnosis as necessary.

Step 2. Create a simple case study. Include age, vocation, hobbies, and the like. If needed, use the *Occupational Therapy Practice Framework* to assist you in designing the case study.

Step 3. Following an initial OT evaluation consisting of ROM, coordination, and strength testing, the occupational therapist requests that you, the OTA, complete the PADL assessment.

Step 4. Which ADL areas might you assess first? Why? Does your ADL assessment take the physical capacities findings into account? And what do you expect the outcome to be?

    a. Will you recommend treatment to follow a top-down approach or a bottom-up approach? Why?

    b. What goals and treatment ideas will you propose to the occupational therapist? Role-play (1) one ADL assessment; (2) conversation between the occupational therapist and the OTA; and (3) one intervention idea.

Step 5. Write a reaction paper or a summary paper of this experience.

Chapter 21

THE HAND

Objectives

Upon completion of this chapter, the reader should be able to:

- Describe the various nerve innervations of the hand muscles.

- Describe the differences between extrinsic and intrinsic muscles.

- Identify the differences between thenar, hypothenar, and deep palm muscles.

- Perform the specific motions for digits 2–5.

- Perform and describe the specific motions of the thumb.

- Describe the actions of each of the muscles listed in this chapter.

Key Words

abductor digiti minimi
abductor pollicis brevis
abductor pollicis longus
adductor pollicis
carpometacarpal
deep palm muscle
distal interphalangeal
extensor digiti minimi
extensor digitorum
extensor hood
extensor indicis

extensor pollicis brevis
extensor pollicis longus
extensor retinaculum
extrinsic muscle
flexor digiti minimi
flexor digitorum profundus
flexor digitorum
   superficialis
flexor pollicis brevis
flexor pollicis longus
hypothenar muscle

interossei muscle
intrinsic muscle
lumbricals
metacarpal phalangeal
midpalm muscle
opponens digiti minimi
opponens pollicis
phalanges
proximal interphalangeal
thenar muscle

INTRODUCTION

After reading the previous chapters, you must realize the dependency that each upper extremity link (shoulder girdle, shoulder joint, elbow joint, wrist) has with one another. The hand is the distal and final link in the ever so important upper extremity open kinetic chain. This terminal point, the hand, allows us to perform fine motor skills such as playing a guitar, throwing darts, and grasping a needle. Conversely, the hand is powerful enough to squeeze over 50 pounds, hold a bowling ball, and carry a suitcase.

The hand consists of five digits: four fingers and the thumb. The fingers and the thumb are discussed separately in this chapter. Although they are similar in some aspects, they have profound differences that deserve special attention. The focus of this chapter is to provide a clear breakdown of the various joints of the hand and fingers, demonstrate and list the differences between the intrinsic and extrinsic muscles of the hand, and realize the simplistic nervous innervation of these specific muscles.

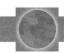

MAJOR LANDMARKS OF THE HAND

The hand involves all of the carpal bones, the metacarpal bones, and the proximal. medial, and distal **phalanges** (Figure 21-1). The most proximal group of bones is the carpal bones. The two rows of four bones include the scaphoid, lunate, triquetrum, pisiform, trapezoid, trapezium, capitate, and hamate. The structure of these bones are discussed in Chapter 20. Moving distally, the fingers and thumb each consist of a long metacarpal bone. The rounded distal end of this bone forms the knuckle portion of the hand. Moving distally once again, the digits 2–5 each have a proximal, middle, and distal plalanx or bone. Interestingly, the thumb, digit 1, only contains a proximal phalanx and a distal phalanx.

NERVOUS INNERVATION

The nerves that innervate the hand are the terminal nerves of the brachial plexus: the radial, median, and ulnar nerves. As their names suggest, these nerves track along the radius and ulna specifically with the median nerve tracking superior to the interosseous membrane. The radial nerve branches distally from the posterior cord, the median nerve from the lateral and medial cord, and the ulnar nerve from the medial cord. Table 21-1 summarizes the nerves innervating the hand.

OTA Perspective

A fracture of the scaphoid is usually caused by hyperextension of the wrist and often occurs at the "waist" of the scaphoid. The physical signs are tenderness and swelling in the anatomical snuffbox. The fracture is often missed, so radiographs are taken. However, if the radiographs are negative initially, they should be repeated at 10 days if there is still suspicion of a fracture. After 10 days the fracture may well be seen. The fracture is immobilized for 10 weeks. Nonunion of the fracture can occur owing to poor blood supply; then internal fixation with a screw may be necessary.

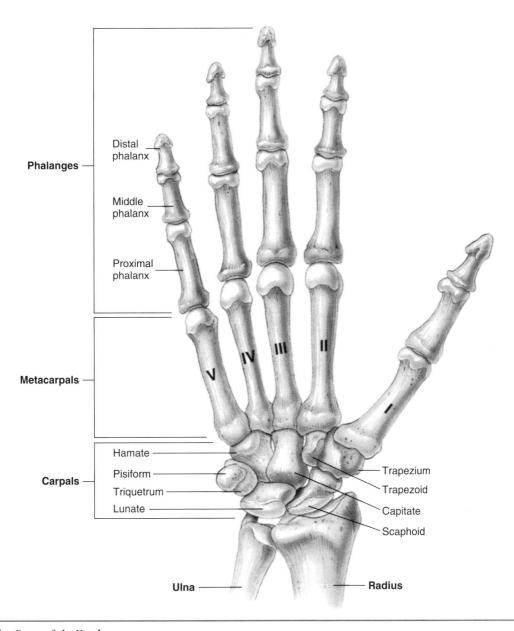

Phalanges
- Distal phalanx
- Middle phalanx
- Proximal phalanx

Metacarpals

Carpals
- Hamate
- Pisiform
- Triquetrum
- Lunate
- Trapezium
- Trapezoid
- Capitate
- Scaphoid

Ulna   **Radius**

Figure 21-1 *Bones of the Hand*

Table 21-1 *Innervation of the Hand*

Nerve	Affected Anterior Muscles	Affected Posterior Muscles
Median	Flexor digitorum superficialis, flexor digitorum profundus (digits 2–3), flexor pollicis longus, flexor pollicis brevis, abductor pollicis brevis, opponens pollicis, first and second lumbricals	None
Radial	None	Extensor digitorum, extensor digiti minimi, extensor indicis, abductor pollicis longus, extensor pollicis brevis, extensor pollicis longus
Ulnar	Flexor digitorum profundus (digits 4–5), abductor pollicis longus, abductor pollicis brevis, flexor digiti minimi, abductor digiti minimi, opponens digiti minimi, palmar interossei, third and fourth lumbricals	Dorsal interossei

MOVEMENT OF THE HAND

The movement of the hand is divided into movements of digits 2–5 and the movements of thumb or digit number 1. Digits 2–5 are more commonly referred to as the index, middle, ring, and pinky fingers respectively. There is a distinct difference between the movements of the fingers and thumb, thus the need for a completely separate discussion.

Digits 2–5 consist of four joints that are listed as follows proximally to distally: **carpometacarpal** (CMC), **metacarpal phalangeal** (MCP), **proximal interphalangeal** (PIP), and the **distal interphalangeal** (DIP) (Figure 21-2).

Carpometacarpal Joint

The CMC joint describes the articulations between the distal row of carpals (trapezoid, trapezium, capitate, hamate) and the bones of fingers II-V. These non-axial joints provide stability to the hand, yet contributes limited flexion and extension of digits 2–4 and flexion, extension, and a slight amount of opposition at digit 5, or the pinky. In addition, the range of motion at the CMC joint increases from the radius side to the ulnar side.

Metacarpal Phalangeal Joint

Moving distally, the next joint to discuss is the metacarpal phalangeal joint (MCP). This joint describes the rounded heads of the metacarpals articulating with the base of the proximal phalanges. These bones have a convex-concave relationship and are commonly referred to as the "knuckles" of the hand. The movements that can occur at this joint are flexion, extension, abduction, and adduction. During abduction and adduction, the middle finger (digit 3) is used as the reference point. On abduction, digits 2, 4, and 5 move away from the middle finger. Conversely, adduction requires those digits to return toward the middle finger.

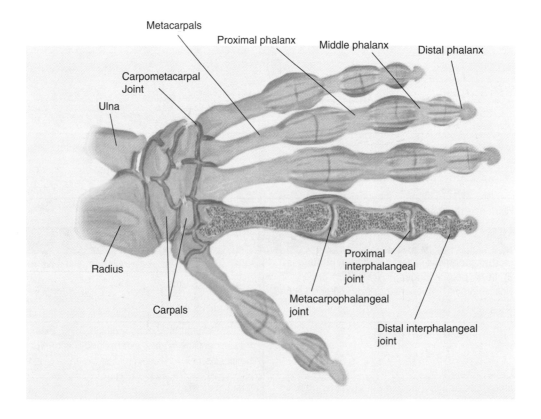

Figure 21-2   *Carpometacarpal Joint*

Proximal Interphalangeal Joint

The proximal interphalangeal joints (PIP) are uniaxial hinge joints that allow flexion and extension. The head of the proximal phalanx and the base of the middle phalanx compose this joint.

Distal Interphalangeal Joint

The distal interphalangeal joints (DIP) are uniaxial hinge joints similar to the PIP joints. They only allow flexion and extension and are composed of the head of the middle phalanx articulating with the base of the distal phalanx.

Thumb

The thumb, or digit 1, has some similarities to the other digits. But because of its own uniqueness it is discussed separately. First, the thumb only consists of three joints instead of the usual four joints that the other digits have. The thumb has a CMC, an MCP, and only one interphalangeal (IP) joint. Second, the thumb can flex, extend, abduct, adduct, and also go through opposition. These motions are discussed later.

Carpometacarpal Joint of the Thumb The CMC joint of the thumb refers to the trapezium bone articulating with the first metacarpal bone (Figure 21-3). This saddle joint allows all five motions of the thumb—flexion, extension, abduction, adduction, and opposition. To understand these motions, use a person standing in the anatomic position as a reference. Flexion occurs in the frontal plane where the thumb sweeps across the palm of the hand. Extension also occurs in the frontal plane with the thumb performing a sweeping motion away from the palm of the hand. Abduction of the thumb occurs in the sagittal plane and takes the thumb "away" from the body. Adduction of the thumb brings the thumb toward the hand. The important action of opposition describes the tip of the thumb moving toward the tips of the fingers, or digits 2–5.

Table 21-2 *Movement of the Hand*

Motion	Plane	Axis	Description
Finger Flexion	Sagittal	Frontal	Moving the finger toward the palm
Finger Extension	Sagittal	Frontal	Return from flexion
Finger Abduction	Frontal	Sagittal	Movement of fingers away from digit 3
Finger Adduction	Frontal	Sagittal	Movement of fingers closer to digit 3
Thumb Flexion	Frontal	Sagittal	Sweeping motion across the palm
Thumb Extension	Frontal	Sagittal	Return to the anatomical position from flexion
Thumb Abduction	Sagittal	Frontal	Movement of the thumb away from palm in the sagittal plane
Thumb Adduction	Sagittal	Frontal	Movement of the thumb toward the palm in the sagittal plane
Opposition	Nonlinear	N/A	Movement of the pollicis toward the digiti minimi
Reposition	Nonlinear	N/A	Return to the anatomical position from opposition

Metacarpal Phalangeal Joint of the Thumb The metacarpal phalangeal joint of the thumb describes the articulation of the head of the first metacarpal and the base of the proximal phalanx. The MCP joint of the thumb allows added range of motion of the thumb in opposition and assists the thumb in grasping objects.

Interphalangeal Joint of the Thumb The IP joint of the thumb describes the articulation of the head of the proximal phalanx and the base of the distal phalanx. The motions occurring at this joint are very similar to the other IP joints of digits 2–5. Table 21-2 summarizes movement in the hand.

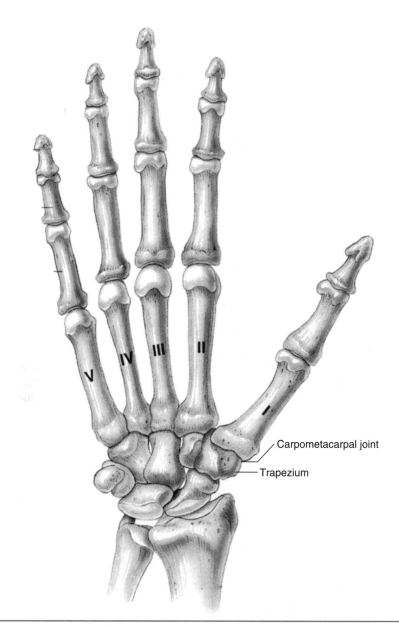

Figure 21-3 *Carpometacarpal Joint of the Thumb*

 STABILITY OF THE HAND

Take a moment to look at your hand and think about the complexity of the arrangement of ligaments, nerves, and muscles. It is amazing to imagine the endless amount of daily tasks our hands allow us to perform and with such great strength and precision. Although there are many ligaments and structures within the hand, only the flexor retinaculum and extensor retinaculum are discussed here.

Flexor Retinaculum

The flexor retinaculum is a band of connective tissue crossing the wrist and hand on the anterior side of the hand (Figure 21-4). This band of connective tissue consists of two ligaments: the palmar carpal and transverse carpal. Superficially, the palmar carpal ligament crosses over the finger flexor tendons. Owing to its superficial location, it acts to contain the finger flexor tendons close to the hand during wrist flexion. The transverse carpal ligament "arches" over the carpal bones, forming somewhat of a tunnel for the median nerve and finger flexors to pass through. This structure has clinical significance because of its contribution to carpal tunnel syndrome. At times, this ligament is cut to relieve the symptoms of this condition.

Extensor Retinaculum

The **extensor retinaculum** is a similar band of connective tissue crossing the wrist on the posterior side (Figure 21-5). The extensor retinaculum has a comparable function to that of its anterior counterpart in that it contains the extensor finger tendons close to the hand during wrist extension.

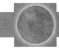 ## MUSCLES OF THE HAND

The following discussion of the hand muscles is divided into the extrinsic muscles and the intrinsic muscles of the hand. The **extrinsic muscles** originate proximally to the carpal bones and exert their influence on hand movement through long tendons. Because these muscles cross the wrist, they have an assistive action at the wrist but have the majority of action on the fingers. These muscles operate the fingers through long tendons, similar to strings of a puppet. Anatomically, this design is ideal for the performance of fine motor skills. The extrinsic muscles on the anterior side of the arm are the flexor digitorum superficialis, flexor digitorum profundus, and flexor pollicis longus. The posterior extrinsic muscles are the extensor digitorum, extensor digiti minimi, extensor indicis, extensor pollicis longus, extensor pollicis brevis, and abductor pollicis longus.

The **intrinsic muscles** are generally smaller and originate within the hand. In other words, their origin is distal to the carpal bones. These muscles assist with fine motor skills and specific movements of the hand. The intrinsic muscles are divided into three groups: **thenar**, **hypothenar**, and **midpalm** or **deep palm muscles**. The thenar muscles are the small muscles that act specifically on the thumb. The hypothenar muscles exert their action mainly on digit 5, or the pinky. Lastly, the midpalm or deep palm muscles are deep within the hand and between the thenar and hypothenar muscles.

Extrinsic Muscle Group

The extrinsic muscles of the hand have long tendons, with the belly located in the forearm region. These muscles aid in the fine motor movements of the fingers.

Anterior Muscles The muscles that act on the anterior surface of the hand are innervated by the median nerve and assist in wrist flexion movements. However, their primary actions are to cause flexion of the digits (2–5) and the pollicis muscle.

Flexor Digitorum Superficialis. The **flexor digitorum superficialis** muscle has a large muscle belly and its tendons extend to digits 2–5 (Figure 21-6). Near the insertion point, the tendons split to insert at the middle phalanges of the fingers. As with all wrist or finger flexors, it lies on the anterior side of the forearm. Because the flexor digitorum superficialis crosses the wrist, it assists in wrist flexion, but, more importantly, it is one of two main finger flexors. It can be palpated on the

OTA PERSPECTIVE

De Quervain's tenosynovitis involves an inflammation of the tendon sheaths of the extensor pollicis brevis and the abductor pollicis longus muscles. The tendons pass under a tight fibrous band just proximal to the radial styloid process, and repeated stress can cause inflammation in this area. Swelling may be seen over the tendons, and movements of the thumb can be painful. Finklestein's test will be positive. Ask the patient to grasp the thumb with the other fingers, then deviate the wrist ulnarly and the symptoms will be reproduced. The inflammation is usually caused by repetitive activities involving the thumb. Treatment includes anti-inflammatory modalities.

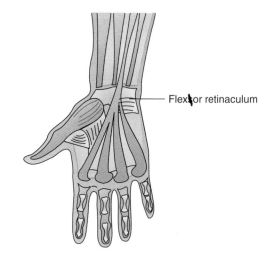

Figure 21-4 *Flexor Retinaculum*

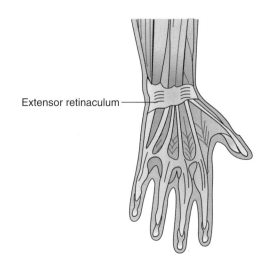

Figure 21-5 *Extensor Retinaculum*

anterior side of the forearm on the ulnar side.

Name:	Flexor Digitorum Superficialis
O:	Medial epicondyle of the humerus, coronoid process, radial tuberosity
I:	Middle phalanges of digits 2–5
N:	Median nerve
A:	Finger flexion, assists in wrist flexion, weak elbow flexion
P:	Ulnar side, anterior forearm

Flexor Digitorum Profundus. The **flexor digitorum profundus** is a deep finger flexor located on the medial and anterior regions of the forearm (Figure 21-7). Its tendons attach at the distal phalanges of the fingers and work synergistically with the flexor digitorum superficialis to flex the fingers. Once again, this muscle is a weak wrist flexor because it crosses the wrist. It can be palpated on the anterior surface of the forearm.

Name:	Flexor Digitorum Profundus
O:	Upper three-fourths of the anterior surface of the ulna and interosseus membrane
I:	Digits 2–5 at the base of the distal phalanges
A:	Flexion of the distal interphalangeal joint, whole finger flexion, wrist flexion
N:	Digits 2 and 3: median nerve; digits 4 and 5: ulnar nerve
P:	Anterior forearm

Flexor Pollicis Longus. The **flexor pollicis longus** is a small muscle located on the anterior surface of the forearm on the distal half (Figure 21-8). The tendon inserts to the distal phalanx of the thumb, running deep to the flexor retinaculum. The flexor pollicis longus flexes the thumb and aids in wrist flexion. It can be palpated on the anterior surface of the thumb.

Name:	Flexor Pollicis Longus
O:	Anterior surface of the radius on the distal half
I:	Distal phalanx of the thumb at the base
N:	Median nerve
A:	Flexion of the thumb; wrist flexion
P:	Anterior surface of the thumb

Posterior Hand Muscles The muscles that act on the anterior surface of the hand are innervated by the radial nerve and have origins on the posterior surface of the forearm. However, their primary actions are to cause extension of the digits (2–5) and the pollicis muscle.

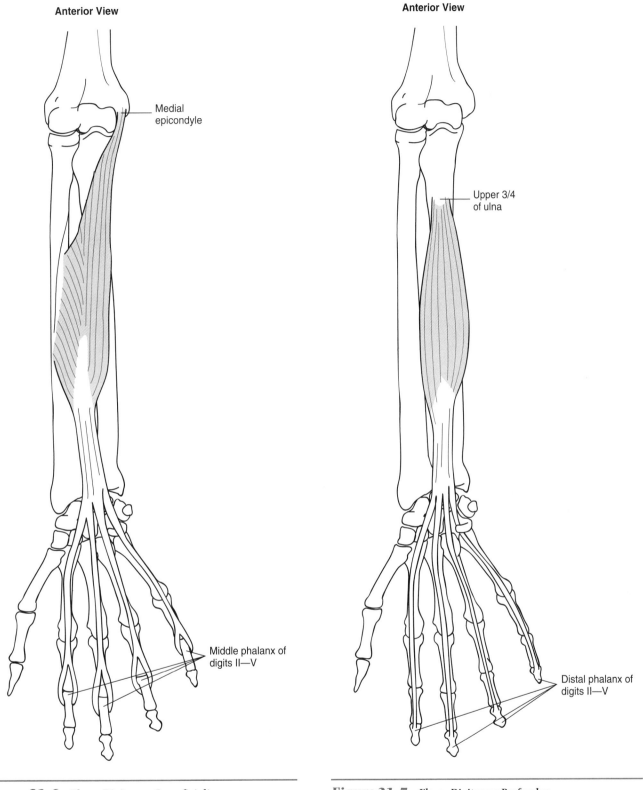

Figure 21-6 *Flexor Digitorum Superficialis*

Figure 21-7 *Flexor Digitorum Profundus*

Extensor Digitorum. The **extensor digitorum** is located on the posterior side of the forearm and extends to digits 2–5 (Figure 21-9). Unlike the finger flexors, which require two separate muscles, the extensor digitorum muscle in the only muscle that extends all four digits. This muscle can also extend the wrist. It can be palpated on the posterior aspect of the forearm and hand.

Anterior View

Posterior View

Lateral epicondyle

Anterior radius

Distal phalanx of digit I

Distal phalanx of digits II-V

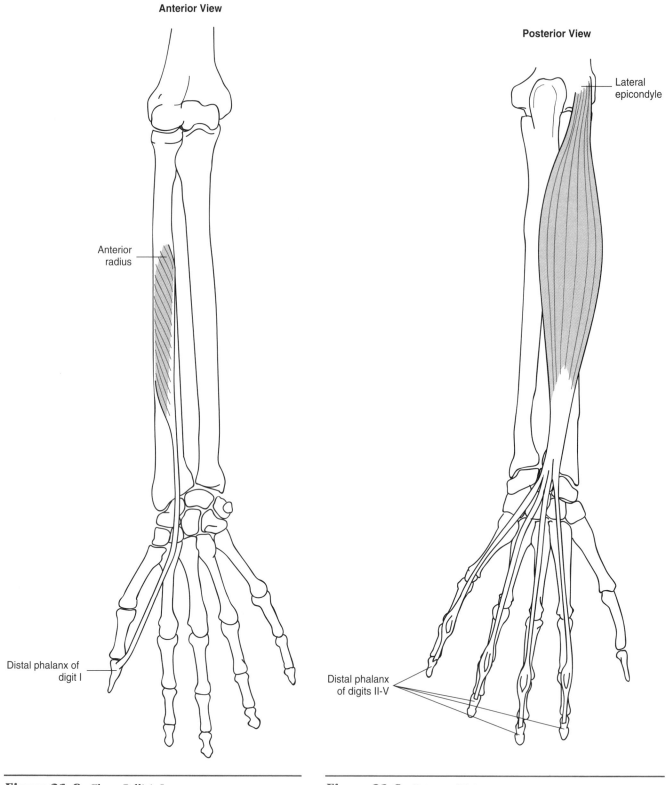

Figure 21-8 *Flexor Pollicis Longus*

Figure 21-9 *Extensor Digitorum*

Name: Extensor Digitorum

O: Lateral epicondyle of the humerus

I: Digits 2–5 at the bases of the second and third phalanges

N: Radial nerve

A: Finger extension, wrist extension

P: Posterior surface of the forearm and hand

The **extensor hood** deserves brief mention here. The extensor muscles of the hand narrow and blend into a broad aponeurosis at the dorsal and distal areas of the hand. This aponeurosis is called the extensor hood.

Extensor Digiti Minimi. The **extensor digiti minimi** is a long, narrow muscle located on the posterior surface of the forearm and joins the extensor expansion at the distal phalanx of digit 5 (Figure 21-10). It extends all of the joints of the pinky finger and acts as a weak wrist extensor. This muscle cannot be palpated.

Name: Extensor Digiti Minimi

O: Lateral epicondyle of the humerus

I: Distal phalanx of digit 5

N: Radial nerve

A: Extension of all joints of digit 5

P: Cannot be palpated

Extensor Indicis. The **extensor indicis** is a fairly small and narrow muscle located on the posterior side of the forearm (Figure 21-11). It acts as the main extensor of the index finger at the metacarpal phalangeal joint and, as with most muscles that cross the wrist, also weakly assists in wrist extension. This muscle is best palpated on the posterior hand just medial to the extensor digitorum tendon of the index finger.

Name: Extensor Indicis

O: Distal third of the posterior ulna

I: Distal phalanx of the index finger at the base

N: Radial nerve

A: Extension of the index finger, weak wrist extension

P: Posterior surface of the hand just medial to the extensor digitorum tendon

Extensor Pollicis Longus. Recall that the word "pollicis" relates to the thumb or digit 1 (Figure 21-12). The **extensor pollicis longus** is a small muscle located on the posterior aspect of the hand. It works with the extensor pollicis brevis to extend the thumb and is best palpated on the posterior aspect of the hand.

Name: Extensor Pollicis Longus

O: Posterior lateral surface of the ulna

I: Distal phalanx of the thumb at the base

N: Radial nerve

A: Extension of the thumb, extension of the wrist

P: Dorsal side of the hand

Extensor Pollicis Brevis. The **extensor pollicis brevis**, like the other hand muscles, is a small, thin muscle located on the posterior side of the forearm and hand (Figure 21-13). Notice the term *brevis*, meaning "short," because this can help you distinguish this muscle from the extensor pollicis longus. This muscle inserts at the proximal phalanx of the thumb. The extensor pollicis brevis works synergistically with the extensor pollicis longus to extend the thumb. It can be palpated on the dorsal side of the hand.

Name: Extensor Pollicis Brevis

O: Posterior surface of the distal radius

I: Proximal phalanx of the thumb on the distal side

N: Radial nerve

A: Extension of the thumb at the metacarpal phalangeal joint, weak wrist extension

P: Dorsal surface of the hand

Abductor Pollicis Longus. The **abductor pollicis longus** is a small muscle located on the posterior aspect of the forearm and hand (Figure 21-14). It acts mainly as an agonist in thumb abduction, as its name implies. It can be palpated on the lateral aspect of the wrist, proximal to the first metacarpal bone.

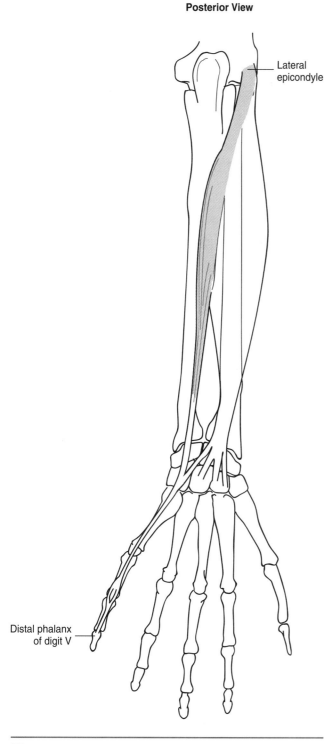

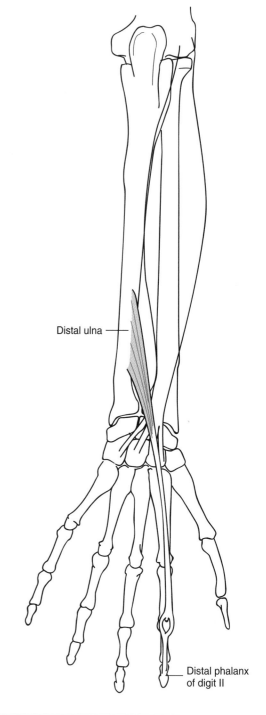

Figure 21-10 *Extensor Digiti Minimi*

Figure 21-11 *Extensor Indicis*

Name:	Abductor Pollicis Longus
O:	Posterior radius and ulna
I:	Base of first metacarpal
N:	Radial nerve
A:	Thumb abduction
P:	Lateral wrist near first metacarpal

Posterior View

Posterior View

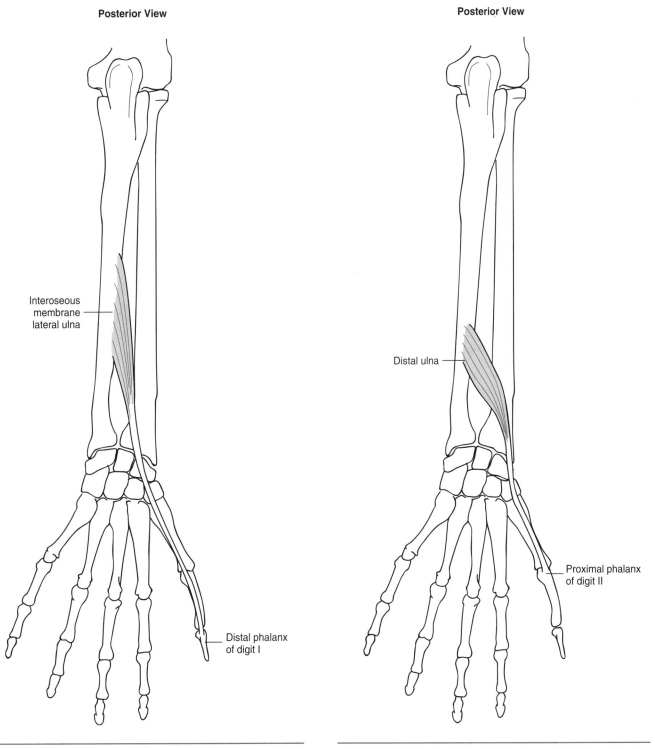

Interoseous
membrane
lateral ulna

Distal ulna

Distal phalanx
of digit I

Proximal phalanx
of digit II

Figure 21-12   *Extensor Pollicis Longus*

Figure 21-13   *Extensor Pollicis Brevis*

Intrinsic Muscle Group

The intrinsic muscles of the hand allow us to perform fine motor movements and are integral to the complexity of the human hand. Because they allow us the luxury of fine motor movement, they are extremely small muscles. Consequently, the origin and insertion of these muscles are not listed here. Instead, we will discuss nervous innervation and the action of each of these muscles and discuss each muscle group based on the part of the hand where their action is exerted. From a learning perspective, students may find it helpful to look for the common denominator of each muscle group. The thenar muscle group acts on the thumb (thus the name "pollicis"). The hypothenar muscle group affects the pinky finger (thus the name "digiti minimi"). Lastly, the deep or midpalm muscles are the ones that do not specifically fit in either the thenar or hypothenar muscle group.

Thenar Muscle Group This small bundle of muscle between the wrist and the base of the thumb consists of the flexor pollicis brevis, abductor pollicis brevis, and opponens pollicis. According to the names of the muscles, one may guess what part of the hand they affect—the thumb! In addition, the median nerve innervates each of these muscles.

Flexor Pollicis Brevis. The **flexor pollicis brevis** is a superficial muscle arising from the flexor retinaculum (Figure 21-15). Because it inserts on the proximal phalanx, it flexes the CMC and MCP joints.

Name:	Flexor Pollicis Brevis
O:	Flexor retinaculum and trapezium bones
I:	The base of the proximal phalanx of the thumb
N:	Median nerve
A:	Thumb flexion
P:	Difficult to palpate

Abductor Pollicis Brevis. The **abductor pollicis brevis** is the most superficial muscle of the group and arises from the flexor retinaculum (Figure 21-16). It attaches to the lateral side of the proximal phalanx of the thumb and, as its name implies, abducts the thumb.

Name:	Abductor Pollicis Brevis
O:	Flexor retinaculum, scaphoid, and trapezium
I:	The base of the proximal phalanx of the thumb
N:	Median nerve
A:	Thumb abduction
P:	Difficult to palpate

Opponens Pollicis. Lying deep to the abductor pollicis brevis is the **opponens pollicis**. This muscle also arises from the flexor retinaculum, in addition to the trapezium. It attaches on the lateral and palmar areas of the first metacarpal (Figure 21-17). This muscle is active in opposition of the thumb.

Name:	Opponens Pollicis
O:	Flexor retinaculum, trapezium bone
I:	The head of the first metacarpal bone
N:	Median nerve
A:	Thumb opposition
P:	Difficult to palpate

Hypothenar Muscle Group Smaller than the thenar muscle group, but equally important, is the hypothenar muscle group. This muscle group consists of three muscles that lie in the region between the wrist and the base of the little finger. These muscles are the flexor digiti minimi, abductor digiti minimi, and opponens digiti minimi. The names of these muscles give a clue to the action they perform and the area where the action is exerted. In this case, these muscles act on the little finger. The ulnar nerve innervates these muscles.

Flexor Digiti Minimi. The **flexor digiti minimi** originates from the flexor retinaculum and the hamate bone (Figure 21-18). Its insertion point at the proximal phalanx allows it to flex the fifth metocarpal phalangeal joint.

Name:	Flexor Digiti Minimi
O:	Flexor retinaculum, hamate bone
I:	Base of the proximal phalanx of the fifth finger
N:	Ulnar nerve
A:	Flexion of the fifth finger
P:	Difficult to palpate

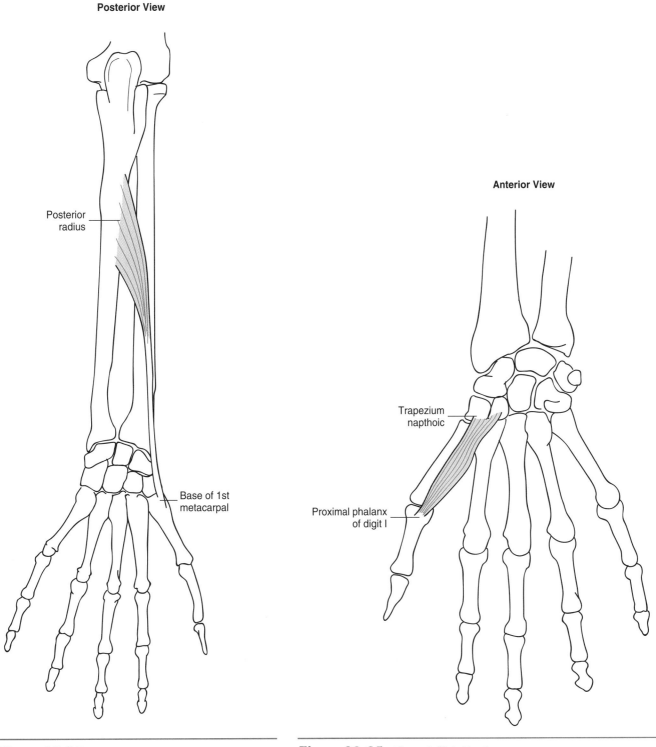

Figure 21-14 *Abductor Pollicis Longus*

Figure 21-15 *Flexor Pollicis Brevis*

Abductor Digiti Minimi. The **abductor digiti minimi** arises from the flexor retinaculum and the pisiform bone and inserts at the base of the proximal phalanx on the ulnar side (Figure 21-19). This muscle abducts the metacarpal phalangeal joint of the little finger.

Name: Abductor Digiti Minimi

O: Pisiform bone

I: Lateral surface of the base of the proximal phalanx of the fifth finger

Anterior View

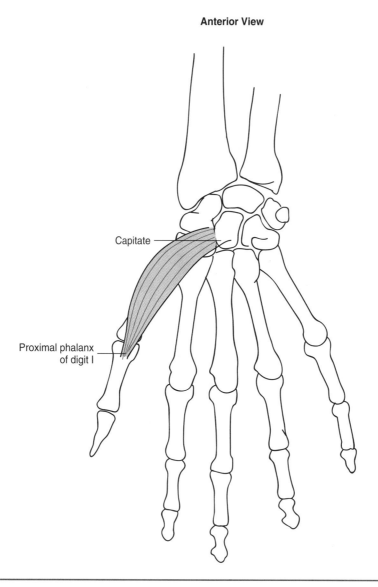

Capitate

Proximal phalanx
of digit I

Figure 21-16 *Abductor Pollicis Brevis*

N:	Ulnar nerve
A:	Abduction of the fifth finger
P:	Difficult to palpate

Opponens Digiti Minimi. The deepest of the three hypothenar muscles, the **opponens digiti minimi** arises from the flexor retinaculum and the hook of the hamate bone. It inserts at the fifth metacarpal bone and, thus, opposes the pinky finger (Figure 21-20).

Name:	Opponens Digiti Minimi
O:	Flexor retinaculum, hamate bone
I:	Lateral surface of the head of the fifth metacarpal bone
N:	Ulnar nerve
A:	Assists with opposition of the fifth finger
P:	Difficult to palpate

Midpalm or Deep Palm Muscle Group This muscle group is located deep within the palm, as the name implies, between the thenar and hypothenar muscle groups. Although there are three muscles included in this group, the interossei

Anterior View

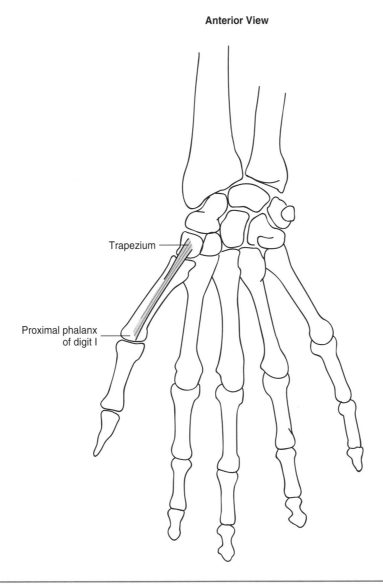

Trapezium

Proximal phalanx
of digit I

Figure 21-17   *Opponens Pollicis*

contain four palmar and dorsal muscles, and the **lumbricals** also contain four muscles. These muscles allow for fine motor control and precise movements of the hand. The ulnar or median nerve innervates these muscles.

Adductor Pollicis. The **adductor pollicis** muscle is located deep within the hand and operates the thumb but is not considered part of the thenar eminence because of its deep location (Figure 21-21). It has a broad origin ranging from the capitate, second metacarpal base, and third metacarpal. It inserts at the base of the proximal phalanx of the thumb. As the name implies, this muscle adducts the thumb. The ulnar nerve innervates this muscle.

Name:	Adductor Pollicis
O:	Trapezium, trapezoid, and metacarpal bones II and III
I:	Medial surface of the base of the proximal phalanx of the first finger
N:	Ulnar nerve
A:	Adduction of the first finger
P:	Difficult to palpate

The Interossei. The **interossei muscle** group originates between the metacarpals and inserts to the base of the proximal phalanges. There are four palmar interossei and four dorsal interossei muscles. The palmar interossei muscles (Figure 21-22) are located deep in the palmar side of the hand and cause adduction at the MCP joint at digits 2–5. Conversely, the

Anterior View

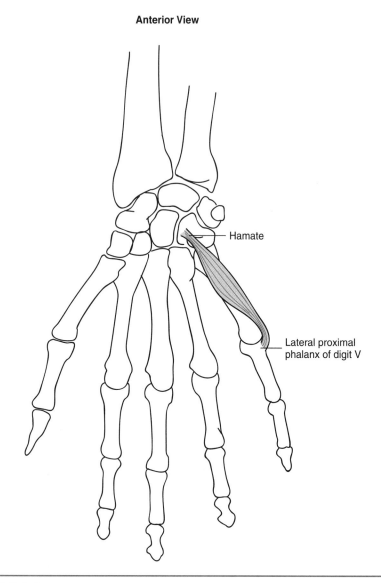

Hamate

Lateral proximal
phalanx of digit V

Figure 21-18 *Flexor Digiti Minimi*

dorsal interossei muscles (Figure 21-22 and Figure 21-23) are located deep in the dorsal side of the hand and abduct digits 2–5. Keep in mind that the middle finger (digit 3) is the point of reference for finger abduction and adduction. The ulnar nerve innervates each of these muscles.

Name:	Interossei
O:	Bilaterally on the base of the metacarpals digits I–V
I:	Base of the proximal phalanx of digits I–V
N:	Ulnar nerve
A:	Abduction away from the middle finger
P:	Difficult to palpate

Lumbricals. The lumbricals are the only muscles within the body that do not have a bony attachment, either origin or insertion (Figure 21-24). They originate and insert on tendons of other muscles. More specifically, they originate on the tendon of the flexor digitorum profundus and insert on the tendon of the extensor digitorum. They flex the MCP joint and extend the IP joints of digits 2–5. The first and second lumbrical muscles are innervated by the median nerve, and the third and fourth lumbricals are innervated by the ulnar nerve.

Name:	Lumbricals
O:	Distal tendon of the flexor digitorum profundus muscle
I:	Lateral, proximal base of the proximal phalanx of digits II–V

Anterior View

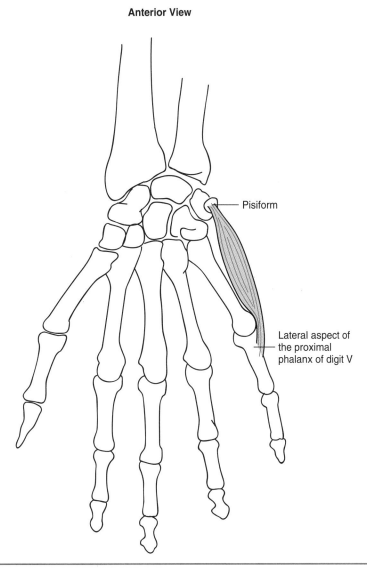

Pisiform

Lateral aspect of
the proximal
phalanx of digit V

Figure 21-19 *Abductor Digiti Minimi*

N:	Median and ulnar nerves
A:	Flex metacarpophalangeal joints and extends IP joints
P:	Difficult to palpate

Muscle Similarities of the Hand

Before we conclude our discussion of hand muscles, let us attempt to find some similarities of this large number of muscles. By studying the origin, insertion, action, and innervation, we can draw some similarities that may assist in learning. First, the finger flexors all are located on the anterior side of the forearm. Most of these muscles are also innervated by the median nerve and also assist in weak wrist flexion because they span the wrist. Next, the extensors of the fingers also contribute to weak wrist extension. In addition, they all are innervated by the radial nerve and are located on the posterior side of the forearm.

Anterior View

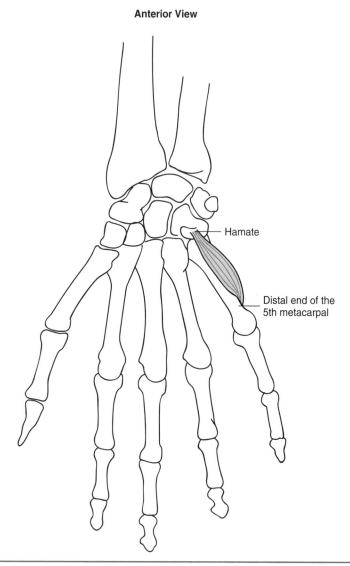

Hamate

Distal end of the
5th metacarpal

Figure 21-20   *Opponens Digiti Minimi*

Anterior View

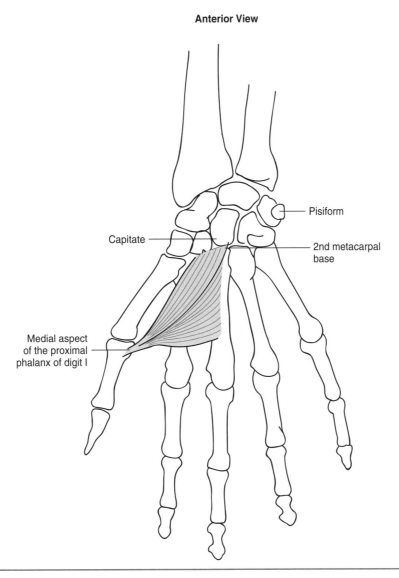

Pisiform

Capitate

2nd metacarpal base

Medial aspect of the proximal phalanx of digit I

Figure 21-21 *Adductor Pollicis*

Anterior View

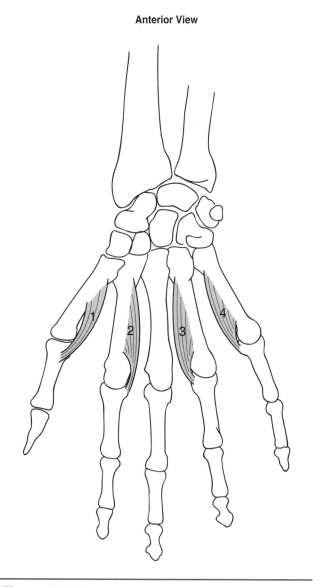

Posterior View

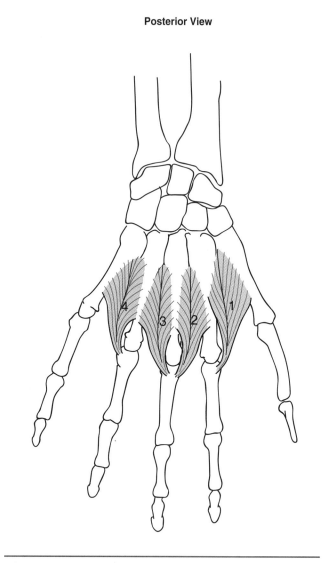

Figure 21-22 *Palmar Interossei*

Figure 21-23 *Dorsal Interossei*

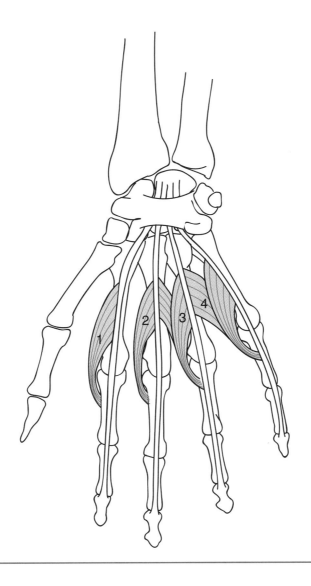

Figure 21-24 *Lumbricals*

KEY CONCEPTS

∎ Refer to Table 21-1 to see the table format for nerve and muscle innervations. In short, the median nerve innervates the following muscles: flexor digitorum superficialis and profundus (digits 2 and 3), flexor pollicis longus and brevis, abductor pollicis brevis, opponens pollicis, and the first and second lumbricals. The radial nerve innervates the extensor digitorum, extensor digiti minimi, extensor indicis, abductor pollicis longus, and extensor pollicis brevis and longus. The ulnar nerve innervates the flexor digitorum profundus (digits 4 and 5) abductor pollicis longus and abductor pollicis brevis, flexor digiti minimi, abductor digiti minimi, opponens digiti minimi, palmar interossei and 3rd and 4th lumbricals.

∎ The muscles of the hand can be categorized into extrinsic and intrinsic muscles. Extrinsic muscles originate proximal to the carpal bones and operate the fingers through long tendons. The intrinsic muscles are smaller and originate within the hand or distal to the carpal bones.

∎ Intrinsic muscles of the hand can be subdivided further into three types: thenar, hypothenar, and deep palm muscles. The thenar muscles exert action on the thumb. The hypothenar muscles exert actions on the pinky finger, and the deep palm muscles do not necessarily fit into either one of the thenar or hypothenar categories.

∎ Use Table 21-2 to study and perform the movements of digits 2–5. These include finger flexion, extension, abduction, and adduction. Practice these movements to gain a solid understanding of the muscles responsible for these movements.

∎ Once again, use Table 21-2 to study and perform the movements of the thumb. These movements include thumb flexion, extension, abduction, adduction, opposition, and reposition.

∎ There are multiple muscles that exert action on the fingers and thumb. In many cases, the name of the muscle provides a clue as to what action it exerts and where. For instance, the extensor digitorum muscle extends the digits, or fingers. This technique can be used to identify and describe the actions of specific muscles. In other cases, it is necessary to memorize specific muscle actions if the name of the muscle does not provide clues.

BIBLIOGRAPHY

Hall-Craggs, E. (1990). *Anatomy as a basis for clinical medicine* (2nd ed.). Baltimore: Urban and Schwarzenberg.

Norkin, C. C., & Levangie, P. K. (2001). *Joint structure and function: A comprehensive analysis* (3rd ed.). Philadelphia: F. A. Davis.

Smith, L. K., Weiss, E. L., & Lehmkuhl, L. (1996). *Brunnstrom's clinical kinesiology* (5th ed.). Philadelphia: F. A. Davis.

Thompson, C. W., & Floyd, R. T. (2000). *Manual of structural kinesiology* (14th ed.) St. Louis, MO: Mosby.

WEB RESOURCES

- For features on A & P, joint injuries, diagnostics, and prevention of hand joint injuries, go to www.nlm.nih.gov/medlineplus/handinjuriesanddisorders.html.
- Orthopedics.hss.edu/services/conditions/hand/sprained_thumb.asp features the etiology, signs and symptoms, and functional treatment of sprained thumbs.
- Go to www.pncl.co.uk/~belcher/trigger.htm for an introduction to trigger finger disorders, a discussion of tenosynovities, and treatment of trigger finger disorders.

(These Web addresses were current as of February 2004.)

REVIEW QUESTIONS

Fill in the Blank

Provide the word(s) or phrase(s) that best completes the sentence.

1. The muscles of the hypothenar group are _____, _____, _____.

2. Muscles that have their origin "within" the hand or distal to the carpals are called _____.

3. The reference point for finger abduction is the _____ digit.

4. Flexion of the thumb occurs in the _____ plane.

5. The bones of the wrist are more specifically called the _____.

Multiple Choice

Select the best answer to complete the following statements.

1. Of the following muscles the _____ does not belong to the thenar muscle group.
   a. opponens pollicis
   b. abductor pollicis brevis
   c. flexor digiti minimi
   d. flexor pollicis brevis

2. The "knuckles" of the hand refer to the bones of the _____ joint.
   a. PIP joint
   b. DIP joint
   c. CMC joint
   d. MCP joint

3. The muscle that flexes all the joints of the finger is the _____ .
   a. flexor digitorum profundus
   b. abductor pollicis
   c. flexor digitorum superficialis
   d. opponens pollicis

4. Abduction of the thumb occurs in the _____ plane.
   a. frontal
   b. transverse
   c. sagittal
   d. vertical

5. Adduction of the fingers occurs in the _____ plane.
   a. sagittal
   b. horizontal
   c. frontal
   d. vertical

Matching

Match each of the following descriptions with the appropriate term.

_____ **1.** Midpalm muscle

_____ **2.** Return from opposition

_____ **3.** Sweeping motion across the palm

_____ **4.** Flexor pollicis brevis, abductor pollicis brevis, Opponens pollicis

_____ **5.** Flexor digiti minimi, Abductor digiti minimi, Opponens digiti minimi

A. Reposition

B. Thumb flexion

C. Hypothenar muscle group

D. Thenar muscle group

E. Adductor pollicis

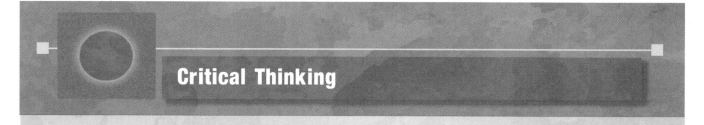

Critical Thinking

1. If a client of yours had damaged the median nerve in an accident, what movements would be affected?

2. Could you teach this client to pick up a pencil? If so, how would you accomplish this? What muscles would not be affected by the damaged median nerve?

3. A typical OT evaluation includes a chart review and an interview. The OT is searching for information that may assist in choosing which assessments to use, what the appropriate goals may be, what the "prior (to the injury, to the hospitalization, or to the OT evaluation) functional status" was, who the client's support system is, and what the discharge plans are. It might be obvious in the case of an elderly client who is living alone and who was just diagnosed with hemiplegia that a more thorough chart review and interview are indicated. Is this the case with other wrist/forearm diagnoses? What information might be necessary for a 40-year-old with a cumulative trauma diagnosis that is likely not necessary for a 10-year-old with a Colles' fracture? Besides the primary diagnosis, what other information seems necessary? And what information might be secondary? Quickly being able to assess the situation, ruling in and out what is pertinent, is vital given the "business of health care" and funding constraints. Learning how to do this, through practice and discussion or reflection with an experienced practitioner, contributes to the process of developing clinical reasoning.

4. Your 55-year-old patient has severe rheumatoid arthritis of the hands. Research and describe the deformities that will occur at each of the joints and the signs and symptoms. At this time she is not an acute flare-up, so describe a heat modality that would be appropriate. Also describe four exercises that you would give her at this time.

5. For each of the following grips, prescribe two different strengthening exercises.

   a. Power grip

   b. Pinch grip

   c. Key grip

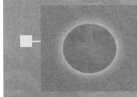

Lab Activities

Lab 21-1: Assessing Nerves in the Hand

Objective: To assess and develop therapy for damaged nerves in the hand.

Equipment Needed: A lab partner, pen/pencil, miscellaneous equipment from a PT/OT laboratory.

Step. 1.   Consider the client described in Critical Thinking question 1. If the client had damaged the median nerve, describe and have partner number 2 perform two low-level exercises you prescribe to initially rehabilitate the muscles involved.

Step 2.   Next have partner 2 describe and have partner 1 perform two different low-level exercises necessary for initial rehabilitation of the involved muscles.

Lab 21-2: Assessing Nerve Damage

Objective: To assess and develop therapy for damaged nerves of the hand.

Equipment Needed: A lab partner, pen/pencil, miscellaneous equipment from a PT/OT laboratory.

Step 1.   Consider a 13-year-old music student who plays the piano. Owing to a devastating accident, she has damage to the ulnar nerve on her left side. Partner 1, imagine partner 2 is the client. Prescribe and have the client perform specific grip strengthening exercises for the muscles involved in the damaged area. Use a variety of equipment to do this.

Step 2.   Partner 2, prescribe and have the client perform specific exercises that will aid in precision movements like advanced piano playing. Use a variety of equipment to do this.

Lab 21-3: Landmarks of the Hand

Objective: To properly locate and palpate the landmarks of the hand.

Equipment Needed: A lab partner, pen/pencil, paper

Step 1.   On your partner, palpate the following landmarks on the hand.
- Anatomical snuffbox
- Scaphoid
- Fourth distal interphalangeal joint
- Hook of hamate
- Pisiform
- Second metacarpal

Lab 21-4: Muscle Testing of the Hand

Objective: To properly locate and assess the function of the muscles of the hand.

Equipment Needed: A lab partner, pen/pencil, paper

Step 1.   On your partner, perform manual testing for the following muscles:
- Lumbricals
- Opponens pollicis
- Abductor pollicis longus
- Extensor digitorum

(continues)

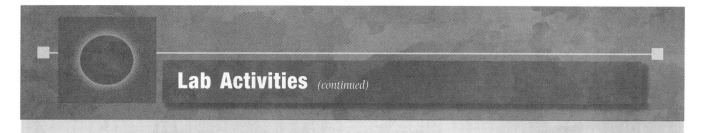

Lab Activities *(continued)*

Lab 21-5: Scaphoid Fracture

Objective: To properly assess and evaluate a fracture of the scaphoid bone.

Equipment Needed: A lab partner, pen/pencil, paper

Step 1.   Your client sustained a fracture of the scaphoid 7 weeks ago. The cast was removed two days ago and there is significant swelling of the forearm and wrist. Perform a massage on the forearm and wrist of your partner in an appropriate manner for this client. Pay particular attention to the positioning of the client and the direction and depth of the massage. What advice would you give the client to manage the swelling at home?

Chapter 22

MOVEMENT ANALYSIS

Objectives

Upon completion of this chapter, the reader should be able to:

- Utilize the charts provided to determine different movements at the major joints during a given human movement.

- Apply the knowledge gained from this text to provide a sound basis for understanding movement analysis.

Key Words

multiplaner

INTRODUCTION

Throughout this chapter, various movements, both athletic and ADL are analyzed from a kinesiology perspective. Each specific joint, muscle action, and muscle causing the action are analyzed on a region-to-region basis. By analyzing **multiplaner** movements such as throwing, students can develop movement analysis skills that can be used with any movement. *Multiplaner* refers to movements that occur in a variety of movement planes (e.g., sagittal, frontal, etc.).

    The first action of throwing a football is very similar to any overhead throwing motion, although there may be minor differences in technique among athletes. The student should also attempt to simulate the throwing motion in front of a mirror or student group to enhance learning.

PHASES OF MOVEMENT: THROWING A FOOTBALL

Most complex activities have multiple sequential "phases" or stages. As the movement progresses from one phase to another, it may occur in various planes. Referring to the first example of a person throwing a football, the throwing motion will be broken down phase by phase (e.g., Phase A-B, Phase B-C, Phase C-D etc.). The movements and actions often stay the same so the word "same" is input into the chart. In addition, the chart provided may help facilitate learning movement analysis.

Phase A to Phase B

At this point in the analysis the quarterback is dropping back to pass and stabilizing his or her body with the lower extremity. Also during this stage, involvement of the upper extremities begins. The throwing arm begins abduction as the quarterback eyes the target. Trunk rotation is also assisted by the nonthrowing arm pulling backward to cause rotation.

Joint	Movement	Prime Mover
Shoulder Girdle	Retraction Upward rotation	Rhomboids Trapezius
Shoulder Joint	Horizontal abduction Abduction	Posterior deltoid Medial deltoid
Elbow	Flexion	Biceps brachii Brachialis
Forearm/Wrist	Neutral position	Wrist flexors Wrist extensors
Hand	Finger flexion (gripping)	Intrinsic/extrinsic Hand muscles
Trunk	Stabilization	All abdominals
Hip	Rt: Abduction, external rotation Lt: Flexion	Tensor fasciae latae Gluteus medius Gluteus minimus Rectus femoris
Knee	Rt: Extension Lt: Flexion	Co-contraction of the quadriceps and hamstrings
Ankle	Rt: Neutral Lt: Neutral	Ankle flexors and extensors

Phase B to Phase C

During this stage, the quarterback "cocks" the throwing arm and rotates the trunk to prepare for increased throwing velocity. After analyzing the diagram provided, it should become evident how important the rotator cuff musculature is in overhead throwing motions.

Joint	Movement	Prime Mover
Shoulder Girdle	Retraction	Rhomboids Trapezius
Shoulder Joint	Abduction External rotation Horizontal abduction	Supraspinatus Infraspinatus Medial deltoid Posterior deltoid
Elbow	Flexion	Biceps brachii Brachialis
Forearm/Wrist	Neutral	Wrist flexors Wrist extensors
Hand	Finger flexion (gripping)	Extrinsic/intrinsic Hand muscles
Trunk	Right to left rotation	Obliques
Hip	Rt: Abduction External rotation Lt: Flexion	Same Same
Knee	Rt: Same Lt: Same	Same Same
Ankle	Rt: Plantar flexion Lt: Neutral	Gastrocnemius Soleus Tibialis anterior Tibialis posterior

Phase C to Phase D

At this stage the quarterback begins forward trunk rotation while the shoulder joint is forced into greater external rotation. It is important to note that involuntary momentum often places the arm into excessive ranges of external rotation during throwing movements. This excessive range of external rotation may not be reached during voluntary joint movements.

Joint	Movement	Prime Mover
Shoulder Girdle	Elevation Retraction	Trapezius Rhomboids
Shoulder Joint	External rotation Abduction	Supraspinatus Infraspinatus Teres minor Medial deltoid Posterior deltoid
Elbow	Flexion	Biceps brachii Brachialis Brachioradialis
Forearm/Wrist	Neutral	Wrist flexors and extensors
Hand	Finger flexion (gripping)	Same
Trunk	Right to left rotation	Obliques

Joint	Movement	Prime Mover
Hip	Rt: External rotation Abduction Lt: Flexion	Tensor fasciae latae Gluteus medius Gluteus minimus Iliopsoas Rectus femoris
Knee	Rt: Extension Lt: Flexion	Quadriceps Quadriceps and hamstrings co-contraction
Ankle	Rt: Plantar flexion Lt: Neutral	Gastrocnemius Soleus Tibialis anterior Gastrocnemius and soleus co-contraction

Phase D to Phase E

At this stage of the movement the throwing movement of the arm and body are in forward motion. The hips are turning forward as the throwing arm comes overhead. The drive caused by a combination of trunk rotation and hip rotation aids in throwing velocity.

Joint	Movement	Prime Movers
Shoulder Girdle	Upward rotation Retraction	Trapezius Rhomboids Serratus anterior
Shoulder Joint	Internal rotation Flexion	Medial deltoid Subscapularis
Elbow	Flexion	Same
Forearm/Wrist	Same	Same
Hand	Same	Same
Trunk	Rotation Flexion	Obliques Rectus abdominus

Hip	Rt: Internal rotation
	  Abduction
	  Extension
	Lt: Flexion
		Gluteus minimus
		Gluteus medius
		Gluteus maximus
		Iliopsoas
		Rectus femoris

Knee	Rt: Extension Lt: Flexion	Quadriceps Quadriceps and hamstrings co-contraction
Ankle	Rt: Plantar flexion Lt: Neutral	Gastrocnemius Soleus Same

Phase E to Phase F

This transition from phase E to phase F causes the release of the football from the hand. At this point, the body is facing forward to improve accuracy and the trunk also contributes to the velocity of the throw.

Joint	Movement	Prime Mover
Shoulder Girdle	Protraction Upward rotation	Same Same
Shoulder Joint	Flexion Internal rotation	Same Same
Elbow	Extension	Triceps
Forearm/Wrist	Neutral to wrist flexion	Wrist flexors
Hand	Flexion to neutral	Finger extensors
Trunk	Slight rotation and flexion	Obliques Rectus abdominus
Hip	Rt: Extension Lt: Flexion	Gluteus maximus Rectus femoris Iliopsoas
Knee	Rt: Flexion Lt: Flexion	Quadriceps Quadriceps and hamstrings co-contraction
Ankle	Rt: Plantar flexion Lt: Neutral	Gastrocnemius Soleus Tibialis anterior Tibialis posterior

Phase F to Phase G

This final stage of the throwing process is the follow-through. Note the shoulder joint performing horizontal adduction along with the trunk performing flexion.

Joint	Movement	Prime Mover
Shoulder Girdle	Protraction	Serratus anterior
Shoulder Joint	Internal rotation Horizontal adduction	Medial deltoid Subscapularis Pectoralis major
Elbow	Extension	Triceps brachii
Forearm/Wrist	Wrist flexion	Wrist flexors
Hand	Neutral	Follow-through
Trunk	Rotation Flexion	Obliques Rectus abdominus
Hip	Rt: Extension Lt: Flexion	Same Same
Knee	Rt: Extension Lt: Flexion	Same Quadriceps and hamstrings co-contraction
Ankle	Rt: Plantar flexion Lt: Neutral	Same Same

OTA Perspective

In order for a movement or action or a task or activity to be OT, it must have meaning and purpose to the recipient of skilled OT services—the client. If the client does not attribute meaning to the action, even if the OT practitioner does, it is not "occupational therapy." When the client is engaged in a task he or she finds purposeful, the performance of that task may provide the means of improving ROM, strength, coordination, or balance (bottom-up approach), or use it to improve hygiene tasks, writing, or singing (top-down approach).

It is an OT skill to analyze activities and to assess occupational performance. This assists in determining which tasks will provide the "just right challenge" to facilitate improved occupational performance. Knowing the reason for the OT intervention, along with other aspects of who the client is and what his or her goals are, provides one "starting place" for accessing occupational performance. Examples include an OT evaluation because of a change in functional status (e.g., client can no longer dress self), a new diagnosis (e.g., juvenile rheumatoid arthritis [JRA]), or following a recent injury (e.g., fall down the steps). The OT practitioner needs to know "who" the client is, and what his or her roles are—grade school student, sibling, little league football player, and the like. Knowing what the prior functional status was might include what the client did (e.g., knowing the client has never played the piano can be just as important as knowing the client enjoys playing several instruments in a local band).

In OT clinical practice, movement analyses, activity or task analysis, or occupational performance analysis are not completed in isolation. Not only does the OT practitioner need to gather more information about the client and the reason for the OT intervention, the OT practitioner needs to research the diagnosis, and recall what she/he has learned about anatomy and physiology, kinesiology, and even communication and interaction skills. And yes, it will all come together!

 ## PHASES OF MOVEMENT: DRINKING A CUP OF COFFEE

Consider a traditional ADL such as example 2, drinking a cup of coffee. Simulate this motion in the mirror to gain a comprehensive understanding of the movements and joints involved in this activity. This movement can be divided into four distinct stages: A (cup resting on the table with the hand on the cup), B (raising the cup to the mouth), C (taking a drink from the cup), D (returning the cup back to the table). Obviously, the movement had to be subdivided into concise and segmented movements although this is a fluid motion for most people. The beginning position for this movement involves the patient's hand on the handle of the coffee cup with the cup on the table (person is seated).

Phase A to Phase B

The starting point for this movement is the person's hand on the cup of coffee. This phase involves the person lifting or raising the cup to the lips.

Joint	Movement	Prime Mover
Shoulder Joint	Abduction Slight flexion	Deltoid (medial head) Deltoid (anterior head)
Elbow Joint	Flexion	Biceps brachii
Wrist/Forearm	Neutral position Slight radial deviation	 Flexor carpi radialis
Hand	Finger/thumb flexion (depending on the type of grip or cup)	Flexor digitorum superficialis Flexor pollicis longus
Neck	Neutral Slight flexion	 Sternocleidomastoid

Phase B to Phase C

This phase involves actually drinking from the cup. There is not a significant amount of motion of the upper body in this phase.

Joint	Movement	Prime Mover
Shoulder Joint	Abduction	Deltoid (medial head)
Elbow Joint	Flexion	Same
Wrist/Forearm	Pronation Slight extension of the wrist	Pronator teres Extensor carpi radialis brevis
Hand	Finger/thumb flexion	Same
Neck	Extension	Splenius capitis

Phase C to Phase D

This phase involves placing the cup of coffee back on the table to the starting position. Pay special attention to the lowering of the cup of coffee and the muscles and muscle actions involved. Recall that sometimes muscles use eccentric actions combined with gravity to accomplish precision tasks or tasks that don't involve great muscle force.

Joint	Movement	Prime Mover
Shoulder Joint	Adduction	Deltoid (Eccentric contraction)
Elbow Joint	Extension	Biceps brachii (Eccentric contraction)
Wrist /Forearm	Return to neutral	Supinator muscle
Hand	Same	Same
Neck	Neutral	Same

OTA Perspective

Using *Uniform Terminology-III* language, an activity analysis of occupational performance areas, components, and contexts of the activities may be intensely examined. It is suggested that an outline of *Uniform Terminology-III* be used to follow this example, because that will assist the OTA student to better comprehend activity analysis from this perspective. Although this language has been replaced by *Occupational Therapy Practice Framework* language, there may be academic sites and clinical practice sites that are continuing to utilize *Uniform Terminology-III*; therefore, an understanding of it is indicated.

1) Performance Components

   a) Sensorimotor Components

   i) Neuromusculoskeletal

   (1) ROM

   (a) using the "throwing a football" example from the text, one might comment: "full ® U/E ROM needed to complete the arc movement of tossing football"

In *Occupational Therapy Practice Framework* language, the client's occupational performance may be analyzed—assessing his or her ability to carry out Activities in the Area of Performance. Again, using an outline of *Occupational Therapy Practice Framework* as a guide to follow the example will assist the OTA student's comprehension.

2) Occupational Performance

   a) Performance Skills and Patterns Used in Performance

   i) Client Factors

   (1) Body Functions

   (a) Neuromusculoskeletal and movement-related functions

   (i) Functions of joints and bones

   1. Mobility of the joint functions (passive ROM)

   2. Stability of the joint functions (postural alignment)

   (ii) Muscle functions

   1. Muscle power functions (strength)

   ii) Motor Skills

   (1) Posture

   (a) Positions (positions arms in relation to the task object…. In this case, the client stabilizes and aligns the body and positions the arm, for throwing the football)

(continues)

(2) **Strength and Effort**

(a) **Lifts (raises or hoists task objects—the football)**

The preceeding are abbreviated examples, not in their entirety, but merely examples used to illustrate how an OT practitioner might take the task of throwing a football and look at it, in part, from a kinesiology perspective. Regardless of which method is used to assess the task, or the client engaged in the task, this analysis is not viewed in isolation. A client interview is indicated, standardized assessments may need to be completed followed by treatment planning and intervention, and a reassessment must be made to determine functional change and outcomes.

KEY CONCEPTS

The method of movement analysis used in this chapter is a simple (and sometimes oversimplified) method of learning and analyzing multiplaner movements. Use this technique to provide an application to the study of kinesiology. Although only two activities are analyzed in this chapter, use this method in a study group or on your own to help you learn. Some other activities to analyze include washing the hair, walking up stairs, or mopping the floor.

- Each of the examples in this chapter uses a chart with the joint involved, movement involved, and prime muscle mover to analyze the muscle movement. Use this chart or perhaps add other variables to the chart such as synergists or antagonists to provide a more complex analysis of human movement.

- Obviously, movement is a freedom that most humans are capable of. The endless list of activities, both simple and complex, that we do on a daily basis and at times take for granted, are only accomplished owing to the amazing structure of the human body. In this text the body is divided into multiple regions, highlighting muscles, structures, and movements. This capstone chapter links most of the chapters in the text in one form or another. Movement analysis can seem like a daunting task at times but it is a very helpful way to gain a greater understanding of kinesiology.

BIBLIOGRAPHY

American Occupational Therapy Association and American Occupational Therapy Foundation. (2002). Occupational therapy practice framework: Domain and process. *American Journal of Occupational Therapy, 56*(6), 609–639.

Hay, J. G. (1993). *The biomechanics of sports techniques* (4th ed.). Upper Saddle River, NJ: Prentice Hall.

REVIEW QUESTIONS

1. Define the term multiplaner.
2. Using every major joint in the body, perform and identify all of the actions allowed at each joint. Use a partner to check yourself.

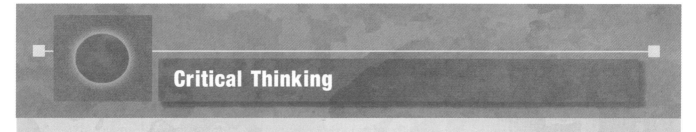

Critical Thinking

1. This is a lot—a study of kinesiology, models of OT practice, clinical reasoning, language styles, and frameworks (e.g., *Occupational Therapy Practice Framework and Uniform Terminology-III*), role delineation between OT and PT and between occupational therapists and OTAs, life span (infant through elderly) considerations, and the disease processes. Do you wonder how it will come together? And when that will happen? Much of the study of OT is accomplished through a mixture of "isolation" (e.g., disease process, anatomy, and physiology) and "interactive" (e.g., this particular text, or studying models of practice in conjunction with diseases or kinesiology—the biomechanical approach, for example). Be patient with yourself, take frequent deep breaths, use both your right and left brain learning abilities, be a "sponge," observe "real life" when the opportunities present themselves, ask questions—enjoy what you are learning!

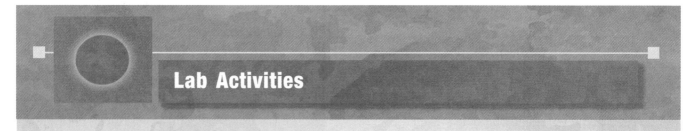

Lab Activities

Lab 22-1: Movement Analysis of Activities

Objective: To analyze movements of specific joints readily used in sport and activity.

Equipment Needed: A lab partner, pen, paper, mirror

Step 1. Using two or three of your favorite activities, perform a movement-by-movement joint analysis on the method used in this chapter.

Lab 22-2: Uniform Terminology-III

Objective: To compare the study of kinesiology to *Uniform Technology-III* language.

Equipment Needed: *Uniform Technology-III* outlines and worksheets, a lab partner, pen, paper

Step 1. Discuss with your partner terms that are utilized in both kinesiology and *Uniform Technology-III*. Make sure that you understand the definitions and, if indicated, can act out the movements.

Step 2. Write down questions or observations you make to discuss with the instructor and your classmates, or in the future with an OT program of student instructor or a fieldwork educator.

Lab 22-3: Occupational Therapy Practice Framework

Objective: To compare the study of Kinesiology to *OT Practice Framework* language

Equipment Needed: A lab partner, pen and paper; *OT Practice Framework* outline or full article: Occupational Therapy Practice Framework: Domain and Process. *American Journal of Occupational Therapy*, 56, 609–639.

Step 1. Discuss with your partner terms that are utilized in both kinesiology and *OT Practice Framework*. Make sure you understand the definitions and, if indicated, can act out the movements.

Step 2. Write down questions or observations you make to discuss with the instructor and your classmates, or in the future with an OT program of student instructor or a fieldwork educator.

GLOSSARY

A

abdominal aponeurosis: a flat sheet of fibrous connective tissue that attaches muscle to bone or other structures; found in the abdominal region

abducens nerve: cranial nerve number 6

abductor digiti minimi: a muscle that acts to abduct the metacarpophalangeal joint of the little finger

abductor pollicis brevis: a superficial muscle that abducts the thumb

abductor pollicis longus: a small muscle on the posterior of the forearm that acts as an agonist in thumb abduction

accessory nerve: the 11th cranial nerve; innervates the sternocleidomastoid and trapezius muscles

acetabulum: the rounded cavity on the external surface of the pelvis that holds the head of the femur

acetylcholine (ACH): a neurotransmitter found in the neuromuscular junction of muscle; takes the action potential from the motor neuron across the synaptic cleft to the sarcolemma

acetylcholinesterase: an enzyme found in the synaptic cleft responsible for breaking down acetylcholine following its release

Achilles tendon: the tendon of the soleus, gastrocnemius, and plantaris muscles located on the back of the heel

acromioclavicular joint: the junction of the acromial end of the clavicle and the acromion process

acromioclavicular ligament: the connective tissue that holds the ac joint together

acromion: a hooklike projection from the lateral aspect of the spine of the scapula

acromion process: a "finger-like" anatomical structure of the scapula. The acromion process is an origin for many muscles of the shoulder joint and provides a strong base of stability for the ligaments of the region. The acromion process is also used as a point of reference for many palpation techniques.

actin filament (F-actin): A double helix structure made up of oval-shaped polymerized proteins

action (of a muscle): the direction of movement of a muscle that can aid in learning its name and where it is located

action potential: a nervous stimulation that causes a muscle contraction

active expiration: the act of forceful expiration with the recruitment of the diaphragm

active inspiration: the act of forceful inspiration with the recruitment of the diaphragm

active insufficiency: the point at which a two-joint muscle can no longer actively contract

adductor brevis: a muscle located on the medial thigh anterior to the adductor longus

adductor longus: a muscle located on the medial thigh posterior to the adductor brevis

adductor magnus: a muscle located on the medial thigh spanning its entire length

adductor pollicis: a small muscle in the hand that is responsible for adduction of the thumb

adductor tubercle: the bony process superior to the medial epicondyle of the femur

adenosine diphosphate (ADP): the broken down form of adenosine triphosphate that is combined with an inorganic phosphate ion to provide the high-energy configuration of the myosin head

adenosine triphosphate (ATP): a high-energy compound that, when broken down, provides energy for the muscle contraction

adrenaline: a stress hormone from the catecholamines group. Adrenaline is often referred to as epinephrine. Adrenaline is a hormone that is produced by the adrenal medula that provides a sympathetic nervous system response.

affective language area: an area of the brain that is associated with the emotional components of verbal communication

afferent: a neuron stimulus that travels toward the next nerve, the spinal cord, or the brain

agonist: the primary mover in a muscle contraction that provides the work in a muscle contraction

all-or-none response: a nerve impulse that is not strong enough to initiate the depolarization process and will not create an action potential

amitotic: division of a cell outside of the nucleus. The letter "a" means "without." True mitosis occurs in the cell nucleus.

amphiarthrosis joint: a type of articulation in which structures are connected by cartilage. The articulation is slightly mobile

477

amygdala: gray matter found in the anterior region of the temporal lobe. The structure plays a role in arousal repsonses

anaerobic glycolysis: the process of breakdown of glycogen

anatomical landmarks: specific structures along the body used as reference points for muscle, bone, and nerve identification purposes

anatomical position: the position that is described as standing erect, feet flat, and the palms facing forward

anatomical pulley: a situation in which a bone is found in a muscle tendon that increases mechanical efficiency

anconeus: a short extensor muscle of the forearm located on the back of the elbow

angle: a bony landmark found on the scapula that provides a large surface area for muscles to attach to

anisotropic band (A band): an area of the sarcomere that does not polarize light

annular ligament: a ring-shaped ligament located in the elbow

annulus fibrosus: the outer portion of the intervertebral disk made up of concentric rings of fibrocartilage

antagonist: the muscle in a contraction that opposes the primary mover. Typically, the antagonist is on the opposite side of the agonist.

anterior: referring to the front side of the body, the abdominal, or the ventral side

anterior cruciate ligament (ACL): a ligament of the knee that extends posteriorly and laterally from the area anterior of the tibia to the posterior portion of the medial surface of the lateral condyle of the femur

anterior inferior iliac spine (AIIS): a bony process inferior to the ASIS.

anterior longitudinal ligament: a broad structure that attaches to the anterior surface of the vertebral bodies and disks

anterior median fissure: an indentation of tissue found on the anterior surface of the spinal cord that helps separate the spinal cord into a left and right half

anterior pelvic tilt: less than a 10-degree angle between the ASIS and PSIS or the ASIS and the pubic symphysis

anterior superior iliac spine (ASIS): a bony process inferior to the crest of the illum

anterolateral: the front and to the side

anteromedial: the front and to the middle

aponeurosis: a band of flat fibrous connective tissue

appendicular: referring to the appendages or extremities

appendicular skeleton: the part of the skeleton that moves around a fixed axial base; a term that pertains to the strucutres of the arms and legs

appositional growth: the growth of bone from the haversian canal in the distal direction

arachnoid mater: middle layer of the meninges of the brain. This is a web-like structure.

arthrokinematics: the movement of the bone surfaces within a joint

arthrosis: referring to the joints

articular capsule: a structure that is continuous with the periosteum and articular cartilage

articular cartilage: hyaline cartilage

ascending nerves: nerves that take stimulation from the periphery to the spinal cord

association fibers: nerve fibers found between sensory and motor nerve fibers

association neuron: central nervous system nerves that sends stimulation from the sensory to motor neurons or other association neurons

astrocytes: star-shaped accessory neurons that assist in the exchange of blood between the capillaries and neurons

atlas: the first cervical vertebrae

ATP-phosphocreatine system: the first energy system used during exercise; provides explosive energy for the first 10 seconds

attachment site: the area where a muscle attaches to a bone

autonomic, or involuntary, system: part of the peripheral nervous system that provides efferent stimulation to the cardiac muscle cells, smooth muscle cells, and glands. Stimulation provided from this system is involuntary.

axial: referring to the spine, ribs, and sternal regions

axial skeleton: the base of support around which appendicular muscles pull for movement

axis: the second cervical vertebra

axon: part of the neuron that takes an efferent impulse from one nerve cell to the next. The axon is found after the nucleus of the neuron.

axonal terminal: the end of the axon where neurotransmitters are stored

axon hillock: a structure prior to the axon that holds an action potential before it fires

B

basal lamina: a structure found at the motor end plate that is permeable to calcium ions following stimulation from an action potential

basal nuclei: gray matter found in the cerebral hemispheres

base: a fixed point around which muscles pull to cause movement

biaxial: two axes

biceps brachii: a muscle located on the anterior humerus crossing the shoulder and elbow joint

biceps femoris: a muscle located on the posterior thigh crossing the hip and knee joint

bipennate muscle: a muscle that has two sides that extends at an angle from a central piece of connective tissue

blood-brain barrier: barrier found between the capillaries and brain tissue that prevents blood from seeping into the brain and affecting brain tissue

border: an anatomical structure of the scapula that provides the linear aspect to its sides

brachialis: a muscle located on the anterior humerus crossing the elbow joint

brachial plexus: a group of nerves that stem from the ventral ramus of the cervical nerves

brachioradialis: a muscle located on the anterolateral surface of the humerus

brainstem: a structure in the brain that contains the pons and the medulla

brevis: short

Broca's area: found in the left hemisphere of the brain and is responsible for speech, movement of the tongue, vocal cords, and lips

Brodmann's areas: found in the cerebral cortex and is divided into 47 areas that are separated into different functions

C

calcaneonavicular ligament: a broad ligament on the plantar surface of the foot providing support to the talus and subtalar joint

calcaneotibial: one of the deltoid ligaments in the foot and ankle

calcaneus: commonly referred to as the heel bone

calcium ion: a chemical ion required for muscle contraction; found in the sarcoplasmic reticulum of muscle and binds to the troponin C molecule during a muscle contraction

canaliculi: a microscopic channel that is found in the osteon of bone and connects two adjacent lacuna

capitate: one of the bones of the wrist

capitulum: a small, rounded end of bone

carbon dioxide: a colorless gas that is heavier than air; a product of the decomposition of carbon and exists in air at 0.03%

cardiac muscle: involuntary, striated cells that form many branches found only in the heart

carpal bones: pertaining to the bones of the wrist

carpi: a singular bone found in the wrist

carpometacarpal: pertaining to the bones of the wrist and fingers

cauda equina: terminal part of the spinal cord where the nerves branch resembling a horse's tail

caudal: pertaining to the tail

caudate nucleus: a specific nuclei of a cell that has a tail

cell body: part of the neuron that contains the cell nucleus

central canal: the haversian canal of the osteon that contains nerve fibers and nutrient arteries that supply blood and stimulus to the bone tissue

central nervous system (CNS): referring to the neurons of the spinal cord and brain

central sulcus: a structure in the brain that separates the frontal lobe from the parietal lobe

central tendon: a flat tendon that is located in the central portion of the diaphragm muscle

cerebellum: found in the posterior region of the brain, and is responsible for coordinating skeletal muscle contractions needed for smooth contractions in the extremities

cerebral aqueduct: a cavity found in the midbrain that connects the third and fourth ventricles

cerebral cortex: gray matter of the cerebral hemisphere

cerebral hemispheres: the two separate parts of the cerebrum; defined as the left and right sides of the brain

cerebrospinal fluid (CSF): fluid that is found in the cavities of the brain and spinal column

cerebrum: refers to the largest part of the brain that contains the cerebral hemispheres and diencephalons

cervical plexus: cervical nerve branches that come together to innervate the muscles of the cervical region

cervical vertebrae: vertebrae that are found in the neck region of the body

choroid plexus: capillary branches that come together and nourish the brain ventricles

circumduction: the action of moving a limb in a cone-shaped figure

clavicle: the S-shaped bone found superior and lateral to the sternum

closed kinetic chain: a situation in which the origin moves toward the insertion during human movement

closed-packed position: a situation in which the ligaments, tendons, and muscles are taut and allow for no movement

coccyx: fused vertebral bones at the inferior part of the vertebral column

commissural fibers: nerve fibers that communicate between the cortial areas of the hemispheres

commissures: a band of nerves that pass through the middle of the spinal cord

compact bone: a bone tissue with no spaces, where layers of lamellae are fitted tightly together; dense bone

concave: a hollow indentation in a bone forming a bowl-like structure

concentric: a contraction of a muscle in which the muscle fiber shortens

condyloid: resembling a condyle

condyloidal joint: biaxial joint found at the metacarpophalangeal joints that provide movements in the sagittal and frontal planes

conoid ligament: an accessory ligament that makes up the acromioclavicular joint whose purpose is to stabilize the clavicle

contractility: the ability to contract or shorten

conus medullaris: referring to the structure at the lower end of the spinal cord

convex: curved evenly or arched

coracoacromial ligament: a ligament spanning the coracoid process to the acromion process

coracobrachialis: a muscle spanning the anterior surface of the chest crossing the anterior shoulder joint

coracoclavicular ligaments: accessory ligaments that make up the acromioclavicular joint whose purpose is to stabilize the clavicle

coracohumeral ligament: connective tissue providing support to the shoulder joint

coracoid process: located on the upper anterior surface of the scapula

coranoid process: the attachment point for the brachialis muscle on the ulna

corpus collosum: nerves that connect the two different cerebral hemispheres together

corpus striatum: a structure that is made up of the lentiform and caudate nucleus

costae: pertaining to a single rib

costal cartilage: hyaline cartilage that attaches a rib to the sternum

costoclavicular: pertaining to the ribs and clavicle

costoclavicular ligament: an accessory ligament that supports the sc joint laterally to the joint capsule

cranial: pertaining to the skull or cranium

cranial nerves: 12 pairs of nerves that are sensory and motor in nature that innervate many of the important structures of the head. The cranial nerves are of great importance because of their roles in the special senses of the brain.

crest: a ridge on a bone

cuboid: like a cube; the outer bone on the medial side of the foot

D

decussation of the pyramids: found in the medulla oblongata where the nerve fibers connect two adjacent pyramid structures

deep: below the surface

deep palm muscle: a group of muscles that lie deep within the hand

deep tendon reflexes: reflexes that maintain muscle tone

deltoid: a muscle located on the lateral shoulder

deltoid ligament: a ligament located on the medial aspect of the ankle

deltoid tuberosity: a rounded process of the humerus on which the deltoid muscle attaches.

dendrite: part of the nerve that abuts adjacent nerves and receives impulses from a synapse and sends the message to the nucleus of the neuron

denticulate ligaments: extensions of the pia mater that anchor the spinal cord to the vertebral column

depolarization: a process in which the nerve changes from a resting state to an active state. The charge goes from negative to positive.

dermatome: areas of the body that are innervated by specific spinal nerves

descending nerves: nerves that take efferent impulses from the centrsal nervous system to the periphery

diaphragm: a muscle located at the superior region of the abdominal cavity

diaphysis: the middle part of long bone

diarthrosis joint: a freely moving articulation

diencephalon: part of the brain that is inferior to the cerebrum that contains the thalmus and hypothalmus

digiti minimi: little toe

distal: refers to an anatomical structure being farther away from the midline of the body than another

distal interphalangeal: the joint between the middle phalanx and the distal phalanx

dopamine: a neurotransmitter found at a synapse in the brain

dorsal: toward the back; opposite of ventral

dorsal horn: the posterior gray matter found in the spinal cord

dorsal radiocarpal ligament: connective tissue on the posterior side of the wrist; attaches from the styloid process of the radius to the lunate and triquetrum bones

dorsal ramus: (plural=*rami*) posterior branch of nerve fibers that are motor in nature

dorsal root: a sensory root of the spinal cord that exits from the dorsal side of the spinal column

dorsal root ganglion: nerve cell body of sensory neurons outside the spinal cord

dorsal scapular nerve: the nerve that innervates the posterior muscles of the shoulder girdle

double limb support: when the weight of the body during gait is supported by both limbs

dura mater: the hard outer layer of the meninge layers

dural sinuses: reservoirs in the dura mater that collect venous blood for return to the heart

dynamic: when the fibers in a particular muscle either shorten or lengthen, they are said to be acting dynamically

E

eccentric: a movement of muscle in which the fibers lengthen

efferent: nerve stimulation that travels away from the brain, spinal cord, or nerve cell structure

elasticity: the ability of tissue to return to its original size after stretching

endomysium: a tissue that covers each individual muscle fiber

endorphins: chemical produced in the brain that is involved in pain perception

endosteum: the deepest bone tissue found lining the medullary cavity of long bone

ependymal cells: nervous system supporting cells with cilia that are responsible for circulating cerebrospinal fluid

epidural space: the region outside the dural space in the meninges

epimysium: the most superficial layer of tissue surrounding the entire muscle

epinephrine: a stress hormone from the catecholamines group. Epinephrine is often referred to as adrenaline. Epinephrine is a hormone produced by the adrenal medulla that provides a sympathetic nervous system repsonse.

epiphyseal structure: part of long bone that is responsible for growth of the long bone; the knobby ends of long bones that articulate with one another, forming a joint

epiphysis: a center for ossification at each end of long bones

erector spinae: the intermediate layer of lower back muscles: iliocostalis, longissimus, and spinalis

excitability: a tissue that is sensitive to stimulation

excursion: the extent of a movement of a body part, such as the extremities

expiration: to exhale air from the lungs

extensibility: the lengthening movement or stretch of a muscle

extensor carpi radialis brevis: a muscle located on the radius crossing the elbow and wrist joints

extensor carpi radialis longus: a muscle located on the radius crossing the elbow and wrist joints

extensor carpi ulnaris: a muscle located on the ulna crossing the elbow and wrist joints

extensor digiti minimi: a long, narrow muscle located on the posterior surface of the forearm that extends all of the joints of the pinky

extensor digitorum: a muscle on the posterior side of the forearm that extends digits 2–5

extensor digitorum longus: a muscle located deep to the tibialis anterior muscle and on the anterolateral surface of the tibia

extensor hallucis longus: a muscle located deep to the extensor digitorum longus muscle

extensor hood: a broad aponeurosis at the dorsal and distal areas of the hand

extensor indicis: a small, narrow muscle located on the posterior side of the forearm that acts as the main extensor of the index finger

extensor pollicis brevis: a small, thin muscle on the posterior side of the forearm and hand that aids in extension of the thumb

extensor pollicis longus: a small muscle on the posterior aspect of the hand that aids in extension of the thumb

extensor retinaculum: a band of connective tissue crossing the wrist on the posterior side

external intercostals: a muscle located between the ribs superficial to the internal intercostals

external oblique: a muscle located in the anterolateral abdominal region superficial to the internal oblique

extrinsic: from or coming from

extrinsic muscle: a muscle located outside an organ that controls its position

F

facial nerve: the seventh cranial nerve that innervates the fine motor muscles of the face

falx cerebelli: part of the dura mater that encapsulates the cerebellum

falx cerebri: part of the dura mater that is found within the longitudinal fissure and separates the two cerebral hemispheres

fasciculi: (singular=*fasciculus*) bundles of muscle fibers surrounded by the perimysium

femoral neck: the portion of the femur that protects the head and increases the surface area for muscles to attach

femoral nerve: the nerve that runs along the femur

femur: the thigh bone

fibula: the lateral thin bone found in the lateral aspect of the leg

fibular head: the proximal end of the fibula that articulates with the tibia

filum terminale: a structure found at the end of the spinal column

first-class lever: where the location of the fulcrum lies between the force and the resistance

first-order neurons: nerves that carry impulses from the most distal part of the body to the spinal cord

flat bone: a bone with a flat appearance

flat-back posture: a posture characteristic of a forward head position with concurrent changes in the cervical and upper thoracic spine

flexor carpi radialis: a muscle located on the anterior radius crossing the elbow and wrist joints

flexor carpi ulnaris: a muscle located on the anterior ulna crossing the elbow and wrist joints

flexor digiti minimi: the muscle originating from the flexor retinaculum and the hamate bone that acts to flex the fifth metacarpophalangeal joint

flexor digitorum longus: a muscle located on the plantar surface of the foot crossing the ankle and phalangeal joints

flexor digitorum profundus: a deep finger flexor on the medial and anterior region of the forearm

flexor digitorum superficialis: a large belly muscle that extends digits 2–5

flexor hallucis longus: a muscle located on the plantar surface of the foot crossing the ankle and phalangeal joints of the great toe

flexor pollicis brevis: a superficial muscle that flexes the CMC and MCP joints

flexor pollicis longus: a small muscle on the anterior surface of the forearm that flexes the thumb and aids in flexion of the wrist

flexor retinaculum: connective tissue spanning from the pisiform and hook of the hamate bone to the trapezium bone; found on the palmar surface of the hand and plantar surface of the foot

footdrop gait: an abnormal gait in which dorsiflexion is needed to help clear the toes during swing and to fight gravity when the foot hits the ground

foramen: an opening in bone for the passage of vessels or nerves

foramen magnum: a hole in the occipital bone that allows the spinal cord to connect with the brain

force: an external influence on an object

force arm: the distance in a lever from the point at which a force is applied to the fulcrum

forced expiration: occurs during conditions when there is an increased physiological demand on the body, as the diaphragm and intercostal muscles are activated, along with a variety of other synergist muscles

forward head posture (FHP): a faulty alignment that is indicated by the position of the head aligned anterior to the ideal position

free dendritic endings: nerve endings that respond to temperature and pain

frontal axis: a pivot point allowing motion only in the sagittal plane

frontal eye fields: part of Broca's area in the brain that controls voluntary eye movements

frontal lobe: the anterior part of the cerebrum responsible for emotional responses

frontal plane: the plane that divides the body into front and back sections

fulcrum: the point on which a lever moves

functional systems: nerve fibers in the brain comprised of various nuclei and fibers that form a network throughout the brain

fundamental position: standing erect, feet flat, and the palms facing toward the sides slightly toward the back

fusiform muscle: cordlike

G

ganglion: (plural=*ganglia*) ganglia a group of nerve cell bodies outside the brain or spinal column

gastrocnemius: a muscle located on the posterior leg crossing the knee and ankle joints

gemellus inferior: one of the six lateral rotator muscles of the hip joint

gemellus superior: one of the six lateral rotator muscles of the hip joint

general interpretation area: "gnostic area" that integrates multiple types of input from many different sensory areas

genu recurvatum: the hyperextension of the knee joint

genu valgus: a condition in which the knees are positioned toward the midline, forming an "L," with the angle of the "L" being the knee and the arms being the femur and tibia; also known as knock knees

genu varus: a condition in which the knees are positioned laterally; also known as bow legs

glenohumeral ligament: a ligament spanning the anterior and lateral shoulder joint

glenoid: a socket appearance

glenoid fossa: the depression on the lateral part of the scapula that forms the ball and socket articulation for the head of the humerus

glenoid labrum: a rim of fibrocartilage that increases the depth of the shoulder joint

glial cells: pertaining to support cells of the nervous system

glide motion: to move in a smooth, frictionless manner

globular actin (G-actin): protein containing adenosine diphosphate that plays a key role in muscle contraction

globus pallidus: part of the brain commonly referred to as the corpus striatum; responsible for starting and stopping movement, coordinating movements, regulating the intensity of movement, and inhibiting unnecessary movement

glossopharyngeal nerve: the ninth cranial nerve; a motor nerve that is responsible for the swallowing action by innervating the tongue and pharynx

gluteus maximus: a muscle located on the posterior hip

gluteus medius: a muscle located on the posterior hip deep to the gluteus maximus

gluteus minimus: a muscle located on the posterior hip deep to the gluteus medius

gnostic area: a part of the brain that processes memories and forms memories

golgi tendon organ: a specific type of proprioceptor nerve found in muscle that inhibits a muscle contraction and causes it to relax at the right time

gomphosis: a conical process that fits into a socket of an immovable joint

gracilis: a muscle located on the medial thigh crossing the hip and knee joints

graded potential: a stimulus that is received by the axon and transmitted to the cell body

gravity: the force of the earth's gravitational pull

gray commissure: a structure that joins the right and left horns of the spinal cord

greater trochanter: the larger and superior bony process of the femur

groove: a narrow depression or furrow

gyri: (singular=*gyrus*) the peak of a fold in the brain

H

hallucis: the great toe

hamate: one of the bones of the wrist.

haversian canal: tiny vascular canals found in osseous tissue

head: a projection on a bone that articulates with another bone

heavy myosin chain: a double helix structure that acts as an arm that extends the myosin toward the active site

Hilton's law: a law that states that "the joints of the body are innervated by the same nerves that innervate the muscles that produce movement at that joint"

hinge joint: a movement that occurs in the sagittal plane around a frontal axis

hippocampus: structure in the brain that stores long-term memories

homeostasis: the constant struggle of the body to remain in the "status quo"

homunculus: a somatotopy of the body characterized by body parts that are disproportional to the body as we know it

humerus: the long bone found in the arm

hyaline cartilage: the true cartilage, which is smooth and covers articular surfaces of bone

hypoglossal nerve: the 12th cranial nerve; a motor nerve that is responsible for the chewing actions, swallowing, and speech by innervating the tongue

hypothalamus: a structure found inferior to the thalamus and is responsible for autonomic functions, emotional response, body temperature regulation, and major endocrine functions

hypothenar muscle: a group of muscles that exert action on the pinky.

I

iliac crest: the crest of the ilium

iliac fossa: a deep, rounded concave surface found on the anterior surface on the ilium of the pelvis

iliacus: a muscle located on the anterior hip

iliocostalis muscle group: made up of three muscles; iliocostalis cervicis, which is a muscle located on the posterior neck region along the spinous processes; iliocostalis lumborum, which is a muscle located on the posterior lumbar region along the spinous processes; iliocostalis thoracis, which is a muscle located on the posterior thoracic region along the spinous processes

iliofemoral ligament: connective tissue on the anterior surface of the hip that attaches to the AIIS and proximal medial region of the femur; also called the Y ligament

iliohypogastric nerve: a nerve located in the abdominal cavity

ilioinguinal nerve: a nerve located in the abdominal cavity deep to the inguinal ligament

iliopsoas muscle: two muscles, the psoas major and iliacus, that cross the hip joint on the anterior surface

ilium: the area on the hip bone that is most superior and runs from anterior and lateral to posterior

inferior: below or underneath

inferior appendicular skeleton: referring to the leg region

inferior border of the rib: the lower portion of each rib

inferior colliculi: structures that play a role in transmission of auditory stimulus to the cortex

inferior extensor retinaculum: a band of fascia located on the anterior portion of the ankle and foot just distal to the superior extensor retinaculum

inferior gluteal nerve: a branch of the sciatic nerve innervating the gluteal muscle group

inferior ramus of pubis: a bony landmark located on the posterior region of the pubis

infra: below or beneath

infraspinatus: a muscle located below the spine of the scapula crossing the posterior shoulder joint

infraspinous fossa: a groove located on the posterior surface of the scapula

inguinal ligament: a ligament located on the anterior hip joint found where the hip bends

inhibitory troponin I (TnI): a troponin molecule that binds the complex to the F-actin.

initial contact: the weight-loading portion of the stance phase

initial swing: the acceleration portion of the swing phase

innervate: to stimulate

insertion: a distal attachment point of a muscle; usually the more moveable part of the muscle

inspiration: to inhale and bring air into the lungs

insula: gray matter found deep within the lateral sulcus

integration center: part of the brain that coordinates all sensory input received

intercarpal joint: a joint composed of the proximal and distal rows of carpal bones; also known as the midcarpal joint

interclavicular: between the clavicles

interclavicular ligament: tissue that connects the superior surface of the manubrium to the superior surface of the sternal end of the clavicles

intercondylar eminence: a prominence between two condyles

intercondylar fossa: a depression between two condyles

intercostal nerve: a nerve that innervates the intercostal muscles

intermediate: between two extremes

intermediate cuneiform: a middle or second cuneiform bone

internal intercostal: a muscle located between the ribs deep to the external intercostal muscles

internal oblique: a muscle located in the anterolateral abdominal cavity deep to the external oblique muscle

internuncial neuron: nerve that performs the same function as the spinal cord

interossei muscle: a group of muscles that act in adduction and abduction of the MCP joint and digits 2–5

interosseous membrane: a fibrous connective tissue that is found in the space between the radius and ulna and the tibia and fibula

interspinales: a group of muscles located along the posterior spine that are responsible for maintaining posture and extension of the back

intertubercular groove: a groove between tubercles

interventricular foramen: specific openings found between the four ventricles in the brain

intrafusal fibers: nerve fibers found in the muscle spindle that respond to muscle stretch and initiate a reflex action

intrinsic: a structure belonging only to a particular body part

intrinsic muscle: a muscle that is located within an organ that helps the organ to function correctly

irregular bone: a bone that does not have a specific shape

ischial tuberosity: the rounded prominence on the ischial bones

ischiofemoral ligament: connective tissue that spans the posterior surface of the hip joint

ischium: the area in the hip bone that is located inferior and posterior

isokinetic: same or controlled speed of movement

isometric: no movement

isotonic: a constant resistance of force in which both eccentric and concentric movements occur

isotropic band (I band): an area of the sarcomere that polarizes light

---

J

joint kinesthetic receptors: receptors in nerves that monitor the amount of stretch in synovial joints

jugular foramen: a hole between the occipital and temporal bones that allows the passage of the jugular vein and cranial nerves

---

K

kinesiology: the study of movements

kinesthesia: receptors in a joint that provide information regarding its position and speed of movement

kinetic chain: the ability of multiple joints to move together through a full range of motion

kyphosis-lordosis posture: a posture characteristic of forward head positioning, hyperextension of the upper cervical spine, flexion of the lower cervical spine, and flexion of the upper thoracic spine

---

L

lacuna: a porous structure in the osteon that houses the osteocyte

lamella: a thin layer of fine bone tissue

lateral: away from the middle, or to the side

lateral aperture: an opening from the fourth ventricle into the subarachnoid space

lateral collateral ligament (LCL): a ligament in the elbow and knee that spans the lateral surface of these joint structures

lateral condyle: the large knuckle-like projection that is found on the lateral surface of the distal end of the fibula

lateral cuneiform: the outside or third cuneiform bone

lateral epicondyle: the side prominence on top of a condyle

lateral epicondyle of the tibia: a rounded prominence on the lateral side of the tibia

lateral fissure: a groove-like structure in the osteon that houses the osteocyte

lateral horns: gray matter in the spinal cord that project in the lateral direction

lateral meniscus: the outside meniscus in the knee

latissimus dorsi: a muscle located on the posterior back region crossing the shoulder joint

length-tension relationship: the direct relationship (to a point) between the length of a muscle or muscle fiber and the tension it is able to develop

lentiform nucleus: part of the brain commonly referred to as the corpus striatum; responsible for starting and stopping movement, coordinating movements, regulating the intensity of movement, and inhibiting unnecessary movement

lesser trochanter: the smaller and inferior bony process of the femur

levator scapula: a muscle located superior to the superior angle of the spine

lever: a rigid bar to which force and resistance are applied

leverage: the mechanical advantage of a lever

lever arm: a rigid bar around which forces are applied to cause movement

lever classes: the three classes of levers

ligament: a strong band of fibrous connective tissue

light myosin chain: the myosin head that is made up of four small polypeptide chains

limbic system: specific regions of the brain that are influenced by behavior and arousal stimulus and contribute to the rest of the body by providing endocrine and sympathetic responses

line: any long narrow mark

linea alba: a white line of connective tissue that runs from the sternum to the pubis down the middle of the abdomen

linea aspera: the long ridge on the posterior surface of the femur

load response: the portion of the stance phase in which the foot is flat on the ground.

long bone: bone that has a structure longer than it is wide

longissimus capitis: a muscle located in the transverse process of the spine in the neck and head region

longissimus muscle group: three muscles within the erector spinae group; longissimus capitis is a muscle located in the transverse processes of the spine in the neck and head region, longissimus cervicis is a muscle located in the transverse processes of the neck region, and longissimus thoracis is a muscle located in the transverse processes of the thoracic region of the back.

longitudinal fissure: a groove-like structure that divides the brain into right and left halves

long thoracic nerve: a nerve that innervates the serratus anterior muscle

longus: referring to a long structure

lumbar: referring to the lumbar vertebrae

lumbar plexus: a group of nerves originating from L4–S4. Because of the common nerve structures with the sacral plexus, these terms usually give rise to the term *lumbosacral plexus.*

lumbosacral plexus: the grouping of nerves that innervate the muscles of the hip and thigh

lumbricals: three muscles in the hand that allow for fine motor control and precise movement of the hand.

lunate: one of the bones of the wrist that makes up the wrist joint

M

magnus: referring to a large structure

mandible: the lower jawbone

manubrium: the most superior portion of the sternum

masseter: a rhomboidal-shaped muscle on the lateral skull; provides movement of the jaw and clenches the teeth

mastoid process: pertaining to the process on the temporal bone

maximus: referring to the largest structure

meatus: a passage way or opening

mechanical advantage: a situation in which the forces applied to a lever increase the efficiency of movement and power of a contraction

mechanical efficiency: the ease at which a muscle moves a given region through space

medial: toward the midline

medial collateral ligament (MCL): a ligament found in the elbow and knee providing medial support for these joint structures

medial condyle: a large knuckle-like projection found on the medial surface of the distal tibia

medial condyle of the tibia: the rounded prominence located toward the midline of the tibia

medial cuneiform: the first cuneiform bone that is located on the medial side of the foot

medial epicondyle: the prominence on top of a condyle located toward the midline of the bone

medial meniscus: the fibrocartilage found toward the midline of the knee

median aperture: an opening from the third ventricle into the subarachnoid space

median pectoral nerve: a nerve within the brachial plexus that innervates the muscles of the shoulder girdle

medius: referring to the middle

medulla oblongata (medulla): located in the inferior brain and is responsible for voluntary movements of muscles, coordinating heart rate, coordinating respiration, and other important muscle functions

medullary cavity: the cavity that contains marrow

Meissner's corpuscles: sensory nerve fibers that respond to discriminative touch

meningeal branch: spinal nerves that are found running through the vertebral canal that innervate the meninges and blood vessels located in the canal

meninges: three separate membranes that cover the brain and spinal column

menisci: a crescent-shaped interarticular fibrocartilage

Merkel's disks: sensory nerve fibers that respond to light touch

metacarpal bones: pertaining to the bones of the hand that lie distal to the carpals

metacarpophalangeal: the joints between the wrist and the fingers

metatarsals: referring to the arch of the foot

microglia: cells of the nervous system that act as macrophages and eat foreign debris

midbrain: part of the brain connecting the pons and cerebellum with the cerebral hemispheres

midcarpal: the area between the two rows of carpal bones

middle cerebellar peduncles: nerve structures that connect the pons to the cerebellum

midline: an imaginary line drawn down the center of the body

midpalm muscle: a group of muscles that lie deep within the hand

midstance: the single limb support period of the stance phase

midswing: the portion of the swing phase when the swing leg is next to the weight-bearing leg of midstance

military-type posture: a posture characteristic of increased lordosis in the lumbar spine, an anterior tilt in the pelvis, and knees slightly hyperextended

minimi: referring to the smallest structure

minimus: referring to muscles of smaller surface area or size

mixed nerves: nerve fibers that carry both sensory and motor impulses to and from the central nervous system

monosynaptic reflex: a reflex that is transmitted only through one synapse

mortise: a socket

motor end plate: the distal end of the motor neuron containing the synaptic structures involved in delivering an action potential to the muscle tissue

motor nerves: nerves that control and direct motor responses

motor neuron: a nerve

multifidus: a muscle located on the posterior lumbar spine that spans from the sacrum and ilium to the spinous processes of the vertebrae just immediately above

multipennate muscle: an oblique muscle fiber arrangement that gives the appearance of many feathers; has many origins that span into one central tendon

multiplaner: movements that occur in a variety of planes

multiple heads: heads that typically originate from their own origin, centralize into a common tendon, and attach into a common insertion

muscle fiber: the cell of the muscle that covers the entire length of the muscle

muscle spindles: structures that are also termed neuromuscular spindles, they are responsible for detecting stretch and providing a reflex if the stretch is too great

myelin: a connective tissue that coats the axon of peripheral nervous system fibers

myofibril: the microscopic unit of the muscle fiber containing the actin and myosin molecules; they are rod-like and span the entire length of the muscle

myosin: the thick filament of the sarcomere

myosin head: structure of the myosin that provides the crossbridge and power stroke; the binding site for ATP for the muscle contraction

myosin tail: a double helix structure that provides the structural base for the mechanical movements of the sarcomere

N

navicular: the medial bone of the ankle just proximal to the cuneiforms

naviculartibial: one of the deltoid ligaments in the foot and ankle

nerve: a structure that carries an electrical impulse throughout the nervous system

neuroglia: support cells of the nervous system

neurolemma: pertaining to the myelin sheath

neurolemmocytes: pertaining to Schwann cells

neuromuscular junction: the junction and structures found between a motor neuron and an adjacent muscle

neuron: referring to a nerve cell

neurotransmitter: a chemical found at a synapse that takes the nervous message/stimulation from either one nerve to the next or a nerve to an affected organ

neutralizer: a muscle contraction that inhibits the contraction of another muscle

nodes of Ranvier: gaps that are found between each Schwann cell along an axon. These structures allow for faster nerve conduction.

nonaxial joint: a joint that does not allow motion in a given plane around a specific axis

notch: a deep indentation at the end of a structure

nuchal ligamentum: a connective tissue spanning from the occipital protuberance along the spinous processes of the cervical spine

nucleus: (plural=*nuclei*) part of a cell responsible for all functions of the cell; also known as the brain of the cell

nucleus pulposus: the inner portion or core of the intervertebral disk made of a soft gel-like substance composed mainly of water

O

oblique: referring to a diagonal structure

oblique muscle: a muscle with a diagonal structure

obturator externus: one of the deep rotator muscles of the hip

obturator foramen: a hole within the ischium through which the obturator nerve runs

obturator internus: one of the deep rotator muscles of the hip

obturator nerve: the nerve that tracks through the obturator foramen and innervates the medial muscles of the hip

occipital lobe: the posterior part of the cerebrum that is responsible for the sense of vision

occipital protuberance: the bony landmark located on the posterior surface of the occipital bone

oculomotor nerve: the third cranial nerve; a motor nerve that is responsible for innervating the muscles of the eye

olecranon fossa: the shallow depression in the humerus where the olecranon articulates

olecranon process: the large process on the proximal end of the ulna that articulates with the humerus to form the elbow joint

olfactory cortex: a part of the brain that processes the sense of smell

olfactory nerves: the first cranial nerve; a sensory nerve that is responsible for the sense of smell

olfactory tract: pairs of nerves that take the nervous stimulation of smell to the olfactory areas of the brain

oligodendoglia: support cells of the central nervous system that form a protective sheath much like myelin of the peripheral nervous system

open kinetic chain: a situation in which the insertion moves toward the origin during human movement

open-packed position: a situation in which the ligaments of a joint are relaxed, allowing mobility of a joint

opponens digiti minimi: a muscle that opposes the pinky

opponens pollicis: a muscle deep to the abductor pollicis that acts in opposition of the thumb

optic chiasma: a region in the brain where the optic nerve fibers cross

optic foramen: a hole in the sphenoid bone that allows the optic nerve to articulate between the eye and the occipital lobe of the cerebrum

optic nerve: the second cranial nerve; a sensory nerve that is responsible for the sense of vision

origin: a more proximal attachment point of a muscle; usually the more stable part of the muscle

osseous tissue: referring to bone tissue

osteo: the combining form showing a relationship to a bone

osteoblast: a type of bone cell responsible for the formation of new bone tissue

osteoclast: a type of bone cell responsible for the breakdown of old bone tissue

osteocyte: a bone cell

osteokinematics: describes the specific joint motion occuring at a joint

osteogenesis: formation of bone

osteon: the functional unit of a bone

oxygen: a colorless, odorless, tasteless gas that is essential for life support

P

pacinian corpuscles: sensory nerve endings that respond to pressure and respond at first only to the pressure

palmar aponeurosis: the connective tissue located on the anterior side of the hand

palmaris longus: a muscle located on the anterior forearm crossing the elbow and wrist joints

palmar radiocarpal ligament: the most important ligament for wrist stability; it attaches from the anterior portion of the distal radius and ulna to the anterior surface of the scaphoid, lunate, and triquetrum bones

parallel muscle: a muscle fiber arrangement in which the fibers span the entire distance of the muscle belly.

parasympathetic system: the division of the autonomic nervous system that controls normal nervous function

parietal lobe: lobe of the brain found posterior to the frontal lobe and anterior to the occipital lobe

passive insufficiency: the contractile excursion movements caused by the agonist muscle

patella: the anterior surface of the kneecap

patellar ligament: the ligament found within the knee

pectineus: a muscle located on the medial hip joint superior to the adductor longus and adductor brevis muscles

pectoralis major: a muscle located on the chest crossing the anterior shoulder joint

pectoralis minor: a shoulder girdle muscle located on the coracoid process and anterolateral ribs

pelvic bone: the bone found in the hip region that has three distinct areas, including the ilium, ischium, and pubic regions

pennation: an oblique feather-shaped muscle's fiber arrangement

pennation angle: a fiber arrangement that runs at an angle or at an oblique direction to the long axis of the bone

perikaryon: the center of the neruron responsible for carrying out cellular processes

perimysium: a tissue that surrounds the muscle fascicle; distinguishes one group of muscle fibers from the next

periosteum: the most superficial layer of bone tissue

peripheral nervous system (PNS): a system that consists of nerve fibers outside the spinal cord

peroneus brevis: a muscle located on the lateral leg crossing the ankle joint

peroneus longus: a muscle located on the lateral leg crossing the ankle joint

peroneus tertius: a muscle located on the lateral leg crossing the ankle joint

phalanges: referring to the fingers

phalanges of the foot: referrring to the toes of the foot

phalanx: any bone of the fingers and toes

phrenic nerve: a nerve located in the cervical region innervating muscles of the abdomen

pia mater: a meshlike meninge that is the deepest of the meninges located on the surface of the brain

pineal gland: an endocrine gland located in the third ventricle that regulates sleep and wake cycles

piriformis: one of the deep rotator muscles of the hip

pisiform: one of the bones in the wrist

pivot joint: the joint that exists as the radioulnar joint where the proximal head of the radius articulates with the radial notch of the ulna

plane: a flat smooth surface that makes a cut through the body or part of it

plantar aponeurosis: a band of connective tissue located on the plantar surface of the foot

plantaris: a muscle located on the posterior knee

plumb line: a piece of string with a weight on the bottom that is suspended from the ceiling

polarized state: a state in which the sodium potassium pump maintains the balance of sodium and potassium inside and outside the cell

polysynaptic reflex: a reflex that travels across more than one synapse

pons: a brain structure found between the medulla oblongata and the cerebral peduncles

pontine nuclei: structures that provide communication between the cerebellum and the cortex

popliteal ligament: a ligament located on the posterior surface of the knee

popliteus: a muscle located on the anterior surface of the knee

postcentral gyrus: responsible for interpreting sensory stimulation from different regions of the body

posterior: refers to a structure located on the backside of the body

posterior cruciate ligament (PCL): the ligament of the interior knee that lies behind the anterior cruciate ligament

posterior inferior iliac spine (PIIS): the bony landmark on the back lower part of the iliac spine

posterior longitudinal ligament: a broad structure that attaches to the posterior surface of the vertebral bodies and disks

posterior median sulcus: an indentation of tissue found on the posterior surface of the spinal cord that helps separate the spinal cord into left and right halves

posterior pelvic tilt: greater than a 10-degree angle between the ASIS and PSIS or the ASIS and the pubic symphysis

posterior superior iliac spine (PSIS): the bony landmark on the back upper part of the iliac spine

posterolateral: referring to the back and to the side

posteromedial: referring to the back and to the middle

postganglionic neuron: a nerve that exists after a ganglion

postsynaptic neuron: the neuron that is receiving an impulse

precentral gyrus: a structure of the brain that houses the primary motor cortex

pre-expiration: the static phase that precedes expiration and follows inspiration

prefrontal cortex: part of the brain that regulates complex thought and learning and translates the impulse into memory and cognition

preganglionic neuron: a nerve that exists before a ganglion

pre-inspiration: the static phase that precedes inspiration

premotor cortex: also known as the primary motor cortex transmits impulses from cerebrum to the spinal cord

preswing: the period in the stance phase when the weight begins to shift to the other extremity

presynaptic neuron: the neuron that is transmitting an impulse

primary sensory cortex: a strucutre located posterior to the central sulcus

prime mover: the muscle that acts to cause movement or motion

process: an outgrowth on a bone or tissue

projection fibers: nerves that allow for communication between the two cerebral hemispheres

pronator quadratus: a muscle of the inferior radioulnar joint located proximal to the wrist joint

pronator teres: a muscle of the superior radioulnar joint located at the elbow

prone: a position that is described as lying in a horizontal plane with the face down (opposite of supine)

proprioception: the ability of the body part to know where it is located in space or in the environment

proprioceptors: nerve fibers that inform the body part where it is located in space or in the environment

proximal: refers to an anatomical structure that is closer to the midline of the body or closer to another structure

proximal interphalangeal: joint between the proximal phalanx and the middle phalanx

pubic symphysis: the cartilage between the pubic bones

pubis: the area on the hip bone located inferior and anterior

pubofemoral ligament: connective tissue that spans from the superior ramus of the pubis to the inferior region of the femoral neck

putamen: part of the brain commonly referred to as the corpus striatum; responsible for starting and stopping movement, coordinating movements, regulating the intensity of movement, and inhibiting unnecessary movement

pyramidal tract: cell bodies that form the premotor cortex

Q

quadratus femoris: one of the deep rotator muscles of the hip

quadratus lumborum: a muscle located on the inferior posterior region

quadriceps gait: an abnormal gait in which the quadriceps needs to contract during the stance phase to extend the knee

R

radi: a word root pertaining to the radius (singular)

radial collateral ligament: connective tissue that originates on the radius and inserts on the scaphoid, trapezium, and first metacarpal

radial notch: the area on the ulna that articulates with the radial bone

radial tuberosity: a large, rough area on the proximal end of the radius

radiocarpal: the joint between the radius and wrist bones

radius: the bone located on the lateral side of the forearm

ramus of the ischium: an area of the ischium that provides additional surface area for the hamstring muscle group

rectus abdominis: a muscle located in the anterior abdominal region

rectus femoris: a muscle located on the anterior femur crossing the hip and knee joints

red nucleus: a nerve structure that helps regulate skeletal muscle contractions

reflex: an unconscious and involuntary neural reaction to a stimulus

repolarization: a process in which the nerve changes from an active state to resting state. The charge goes from positive back to negative.

resistance: a force that is applied to a lever in the opposite direction of the force

resistance arm: the distance that a resistance is applied to a lever from the fulcrum

resting or membrane potential: a state that occurs when the nerve fiber is at rest and normal resting levels of sodium and potassium exist

reticular activating system (RAS): nerve structures that filter out unwanted and irrelevant stimulus being received by the brain

reticular formation: a network of neurons found throughout the brainstem

retinaculum: a band of connective tissue

reversal of muscle pull: the action that results when insertion becomes fixed and the origin moves towards the insertion

rhomboid: an oblique parallelogram shape

rhomboidal muscle: a muscle that is shaped like a parallelogram

roll motion: occurs when one point of a moving articulation is in contact with the joint surface of a fixed joint

rotatores: muscles of the back region

Ruffini's corpuscles: sensory nerve fibers that respond to deep pressure and monitor stretching of a muscle

S

sacral plexus: a group of nerves originating from L4–S4. Because of the common nerve structures with the lumbar plexus, these terms ususally give rise to the term *lumbosacral plexus.*

sacrum: the fourth region of the vertebral column located posterior between the two pelvic bones

saddle joint: a joint only located between the trapezium bone and the first metacarpal bone, with movements occurring in both the sagittal and frontal planes around the frontal and sagittal axes, respectively

sagittal axis: a pivot point allowing motion only in the frontal plane

sagittal plane: the plane through the body that divides it into right and left sections

sarcolemma: the cell membrane of the muscle fiber

sarcomere: the functional unit of muscle; contains the contractile units of muscle used in the muscle contraction

sarcoplasm: the cytoplasm of the muscle fibers; gel-like fluid that suspends the myofibrils and structural components of the muscle cell

sarcoplasmic reticulum: an organelle of the sarcolemma responsible for the storage of calcium ions

sartorius: a muscle located on the anterior thigh crossing the hip and medial knee joints

scalenes: muscles of the neck and thoracic region spanning from the transverse processes of the spinous processes of the spine below to the transverse processes above

scaphoid: one of the bones of the wrist that makes up the wrist joint

scapula: the shoulder blade

scapulohumoral rhythm: related movements between the scapula and humerus

Schwann cells: support cells of the myelin sheath responsible for forming and laying down myelin

sciatic nerve: the largest nerve in the body that runs from the sacral plexus down the back of the thigh

sciatic notch: an indentation of the pelvis forming a passageway for the sciatic nerve

second-class lever: where the resistance lies closer to the fulcrum than the force

second-order neurons: nerves that carry an impulse from the spianl cord to the thalmus

semimembranosus: a muscle located on the posteromedial region of the thigh

semispinalis capitis: muscles located along the spinous processes near the head

semispinalis cervicis: muscles located along the spinous processes along the neck

semitendinosus: a muscle located in the posteromedial thigh

sensory nerves: nerves that transmit sensory input

sensory receptors: nerve fibers that send nerve impulse toward the central nervous system when stimulated

septa: (singular=*septum*) a term describing walls that divide multiple cavities

septum pellucidum: a tissue that separates the lateral ventricles

serotonin: a neurotransmitter found in different synapses in the brain

serratus anterior: a jagged muscle located on the lateral rib region

sesamoid: a bone that is usually found within a muscle; the best example of a sesamoidal bone is the patella, which is found in the rectus femoris muscle

Sharpey's fibers: a fibrous connective tissue that holds the endosteum to the compact bone

short bone: bone that is cube shaped and is as long as it is wide

shoulder girdle: a muscle group that causes movements around the sternoclavicular joint

single limb support: when the weight of the body during gait is supported by one limb only

skeletal muscle: a voluntary muscle arranged in long rod-like bundles of fibers with a striated appearance

skull: referring to the bones of the head

smooth muscle: a muscle that has a simple shape, unmarked by any striations, and running parallel to the long axis of a particular organ; smooth muscles are not under conscious control

sodium-potassium pump: the nerve function of maintaining the balance between sodium and potassium

soleus: a muscle of the posterior leg crossing the ankle joint

soma: cells that pertain to the body

somatic, or voluntary, system: part of the peripheral nervous system that controls voluntary movements of the skeletal muscles

somatosensory association area: its function is to integrate nerve stimulus with regard to temperature and touch into meaningful information

somatotopy: a map encoded into the brain of every corresponding area on the primary motor cortex

spinal cord: a column of nerve tissue that spans the spinal column from the brain to the second lumbar vertebra

spinal dural sheath: the hard covering of the spinal cord

spinal ganglion: also called dorsal root ganglion. Spinal ganglia are nerve bodies of sensory nerves of the dorsal horn of the spinal cord. Neuron cell bodies lie outside the dorsal horn.

spinalis muscle group: made up of three muscles; spinalis capitis, which is a muscle located in the neck that causes movements of the head; spinalis cervicis, which is a muscle located in the neck region that causes movements of the neck; and spinalis thoracis, which is a muscle located in the thoracic region causing movement of the chest

spinal nerves: nerves that originate at the spinal cord

spine: a sharp process on a bone

spine of the scapula: a projection on the posterior surface of the scapula

spin motion: occurs when the articulation of one joint rotates around a single axis of the second articulation

spinous process: a bony prominence on the posterior side of each vertebra

splenius capitis: a muscle located in the neck region spanning from the spinous processes of the thoracic vertebrae to the head

splenius cervicis: a muscle located in the neck region spanning from the spinous processes of the lower cervical vertebrae to the spinous process of C1

spongy: elastic porous mass

spongy bone: trabecular bone that is porous in nature and resembles a sponge

stabilizer: a muscle that when contracted assists other muscles by fixing a specific joint in place

stance phase: the part of the gait cycle when one extremity makes initial contact with the ground and continues as long as the same extremity remains in contact with the ground

static stretching: a movement in which the muscle length stays the same yet responds to tension

sternal body: the middle, plate-like, region of the sternum

sternoclavicular joint: the joint between the sternum and clavicle

sternoclavicular ligaments: connective tissue that provide anterior and posterior support for the SC joint

sternocleidomastoid: a muscle located on the anterolateral neck

sternum: the bone found in the center of the anterior thoracic cavity. The heart is deep to the sternum.

stimuli: (singular=*stimulus*) substances or signals that cause the response of a body system

strap: a band of tissue

strap muscle: a muscle with a strap-like or band-like structure

stretch reflex: a reflex that maintains muscle tone

styloid process: the pointed distal end on the lateral side of the radius

stylomastoid foramen: a hole located between the mastoid and styloid processes that allows the facial nerve to leave the skull

subarachnoid space: the hollow area found deep to the arachnoid space

subcostal nerve: a nerve located along the ribs that provides innervation for the intercostal muscles

subscapular: referring to below the scapula

subscapular fossa: the groove located on the anterior surface of the scapula

subscapularis: a muscle located on the anterior surface of the scapula

substantia nigra: band-like nuclei found inferior to the medulla and part of the basal nuclei of the cerebral hemispheres

sulci: (singular=*sulcus*) the valley of a fold in the brain

superficial: referring to the surface

superior: higher than or above another structure

superior border of the rib: the top border of each rib

superior cerebellar peduncles: the ventral part of the midbrain

superior colliculi: structures that allow the head and eyes to track movement

superior extensor retinaculum: a band of connective tissue superior to the inferior extensor retinaculum

superior flexor retinaculum: a ligament that attaches the lateral malleous of the fibula to the calcaneous

superior gluteal nerve: a nerve branching from the sciatic nerve that innervates the gluteal muscles

superior orbital fissure: a hole in the bone that allows the optic nerve to enter the skull

supine: lying horizontal on the back with the face toward the ceiling (opposite of prone)

supra: an anatomical direction referring to "above"

supraspinatus: a muscle located superior to the spine of the scapula and crosses the posterior shoulder joint

supraspinous fossa: the groove located on the posterior surface of the scapula

suture: the line between two immovable bones

suture joint: a joint that is found where two cranial bones come together

swayback posture: a posture characteristic of an elongated thoracic spine displaced posterior to the plumb line with the lumbar spine in decreased lordosis

swing phase: the part of the gait cycle in which the toe of the extremity leaves the ground and does not end until the heel of the same extremity hits the ground

sympathetic ganglia or sympathetic chain: also called the paravertebral ganglia; located laterally to each lateral aspect of the spinal cord that exert sympathetic influence

sympathetic system: the nervous system response to stressful situations; also known as the fight or flight system

symphysis joint: the fusion line between two bones that is made up of fibrocartilage

synapse: the junction between two adjacent nerves

synaptic cleft: the junction found between a motor neuron and an innervated muscle

synaptic vesicle: a membranous sac structure found at the motor end plate that houses acetylcholine

synarthrotic joint: immovable joints

synchondrosis joint: an immovable joint that has cartilage between the two bones of the extremities

syndesmosis: a joint articulation that is held together by ligaments

syndesmosis joint: a structure that supports the nonmovable joints between the bones

synergist: to enhance the movement of another structure

synovial fluid: the lubricating fluid in the joint

T

talotibial: one of the deltoid ligaments in the foot and ankle

talus: the ankle bone that articulates with the tibia, fibula, calcaneus, and navicular bone

tarsals: the seven bones of the ankle and foot

telondendria: neurons that possess numerous axon branches

temporalis: a muscle located in the head that crosses the jaw

temporal lobe: a structure of the brain located inferior to the parietal lobe responsible for auditory processing

tendon: a fibrous band of tissue that connects a muscle to a bone

tenon: peg-shaped

tenon-mortise: peg and socket

tensor fasciae latae: a muscle located on the anterolateral thigh that crosses the hip and knee joint via the iliotibial band

tentorium: part of the dura mater that is between the cerebrum and cerebellum

teres major: a muscle located on the scapula that spans the shoulder joint from the anterior to the posterior

teres minor: a muscle located on the scapula that spans the posterior shoulder joint

terminal cisternae: muscle fiber organelles that are an extension of the sarcoplasmic reticulum; responsible for increasing sarcoplasmic concentrations of calcium ions

terminal ganglia: autonomic ganglia located near major organs, for example, the heart

terminal nerves: nerves of the brachial and lumbosacral plexus that end in a specific region

terminal stance: the period in the stance phase when the foot prepares to leave the ground

terminal swing: the portion of the swing phase when the swing leg starts to slow down to prepare for weight loading

thalamus: gray matter found in the diencephalons that is responsible for coordination of sensory impulses from the eyes and ears

thenar muscle: a group of small muscles that act specifically on the thumb

third-class lever: where the force lies closer to the fulcrum than the resistance

third-order neurons: nerve fibers that extend from the thalamus to the cerebrum

third ventricle: the third chamber found in the brain

thoracic: pertaining to the chest cavity or region

thoracic cavity: the space above the diaphragm and below the neck

thoracolumbar fascia: a band of connective tissue that spans the lumbar and thoracic vertebrae

tibia: the large bone in the lower leg

tibialis anterior: a muscle located on the anterior leg that crosses the anterior ankle joint

tibialis posterior: a muscle located on the posterior leg that crosses the posterior ankle joint

tibial nerve: a branch of the sciatic nerve that tracks along the leg in posterior direction

tibial plateau: a band of bone on the superior aspect of the tibia that separates the medial and lateral menisci from one another

tibial tuberosity: the rounded process on the proximal tibia

torque: a force that produces rotary motion

trabecular bone: the network of bone tissue that makes up the cancellous structure of bone

tract: a group of nerve fibers that carries an impulse from the brain to the spinal cord

transverse abdominal aponeurosis: a band of connective tissue located in the anterior abdominal region

transverse plane: the plane that divides the body into top and bottom parts

transverse process: a bony prominence on the lateral sides of each vertebra

transverse tubule: a muscle fiber organelle that extends from the sarcolemma deep into the myofibrils; responsible for delivering the action deep into the myofibrils

transversospinalis muscle group: the deep layer of lower back muscles; interspinalis, multifidus, and rotatores

transversus abdominis: a muscle of respiration located in the abdominal region located deep to the rectus abdominis, external oblique, and internal oblique muscles

trapezium: one of the bones of the wrist

trapezius: a shoulder girdle muscle located in the superior back region

trapezoid: one of the bones of the wrist

trapezoid ligament: accessory ligament that makes up the acromioclavicular joint whose purpose is to stabilize the clavicle

Trendelenberg gait: an abnormal gait in which the hip abductors are responsible for stabilizing the pelvis during the stance phase

triangular muscle: a muscle shape that has a broad origin and a narrow insertion

triaxial joint: a joint that allows motion in three planes

triceps brachii: a muscle located on the posterior humerus and crosses the shoulder and elbow joint

trigeminal nerve: the fifth cranial nerve; innervates the masseter and temporalis muscles of the head

triquetrum: one of the bones of the wrist that makes up the wrist joint

trochanter: one of the two bony processes of the femur

trochlea: the smooth articular surface of a bone on which another bone glides

trochlear nerve: the fourth cranial nerve, which is a motor nerve, that causes the eye to move laterally

trochlear notch: a bony indentation of the ulna that articulates with the trochlear process on the humerus

tropomyosin: a long-stranded structure that wraps around the entire length of the F-actin; covers the active site on each G actin molecule

troponin A: a complex of three molecules that is responsible for the mechanical events that occur on the actin myofilament

troponin C (TnC): a troponin molecule that has a specific binding site for calcium ions

troponin complex: a series of three protein structures bound to the G-actin and tropomyosin positioned next to the active site on the G-actin molecules

troponin T (TnT): a troponin molecule that is attached to the tropomyosin; during a contraction, the molecule tugs on the tropomyosin strand

tubercle: a small rounded elevation on a bone

U

ulna: the smaller and medial bone in the forearm

ulnar collateral ligament: connective tissue that originates on the ulna and passes to the pisiform and triquetrum

ulnar tuberosity: a small rough area on the ulna that provides an attachment point for the brachialis muscle

uniaxial: one axis

uniaxial joint: the movement around one axis in one plane

unipennate muscle: the oblique muscle fiber arrangement shaped similarly to a feather that has been cut in half along the central tendon

V

vagus nerve: the 10th cranial nerve; a motor nerve responsible for innervating muscles involved in swallowing in addition to innervating the heart and the digestive system

vastus intermedius: a muscle located on the anterior thigh deep to the rectus femoris crossing the knee joint

vastus lateralis: a muscle located on the anterolateral thigh lateral to the rectus femoris muscle crossing the knee joint

vastus medialis: a muscle located on the anteromedial thigh medial to the rectus femoris muscle crossing the knee joint

ventral: toward the belly; opposite of dorsal

ventral horn: the anterior gray matter found in the spinal cord

ventral ramus: (plural=*rami*) anterior branch of nerve fibers that are sensory in nature

ventral root: the anterior nerve ganglia that send motor stimulation to affected somatic muscles

ventricles: chambers found in the brain that contain cerebrospinal fluid for nourishment of the brain and spinal cord

vertebral: pertaining to the vertebral column or vertebra

vertebral column: referring to the sections of the vertebrae as a whole

vertical axis: perpendicular to the horizontal axis

vestibulocochlear nerve: the eighth cranial nerve; a sensory nerve that is reponsible for the sense of equilibrium and hearing

Volkmann's canal: vascular canals found in compact bone

W

Wernicke's area: part of the brain that interprets words and sounds in the process of communication

X

xyphoid process: the bony process at the distal end of the sternum

Z

Z disk: sarcolemmal structure that binds the actin to the sarcomere; also defines the sarcomere

INDEX

D

J

K

L

M

O

P